ECG Interpretation

made
Incredibly
Easy! ®

Eighth Edition

ECG Interpretation

made Incredibly Easy!

Eighth Edition

Clinical Editor

Carolynn Spera Bruno, PhD, APRN, MSN, CNS, FNP-C
Clinical Associate Professor
New York University Rory Meyers College of Nursing
New York, New York

Wolters Kluwer

Philadelphia • Baltimore • New York • London
Buenos Aires • Hong Kong • Sydney • Tokyo

Vice President and Publisher: Julie K. Stegman
Senior Acquisitions Editor: Joyce Berendes
Director of Nursing Education and Practice Content: Jamie Blum
Senior Development Editor: Jacquelyn Saunders
Editorial Coordinator: Remington Fernando
Editorial Assistant: Sara Thul
Marketing Manager: Amy Whitaker
Production Project Manager: Matthew West
Manager, Graphic Arts & Design: Stephen Druding
Manufacturing Coordinator: Bernard Tomboc
Prepress Vendor: S4Carlisle Publishing Services

Eighth Edition

Library of Congress Cataloging-in-Publication Data

ISBN-13: 978-1-975236-10-6
ISBN-10: 1-975236-10-6

Library of Congress Control Number: 2024941185

---

shop.lww.com

QUADM0924

Dedication

To Christopher, Abigail, Dr. Stephen, and Sarah.

Philippians 4:13

Contributors

Jennifer Browning, MS, AGACNP-BC
Nurse Practitioner
Department of Cardiac Electrophysiology,
  NYU Langone Heart Rhythm Center
NYU Langone Health
New York, New York

Abigail E. Bruno, MSN, PMHNP-BC
Senior Nurse Clinician
Department of Non-Invasive Cardiology
NYU Langone Health
New York, New York

Carolynn Spera Bruno, PhD, APRN, MSN, CNS, FNP-C
Clinical Associate Professor and Nurse
  Practitioner
New York University Rory Meyers College
  of Nursing and
Department of Cardiac Electrophysiology,
  NYU Langone Health
New York, New York

Melissa Clemente, ANP-BC, GNP
Nurse Practitioner
Department of Cardiac Electrophysiology,
  NYU Langone Heart Rhythm Center
NYU Langone Health
New York, New York

Natalie L. Cohen, DNP, AGACNP-BC
Nurse Practitioner
Leon H. Charney Division of Cardiology,
  Department of Medicine
NYU Langone Health
New York, New York

Anna Davidov, FNP-C
Nurse Practitioner
Department of Cardiac Electrophysiology,
  NYU Langone Heart Rhythm Center
NYU Langone Health
New York, New York

Svetlana Musheyev, ACNP-BC
Nurse Practitioner
Department of Cardiac Electrophysiology,
  NYU Langone Heart Rhythm Center
NYU Langone Health
New York, New York

Marianne Paruch, RN, MBA
Administrative Director
Department of Cardiac Electrophysiology
  and Pediatric Interventional Cardiology
NYU Langone Health
New York, New York

Kristina Rogers, AGPCNP-BC
Nurse Practitioner
Department of Cardiac Electrophysiology,
  NYU Langone Heart Rhythm Center
NYU Langone Health
New York, New York

Shubnum Singh, ANP, CCRN
Nurse Practitioner
Department of Cardiology
Good Samaritan Hospital
New York, New York

Jane Smyth-Melsky, RN, CCDS
Cardiac EP Device Manager
Department of Cardiac Electrophysiology,
  NYU Langone Heart Rhythm Center
NYU Langone Health
New York, New York

Foreword

This is a terrific text that will accomplish several learning objectives including:

1. It will teach the rationale behind arrhythmias.
2. It will provide helpful practice questions that reinforce your knowledge and learning outcomes.
3. It will serve to encourage your acquisition of important electrocardiographic (ECG) skills.

Try these recurring logos on for size:

Ages and stages identifies variations in ECGs related to patient age.

Now I get it offers crystal-clear explanations of complex procedures, such as how to use an automated external defibrillator.

Don't skip this strip identifies arrhythmias that have the most serious consequences.

Mixed signals provides tips on how to solve the most common problems in ECG monitoring and interpretation.

I can't waste time highlights key points you need to know about each arrhythmia for quick reviews.

These icons will serve as markers to explain key concepts, provide important care reminders, and offer reassurance in a relaxed manner along with a bit of humor that will teach and entertain in a way that no other resource can.

I hope you find this book helpful. Best of success throughout your career!

Contents

Part I

ECG fundamentals

Cardiac anatomy and physiology

Just the facts

In this chapter, you'll learn:

- the location and structure of the heart
- the layers of the heart wall
- the flow of blood to and through the heart and the structures involved in this flow
- phases of the cardiac cycle
- properties of cardiac cells
- details of cardiac impulse conduction and their relationship to arrhythmias.

> The mediastinum is home to the heart.

HOME SWEET HOME

A look at cardiac anatomy

Cardiac anatomy includes the location of the heart; the structure of the heart, heart wall, chambers, and valves; and the layout and structure of coronary circulation. A thorough understanding of the various heart structures and their relationship to cardiac electrophysiology, as well as the management of cardiac arrhythmias, is essential.

Outside the heart

The heart is a cone-shaped, muscular organ. It's located in the chest, behind the sternum in the mediastinal cavity (or mediastinum) lying between the lungs and in front of the spine. The heart lies tilted in this area like an *upside-down* triangle. The top of the heart, or its **base**, lies just below the second rib; the bottom of the heart, or its **apex**, tilts forward and down, toward the left side of the body resting on the diaphragm. (See *Location of the pediatric heart*.)

The heart varies in size depending on the person's body size, but the organ is roughly 5″ (12.5 cm) long and 3½″ (9 cm) wide, or about the size of the person's fist. The heart's weight, typically 9 to 12 oz (255 to 340 g), varies depending on the person's size, age, sex assigned at birth, and athletic conditioning. An athlete's heart usually weighs more than

Ages and stages

Location of the pediatric heart

The heart of an infant is positioned more horizontally in the chest cavity than that of the adult. As a result, the apex is at the fourth left intercostal space. Until age 4, the apical impulse is located to the left of the midclavicular line. By age 7, the heart is situated in the same position as the adult heart.

that of the average person, and the heart of an older adult weighs less. (See *The older adult heart.*) There are differences in male and female cardiovascular anatomy and physiology. A smaller heart and coronary vessels are seen in females versus males. Varying levels of estrogen may be the reason for variants in cardiac disease.

Layer upon layer

The heart's wall is made up of three layers: the epicardium, myocardium, and endocardium. (See *Layers of the heart wall.*) The epicardium, the outer layer (and the visceral layer of the serous pericardium), is made up of squamous epithelial cells overlying connective tissue. The myocardium, the middle layer, makes up the thickest portion of the heart's wall. This layer of muscle tissue contracts with each heartbeat. The endocardium, the heart's innermost layer, contains endothelial tissue with small blood vessels and bundles of smooth muscle.

Layers of the heart wall

This cross section of the heart wall shows its various layers.

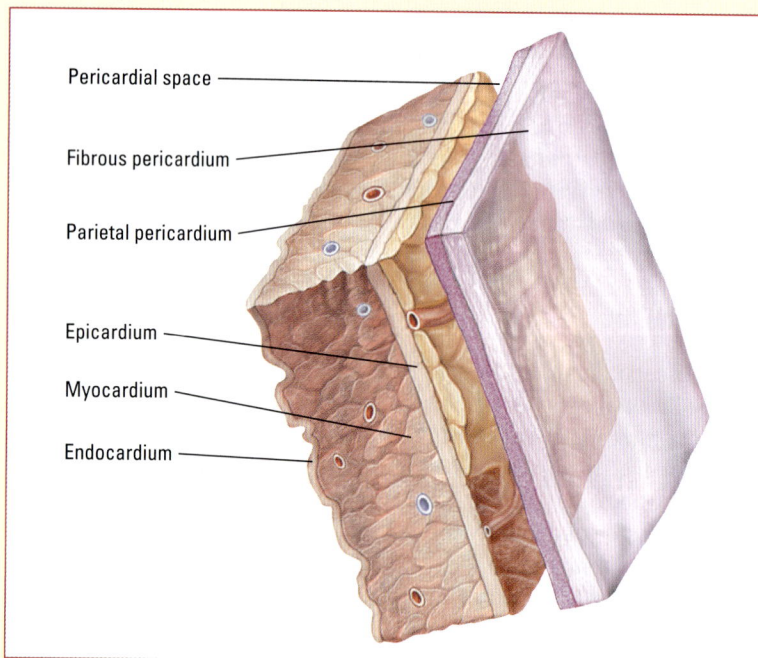

Pericardial space

Fibrous pericardium

Parietal pericardium

Epicardium

Myocardium

Endocardium

Ages and stages

The older adult heart

As a person ages, the heart usually becomes slightly smaller and loses its contractile strength and efficiency (although exceptions occur in people with hypertension or heart disease). By age 70 for many people, cardiac output at rest has diminished by 30% to 35%.

Irritable with age

As the myocardium of the aging heart becomes more irritable, extra systoles may occur, along with sinus arrhythmias and sinus bradycardias. In addition, increased fibrous tissue infiltrates the sinoatrial (SA) node and internodal atrial tracts, which may cause atrial fibrillation and flutter.

A layer of connective tissue called the *pericardium* surrounds the heart and acts as a tough, protective sac. It consists of the fibrous pericardium and the serous pericardium. The fibrous pericardium, composed of tough, white, fibrous tissue, fits loosely around the heart protecting it. The fibrous pericardium attaches to the great vessels, diaphragm, and sternum. The serous pericardium, the thin, smooth, inner portion, has two layers:
- the parietal layer, which lines the inside of the fibrous pericardium
- the visceral layer, which adheres to the surface of the heart

Between the layers
The pericardial space separates the visceral and parietal layers and contains 10 to 20 mL of thin, clear pericardial fluid that lubricates the articulation of these two surfaces and cushions the heart. Excess pericardial fluid, a condition called *pericardial effusion*, compromises the heart's ability to pump blood.

Inside the heart
The heart contains four chambers—two atria and two ventricles. (See *Inside a normal heart*, page 6.) The right and left atria serve as volume reservoirs for blood pumped into the ventricles. The right atrium receives deoxygenated blood returning from the body through the inferior and superior vena cava and from the heart through the coronary sinus. The left atrium receives oxygenated blood from the lungs through the four pulmonary veins. The interatrial septum divides the chambers and helps them to contract. Contraction of the atria forces blood into the ventricles below. Although much emphasis is placed on left heart function, the right ventricle acts as a key contributor to hemodynamic stability.

I rest on the diaphragm.

Pump up the volume
The right and left ventricles serve as important chambers of the heart known for their pumping ability. The right ventricle receives blood from the right atrium and pumps it through the pulmonary arteries to the lungs, where it picks up oxygen and drops off carbon dioxide. The left ventricle receives oxygenated blood from the left atrium and pumps it through the aorta and then out to the rest of the body. The interventricular septum separates the ventricles and also helps them to contract.

The chamber wall's thickness depends on the amount of high-pressure work the chamber performs. Because the atria collect blood and pump it to nearby ventricles, their walls are considerably thinner than the walls of the ventricles. Likewise, the left ventricle has a

Inside a normal heart

This illustration shows the anatomy of a normal heart.

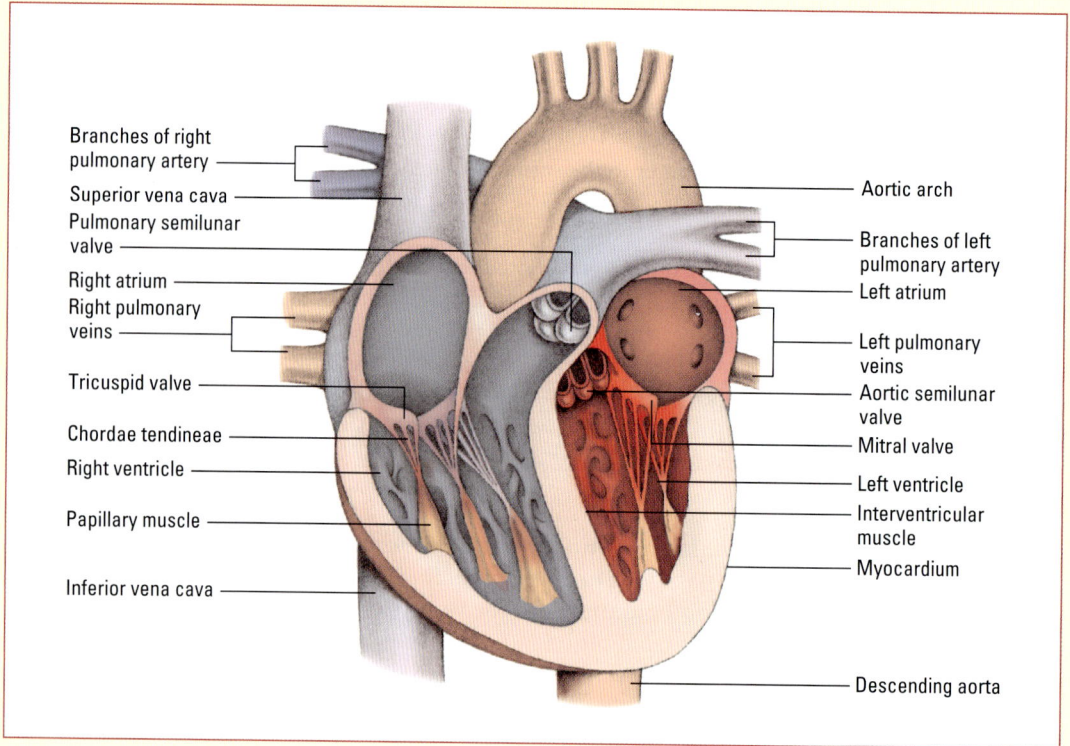

Branches of right pulmonary artery

Superior vena cava

Pulmonary semilunar valve

Right atrium

Right pulmonary veins

Tricuspid valve

Chordae tendineae

Right ventricle

Papillary muscle

Inferior vena cava

Aortic arch

Branches of left pulmonary artery

Left atrium

Left pulmonary veins

Aortic semilunar valve

Mitral valve

Left ventricle

Interventricular muscle

Myocardium

Descending aorta

thicker wall as compared to the right ventricle because the left ventricle pumps blood against a higher pressure gradient, the body's arterial circulation; whereas the right ventricle pumps blood against the lower pressures in the lungs.

One-way valves

The heart contains four valves—two atrioventricular (AV) valves (tricuspid and mitral) and two semilunar valves (aortic and pulmonic). The valves open and close in response to changes in pressure within the chambers to which they connect. In fact, when the AV valves close, the semilunar valves open and vice versa. Heart valves serve as one-way doors that keep blood flowing through the heart in a forward direction.

When the valves close, they prevent backflow or *regurgitation*, of blood from one chamber to another. The closing of the valves creates the heart sounds that are heard through a stethoscope.

The two AV valves, located between the atria and the ventricles, are called the *tricuspid* and *mitral valves*. The tricuspid valve is located between the right atrium and the right ventricle. The mitral valve is located between the left atrium and the left ventricle.

Cardiac cords

The mitral valve has two cusps, or *leaflets*, and the tricuspid valve has three. The cusps are anchored to the papillary muscles in the heart wall by fibers called *chordae tendineae*. These cords work together to prevent the cusps from bulging backward into the atria during ventricular contraction. If damage occurs, blood can flow backward into a chamber, resulting in a heart murmur.

Under pressure

The semilunar valves are the pulmonic valve and the aortic valve. These valves are called *semilunar* because the cusps resemble three half-moons. Because of the high pressures exerted on the valves, their structure is much simpler than that of the AV valves.

The semilunar valves open as a result of a higher pressure gradient within the ventricles and close because of the back pressure of blood in the pulmonary arteries and aorta, which exert pressure to close the cusps. The pulmonic valve, located where the pulmonary artery meets the right ventricle, permits blood to flow from the right ventricle to the pulmonary artery and prevents blood backflow into that ventricle. The aortic valve, located where the left ventricle meets the aorta, allows blood to flow from the left ventricle to the aorta and prevents blood backflow into the left ventricle.

When valves close, heart sounds are heard.

Blood flow through the heart

Understanding how blood flows through the heart is critical to understanding the heart's overall functions and how changes in electrical activity affect peripheral blood flow. Deoxygenated blood from the body returns to the heart through the inferior and superior venae cavae and empties into the right atrium. From there, blood flows through the tricuspid valve into the right ventricle.

Circuit city

The right ventricle pumps blood through the pulmonic valve into the pulmonary arteries and then into the lungs. From the lungs, blood flows through the pulmonary veins and empties into the left atrium, which completes a circuit known as *pulmonary circulation*.

When pressure rises to a critical point in the left atrium, the mitral valve opens and blood flows into the left ventricle. The left ventricle then contracts and pumps blood through the aortic valve into the aorta and then throughout the body. Blood returns to the right atrium through the veins, completing a circuit known as *systemic circulation.*

Getting into circulation

Like the brain and all other organs, the heart needs an adequate supply of blood to survive. The coronary arteries, which lie on the surface of the heart, supply the heart muscle with blood and oxygen. Damaged heart tissue caused by a blockage in a coronary artery, for example, in myocardial infarction (MI), was once thought irreparable. However, recent research has demonstrated the heart is able to repair. The "Singheart" RNA molecule may stimulate damaged cells to regenerate or "self-heal." This could be especially helpful to those with heart failure. With an improved understanding of coronary anatomy and blood flow, you will be able to predict which areas of a patient's heart correspond to a blocked coronary artery. This will be useful in anticipating the patient's cardiac care and overall management.

Open that ostium

The coronary ostium, an opening in the aorta that feeds blood to the coronary arteries, is located near the aortic valve. During systole, when the left ventricle is pumping blood through the aorta and the aortic valve is open, the coronary ostium is partially covered. During diastole, when the left ventricle is filling with blood, the aortic valve is closed and the coronary ostium is open, enabling blood to fill the coronary arteries.

With a shortened diastole that occurs during periods of tachycardia, less blood flows through the ostium into the coronary arteries. Tachycardia can impede coronary blood flow because contraction of the ventricles squeezes the arteries and lessens blood flow through them.

Knowing about coronary blood flow can help me predict which areas of the heart would be affected by a blockage in a particular coronary artery.

That's right, coronary

The right coronary artery and the left coronary artery (also known as the *left main artery*) originate as a single branch off the ascending aorta from the area known as the *sinuses of Valsalva.* The right coronary artery supplies blood to the right atrium, the right ventricle, and part of the inferior and posterior surfaces of the left ventricle. In about 50% of the population, the artery also supplies blood to the SA node. The bundle of His and the AV node also receive their blood supply from the right coronary artery.

What's left, coronary?

The left coronary artery runs along the surface of the left atrium, where it splits into two major branches: the left anterior descending artery and the left circumflex artery. The left anterior descending artery runs down the surface of the left ventricle toward the apex and supplies blood to the anterior wall of the left ventricle, the interventricular septum, the right bundle branch, and the left anterior fasciculus of the left bundle branch. The branches of the left anterior descending artery—the septal perforators and the diagonal arteries—help supply blood to the walls of both ventricles.

Circling circumflex

The circumflex artery supplies oxygenated blood to the lateral walls of the left ventricle, the left atrium and, in about half of the population, the SA node. In addition, the circumflex artery supplies blood to the left posterior fasciculus of the left bundle branch. This artery circles the left ventricle and provides blood to the ventricle's posterior portion.

Circulation, guaranteed

When two or more arteries supply the same region, they usually connect through anastomoses, junctions that provide alternative routes of blood flow. This network of smaller arteries, called *collateral circulation,* provides blood to capillaries that directly feed the heart muscle. Collateral circulation commonly becomes well developed; and in the event that a major coronary artery becomes occluded with plaque, the collateral circulation can continue to supply blood to the heart.

Veins in the heart

The heart has veins just like other parts of the body. Cardiac veins collect deoxygenated blood from the capillaries of the myocardium. The cardiac veins join to form an enlarged vessel called the *coronary sinus,* which returns blood to the right atrium, where it continues through the circulation.

A look at cardiac physiology

This discussion of cardiac physiology includes descriptions of the cardiac cycle, how the cardiac muscle is innervated (distribution/supply of nerves), how the depolarization–repolarization cycle operates, how impulses are conducted, and how abnormal impulses work. (See *Events of the cardiac cycle,* page 10.)

Events of the cardiac cycle

The cardiac cycle consists of the following five events:

• *Isovolumetric ventricular contraction:* In response to ventricular depolarization, tension in the ventricles increases. The rise in pressure within the ventricles leads to closure of the mitral and tricuspid valves. The pulmonic and aortic valves stay closed during the entire phase.

• *Ventricular ejection:* When ventricular pressure exceeds aortic and pulmonary arterial pressure, the aortic and pulmonic valves open and the ventricles eject blood.

• *Isovolumetric relaxation:* When ventricular pressure falls below pressure in the aorta and pulmonary artery, the aortic and pulmonic valves close. All valves are closed during this phase. Atrial diastole occurs as blood fills the atria.

• *Ventricular filling:* Atrial pressure exceeds ventricular pressure, which causes the mitral and tricuspid valves to open. Blood then flows passively into the ventricles. About 70% of ventricular filling takes place during this phase.

• *Atrial systole:* Known as the *atrial kick,* atrial systole (coinciding with late ventricular diastole) supplies the ventricles with the remaining 30% of the blood for each heartbeat.

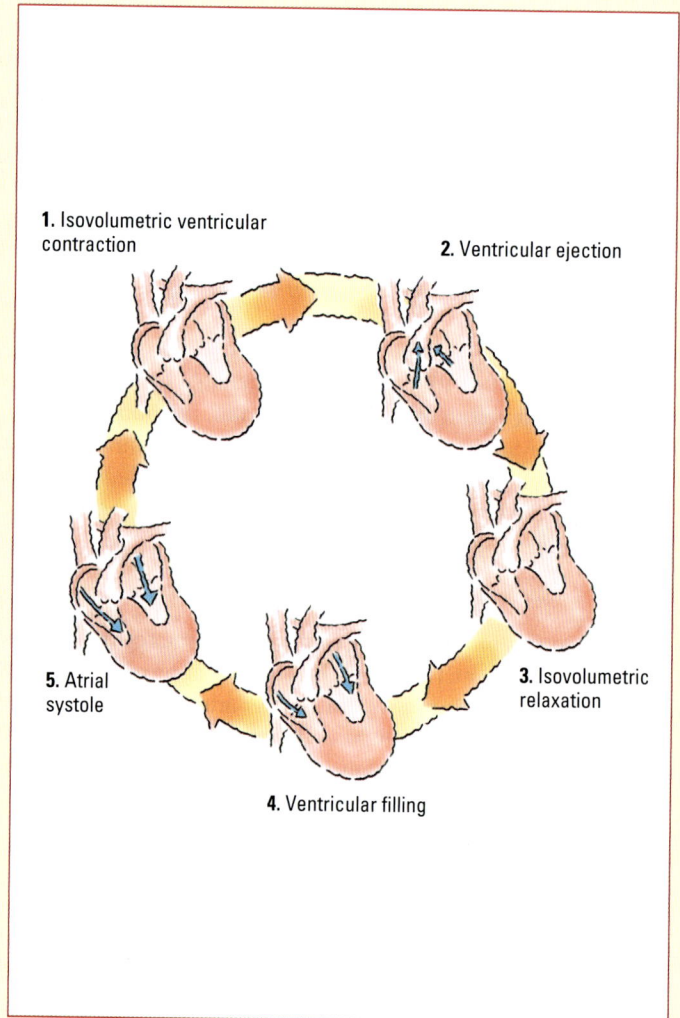

1. Isovolumetric ventricular contraction

2. Ventricular ejection

3. Isovolumetric relaxation

4. Ventricular filling

5. Atrial systole

Cardiac cycle dynamics

During one heartbeat, ventricular diastole (relaxation) and ventricular systole (contraction) occur.

During diastole, the ventricles relax, the atria contract, and blood is forced through the open tricuspid and mitral valves. The aortic and pulmonic valves are closed.

During systole, the atria relax and fill with blood. The mitral and tricuspid valves are closed. Ventricular pressure rises, which forces open to open the aortic and pulmonic valves. The ventricles then contract, and blood flows through the circulatory system.

Atrial kick

The atrial contraction, or atrial kick, contributes about 30% of the cardiac output—the amount of blood pumped by the ventricles in 1 minute. (See *Quick facts about circulation*.) Certain arrhythmias, such as atrial fibrillation, can cause a loss of atrial kick and a subsequent drop in cardiac output. Tachycardia also affects cardiac

Understanding preload, afterload, and contractility

To better understand preload, afterload, and contractility, think of the heart as a balloon.

Preload

Preload is the passive stretching of muscle fibers in the ventricles. This stretching results from blood volume in the ventricles at end diastole. According to Starling's law, the more the heart muscles stretch during diastole, the more forcefully they contract during systole. Think of preload as the balloon stretching as air is blown into it. The more air, the greater the stretch.

Contractility

Contractility refers to the inherent ability of the myocardium to contract normally. Contractility is influenced by preload. The greater the stretch, the more forceful the contraction—or, the more air in the balloon, the greater the stretch and the farther the balloon will fly when air is allowed to expel.

Afterload

Afterload refers to the pressure that the ventricular muscles must generate to overcome the higher pressure in the aorta and force the blood out of the heart. *Resistance* is the knot on the end of the balloon, which the balloon has to work against to get the air out.

Quick facts about circulation

- It would take about 25 capillaries laid end to end to fill 1″ (2.5 cm).
- The body contains about 10 billion capillaries.
- On average, it takes a red blood cell less than 1 minute to travel from the heart to the capillaries and back again.

output by shortening diastole and allowing less time for the ventricles to fill. Less filling time means less blood will be ejected during ventricular systole and less will be sent through the circulation.

A balancing act

The cardiac cycle produces cardiac output, which is the amount of blood the heart pumps in 1 minute. It's measured by multiplying heart rate times stroke volume. (See *Understanding preload, afterload, and contractility*, page 11.) The term *stroke volume* refers to the amount of blood ejected with each ventricular contraction.

Normal cardiac output is 4 to 8 L/min, depending on body size. The heart pumps as much blood as the body requires. Three factors affect stroke volume—preload, afterload, and myocardial contractility. A balance of these three factors produces optimal cardiac output.

Preload

Preload is the stretching of muscle fibers in the ventricles and is determined by the pressure and amount of blood remaining in the left ventricle at the end of diastole.

Afterload

Afterload is the amount of pressure the left ventricle must work against to pump blood into the circulation. The greater this resistance, the more the heart works to pump out blood.

Contractility

Contractility is the ability of muscle cells to contract after depolarization. This ability depends on how much the muscle fibers are stretched at the end of diastole. Overstretching or understretching these fibers alters contractility and the amount of blood pumped out of the ventricles. To better understand this concept, imagine that you are trying to shoot a rubber band across the room. If the rubber band isn't stretched enough, it won't go far when launched. Conversely, if the rubber band is overstretched, it will snap. However, a rubber band that is stretched to just the right amount will launch as far as you need it to go.

Nerve supply to the heart

The heart is supplied by the two branches of the autonomic nervous system—the sympathetic, or *adrenergic*, and the parasympathetic, or *cholinergic*.

The sympathetic nervous system is basically the heart's accelerator. Two sets of chemicals—norepinephrine and epinephrine—are highly influenced by this system. These chemicals increase heart rate, automaticity, AV conduction, and contractility.

Contractility is the heart's ability to stretch—like a balloon!

Braking the heart

The parasympathetic nervous system, on the other hand, serves as the heart's brakes. The vagus nerve carries impulses that slow heart rate and the conduction of impulses through the AV node and ventricles. Stimulating this system releases the chemical acetylcholine, slowing the heart rate.

The vagus nerve is stimulated by baroreceptors, specialized nerve cells in the aorta, and the internal carotid arteries. Conditions that stimulate the baroreceptors also stimulate the vagus nerve.

For example, a stretching of the baroreceptors, which can occur during periods of hypertension or when applying pressure to the carotid artery, stimulates the receptors. In a maneuver called *carotid sinus massage*, baroreceptors in the carotid arteries are purposely activated in an effort to slow a rapid heart rate.

Transmission of electrical impulses

The heart is unable to pump unless an electrical stimulus occurs first. Generation and transmission of electrical impulses depend on four characteristics of cardiac cells:

- *Automaticity* refers to a cell's ability to spontaneously initiate an impulse. Pacemaker cells possess this ability.
- *Excitability* results from ion shifts across the cell membrane and indicates how well a cell responds to an electrical stimulus.
- *Conductivity* is the ability of a cell to transmit an electrical impulse to another cardiac cell.
- *Contractility* refers to how well the cell contracts after receiving a stimulus.

"De"-cycle and "re"-cycle

As impulses are transmitted, cardiac cells undergo cycles of depolarization and repolarization. (See *Depolarization–repolarization cycle*, page 14.) Cardiac cells at rest are considered polarized, meaning that no electrical activity takes place. Cell membranes separate different concentrations of ions, such as sodium and potassium, and create a more negative charge inside the cell. This is called the *resting potential*. After a stimulus occurs, ions cross the cell membrane and cause an action potential, or cell depolarization. Researchers have discovered a "calcium-sensing gate," which initiates calcium waves responsible for calcium-triggered arrhythmias. This discovery may aid in the development of new drug treatments. When a cell is fully depolarized, it attempts to return to its resting state in a process called *repolarization*. Electrical charges in the cell reverse and return to normal.

Memory jogger

To help you remember the difference between depolarization and repolarization, think of the **R** in repolarization as standing for **REST**. Remember that repolarization is the resting phase of the cardiac cycle.

Those impulses really get around!

Depolarization–repolarization cycle

The depolarization–repolarization cycle consists of the following phases:

Phase 0:
Rapid depolarization
- Sodium (Na^+) moves rapidly into cell
- Calcium (Ca^{++}) moves slowly into cell

Phase 1:
Early repolarization
- Sodium channels close

Phase 2:
Plateau phase
- Calcium continues to flow in
- Potassium (K^+) continues to flow out

Phase 3:
Rapid repolarization
- Calcium channels close
- Potassium flows out rapidly
- Active transport via the sodium–potassium pump begins restoring potassium to the inside of the cell and sodium to the outside of the cell

Phase 4:
Resting phase
- Cell membrane is impermeable to sodium
- Potassium moves out of the cell

A cycle of depolarization–repolarization consists of five phases—0 through 4. The action potential is represented by a curve that shows voltage changes during the five phases. (See *Action potential curve*, page 15.)

Many phases of the curve

During phase 0, the cell receives an impulse from a neighboring cell and is depolarized.

Phase 1 is marked by early, rapid repolarization.

Phase 2, the plateau phase of the ST segment, is a period of slow repolarization. During phases 1 and 2 and at the beginning of phase

Action potential curve

An action potential curve shows the electrical changes in a myocardial cell during the depolarization–repolarization cycle. This graph shows the changes in a nonpacemaker cell.

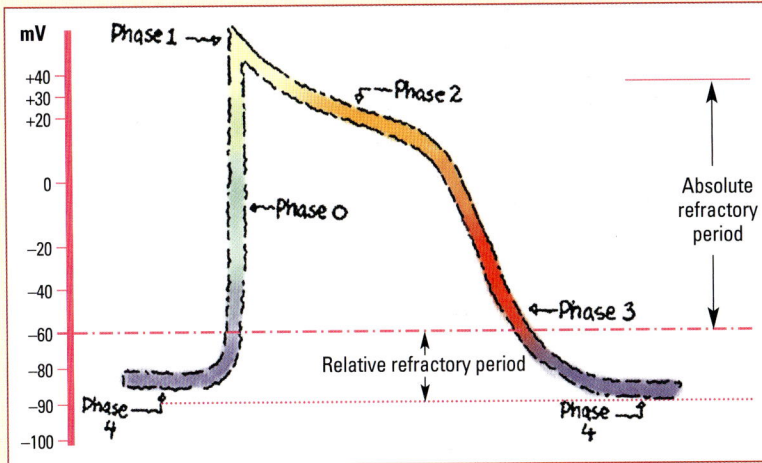

3, the cardiac cell is said to be in its absolute refractory period. During that period, no stimulus, no matter how strong, can excite the cell.

Phase 3, the rapid repolarization phase denoted by the T wave, occurs as the cell returns to its original state. During the last half of this phase, when the cell is in its relative refractory period, a very strong stimulus can depolarize it.

Phase 4 is the resting phase of the action potential. By the end of phase 4, the cell is ready for another stimulus.

All that electrical activity is represented on an electrocardiogram (ECG). Keep in mind that electrical activity of the heart seen on the ECG precedes muscular contraction and pumping of the heart. Therefore, the ECG represents electrical activity only, not actual pumping of the heart.

Pathway through the heart

After depolarization and repolarization occur, the resulting electrical impulse travels through the heart along a pathway called the *conduction system*. (See *The cardiac conduction system*, page 16.)

The cardiac conduction system

Specialized fibers propagate electrical impulses throughout the heart's cells, causing the heart to contract. This illustration shows the elements of the cardiac conduction system.

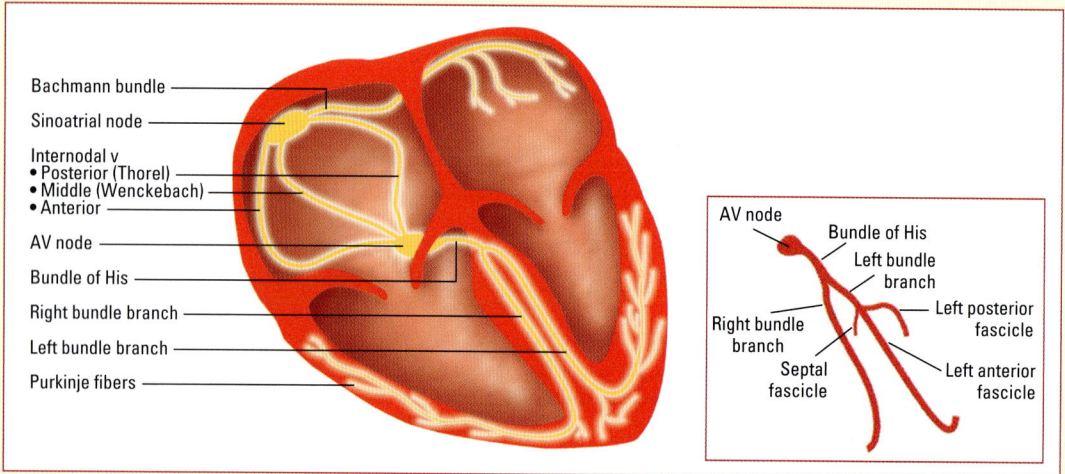

Impulses travel out from the SA node and through the internodal tracts and Bachmann bundle to the AV node. From there, they travel through the bundle of His, the bundle branches, and lastly to the Purkinje fibers.

Setting the pace

The SA node is located in the upper right corner of the right atrium, where the superior vena cava joins the atrial tissue mass. The SA node is the heart's primary pacemaker, generating impulses 60 to 100 times/min. When initiated, normal electrical conduction causes impulses to follow a specific pathway through the heart.

Bachmann bundle of nerves

Impulses from the SA node next travel through Bachmann bundle—tracts of tissue extending from the SA node to the left atrium. Impulses are thought to be transmitted throughout the right atrium through the anterior, middle, and posterior internodal tracts. Impulse transmission through the right and left atria occurs so rapidly that the atria contract almost simultaneously.

AV: The gatekeeper

The AV node, located in the inferior right atrium near the ostium of the coronary sinus, functions like a gatekeeper by delaying the impulses coming from the SA node. Although the nodal tissue itself has no pacemaker cells, the tissue surrounding it (called *junctional tissue*) contains pacemaker cells that can fire at a rate of 40 to 60 times/min.

The AV node's main function is to delay impulses by 0.04 seconds to keep the ventricles from contracting too quickly. This delay allows the ventricles to complete their filling phase as the atria contract. It also allows the cardiac muscle to stretch to its fullest for peak cardiac output.

Branch splitting

The bundle of His, a tract of tissue extending into the ventricles next to the interventricular septum, resumes the rapid conduction of the impulse through the ventricles. The bundle eventually divides into the right and left bundle branches.

The right bundle branch extends down the right side of the interventricular septum and through the right ventricle. The left bundle branch extends down the left side of the interventricular septum and through the left ventricle.

The left bundle branch then splits into two branches, or fasciculi: the left anterior fasciculus, which extends through the anterior portion of the left ventricle, and the left posterior fasciculus, which runs through the lateral and posterior portions of the left ventricle. Impulses travel much faster down the left bundle branch (which feeds the larger, thicker walled left ventricle) than the right bundle branch (which feeds the smaller, thinner walled right ventricle).

The difference in the conduction speed allows both ventricles to contract simultaneously. The entire network of specialized nervous tissue that extends through the ventricles is known as the *His–Purkinje system*.

Those perky Purkinje fibers

Purkinje fibers extend from the bundle branches into the endocardium, deep into the myocardial tissue. These fibers conduct impulses rapidly through the muscle to assist in its depolarization and contraction.

Purkinje fibers can also serve as a pacemaker and are able to discharge impulses at a rate of 20 to 40 times/min, sometimes even more slowly. (See *Pacemakers of the heart*, page 18.) Purkinje fibers are typically activated as a pacemaker only in special circumstances, when conduction through the bundle of His becomes blocked or a higher pacemaker (SA or AV node) fails to generate an impulse. (See *Pediatric pacemaker rates*, page 18).

Pacemakers of the heart

Pacemaker cells in lower areas, such as the junctional tissue and the Purkinje fibers, normally remain dormant because they receive impulses from the SA node. However, when an impulse is not received from these areas, such as when the SA node is damaged from a MI, then the junctional tissue or Purkinje fibers will generate an impulse.

Firing rates

This illustration shows intrinsic firing rates of pacemaker cells located in three critical areas of the heart.

SA node, 60–100/min

AV junction, 40–60/min

Purkinje fibers, 20–40/min

Ages and stages

Pediatric pacemaker rates

In children younger than age 3, the AV node may discharge impulses at a rate of 50 to 80 times/min; the Purkinje fibers may discharge at a rate of 40 to 50 times/min.

Abnormal impulses

Now that you understand how the heart generates a normal impulse, let's look at some causes of abnormal impulse conduction, including automaticity, backward conduction of impulses, reentry abnormalities, and ectopy.

When the heart goes on "manual"

Automaticity is a special characteristic of pacemaker cells that generate impulses automatically, without being stimulated to do so. If a cell's automaticity is increased or decreased, an arrhythmia can occur. Tachycardia, for example, is commonly caused by an increase in the automaticity of pacemaker cells below the SA node. Likewise, a decrease in automaticity of cells in the SA node can cause the development of bradycardia or an escape rhythm (a compensatory beat generated by a lower pacemaker site).

Out of synch

Impulses that begin below the AV node can be transmitted backward toward the atria. This backward, or retrograde, conduction usually takes longer than normal conduction and can cause the atria and ventricles to beat out of synch.

Coming back for more

Sometimes, impulses cause depolarization twice in a row at a faster than normal rate. Such events are referred to as *reentry events*. In reentry, impulses are delayed long enough that cells have time to repolarize. In these cases, the active impulse reenters the same area and produces another impulse.

That's a wrap!

Cardiac anatomy and physiology review

The heart's valves
- *Tricuspid*: AV valve between the right atrium and the right ventricle
- *Mitral*: AV valve between the left atrium and the left ventricle
- *Aortic*: Semilunar valve between the left ventricle and the aorta
- *Pulmonic*: Semilunar valve between the right ventricle and the pulmonary artery

Blood flow
- Deoxygenated blood from the body returns to the right atrium and then flows to the right ventricle.
- The right ventricle pumps blood into the lungs where it's oxygenated. Then the blood returns to the left atrium and flows to the left ventricle.
- Oxygenated blood is pumped to the aorta and the body by the left ventricle.

Coronary arteries and veins
- *Right coronary artery*: Supplies blood to the right atrium and ventricle and part of the left ventricle
- *Left anterior descending artery*: Supplies blood to the anterior wall of the left ventricle, interventricular septum, right bundle branch, and left anterior fasciculus of the left bundle branch
- *Circumflex artery*: Supplies blood to the lateral walls of the left ventricle, left atrium, and left posterior fasciculus of the left bundle branch
- *Cardiac veins*: Collect blood from the capillaries of the myocardium
- *Coronary sinus*: Returns blood to the right atrium

Cardiac cycle dynamics
- *Atrial kick*: Atrial contraction, contributing about 30% of the cardiac output
- *Cardiac output*: The amount of blood the heart pumps in 1 minute, calculated by multiplying heart rate times stroke volume
- *Stroke volume*: The amount of blood ejected with each ventricular contraction (it's affected by preload, afterload, and contractility)
- *Preload*: The passive stretching exerted by blood on the ventricular muscle at the end of diastole
- *Afterload*: The amount of pressure the left ventricle must work against to pump blood into the aorta
- *Contractility*: The ability of the heart muscle cells to contract after depolarization

Innervation of the heart
Two branches of the autonomic nervous system supply the heart:
- *Sympathetic nervous system*: Increases heart rate, automaticity, AV conduction, and contractility through the release of norepinephrine and epinephrine
- *Parasympathetic nervous system*: Vagus nerve stimulation reduces heart rate and AV conduction through the release of acetylcholine.

Transmission of electrical impulses
Generation and transmission of electrical impulses depend on the following cell characteristics:

Cardiac anatomy and physiology review *(continued)*

- *Automaticity.* A cell's ability to spontaneously initiate an impulse, such as found in pacemaker cells
- *Excitability.* How well a cell responds to an electrical stimulus
- *Conductivity.* The ability of a cell to transmit an electrical impulse to another cardiac cell
- *Contractility.* How well the cell contracts after receiving a stimulus

Depolarization–repolarization cycle
Cardiac cells undergo the following cycles of depolarization and repolarization as impulses are transmitted:
- *Phase 0: Rapid depolarization*—the cell receives an impulse from a nearby cell and is depolarized.
- *Phase 1: Early repolarization*—early rapid repolarization occurs.
- *Phase 2: Plateau phase*—a period of slow repolarization occurs.
- *Phase 3: Rapid repolarization*—the cell returns to its original state.
- *Phase 4: Resting phase*—the cell rests and readies itself for another stimulus.

Cardiac conduction
- The electrical impulse begins in the SA node and travels through the internodal tracts and Bachmann bundle to the AV node.
- From the AV node, the impulse travels down the bundle of His, along the bundle branches, and through the Purkinje fibers.

Intrinsic firing rates
- *SA node*: 60 to 100 times/min
- *AV junction*: 40 to 60 times/min
- *Purkinje fibers:* 20 to 40 times/min

Abnormal impulses
- *Automaticity.* The ability of a cardiac cell to initiate an impulse on its own
- *Retrograde conduction.* Impulses that are transmitted backward toward the atria
- *Reentry.* When an impulse follows a circular, rather than the normal, conduction path

Repeating itself

An injured pacemaker (or nonpacemaker) cell may partially depolarize, rather than fully depolarizing. Partial depolarization can lead to spontaneous or secondary depolarization, which involves repetitive ectopic firings called *triggered activity.*

The resultant depolarization is called *afterdepolarization.* Early afterdepolarization occurs before the cell is fully repolarized and can be caused by hypokalemia, slow pacing rates, or drug toxicity. If it occurs after the cell has been fully repolarized, it's called *delayed afterdepolarization.* These problems can be caused by digoxin toxicity, hypercalcemia, or increased catecholamine release. Atrial or ventricular tachycardia may result. You'll learn more about these and other arrhythmias in later chapters.

Quick quiz

1. The term *automaticity* refers to the ability of a cell to:
    A. initiate an impulse on its own.
    B. send impulses in all directions.
    C. block impulses formed in areas other than the SA node.
    D. generate an impulse when stimulated.

Answer: A. Automaticity, the ability of a cell to initiate an impulse on its own, is a unique characteristic of cardiac cells.

2. Parasympathetic stimulation of the heart results in:
    A. increased heart rate and decreased contractility.
    B. increased heart rate and faster AV conduction.
    C. decreased heart rate and slower AV conduction.
    D. decreased heart rate and increased contractility.

Answer: C. Parasympathetic stimulation of the vagus nerve causes a decrease in heart rate and slowed AV conduction.

3. The normal pacemaker of the heart is the:
    A. SA node.
    B. AV node.
    C. bundle of His.
    D. Purkinje fibers.

Answer: A. The SA node is the normal pacemaker of the heart, firing at an intrinsic rate of 60 to 100 times/min.

4. The impulse delay produced by the AV node allows the atria to:
    A. repolarize simultaneously.
    B. contract before the ventricles.
    C. send impulses to the bundle of His.
    D. complete their filling.

Answer: B. The 0.04-second delay allows the atria to contract and the ventricles to completely fill, which optimizes cardiac output.

5. The coronary arteries fill with blood during:
    A. atrial systole.
    B. atrial diastole.
    C. ventricular systole.
    D. ventricular diastole.

Answer: D. The coronary arteries and the ventricles fill with blood during diastole. The aortic valve is closed at that time, so it no longer blocks blood flow through the coronary ostium into the coronary arteries.

6. When stimulated, baroreceptors cause the heart rate to:
   A. increase.
   B. decrease.
   C. stay the same.
   D. become irregular.

Answer: B. Baroreceptors, when stimulated, cause the heart rate to decrease.

7. The two valves called the *semilunar valves* are the:
   A. pulmonic and tricuspid valves.
   B. pulmonic and aortic valves.
   C. aortic and mitral valves.
   D. aortic and tricuspid valves.

Answer: B. The pulmonic and aortic valves are semilunar.

8. Passive stretching exerted by blood on the ventricular muscle at the end of diastole is referred to as:
   A. preload.
   B. afterload.
   C. the atrial kick.
   D. cardiac output.

Answer: A. Preload is the passive stretching exerted by blood on the ventricular muscle at the end of diastole. It increases with an increase in venous return to the heart.

9. A patient admitted with an acute MI has a heart rate of 36 beats/min. Based on this finding, which area of the heart is most likely serving as the pacemaker?
   A. SA node.
   B. AV node.
   C. Bachmann bundle.
   D. Purkinje fibers.

Answer: D. If the SA node (which fires at a rate of 60 to 100 times/min) and the AV node (which takes over firing at 40 to 60 times/min) are damaged, the Purkinje fibers take over firing at a rate of 20 to 40 times/min.

Scoring

★★★ If you answered all nine questions correctly, hooray!

★★ If you answered six to eight questions correctly, way to go!

★ If you answered fewer than six questions correctly, take heart. Just review this chapter and you'll be up to speed.

Selected references

Buddiga, P. (2014). *Cardiovascular system anatomy*. Medscape. Retrieved November 20, 2014, from http://emedicine.medscape.com/article/1948510-overview

Hai, J. J., Lachman, N., Syed, F. F., Desimone, C. V., & Asirvatham, S. J. (2014). The anatomic basis for ventricular arrhythmia in the normal heart: What the student of anatomy needs to know. *Clinical Anatomy, 27*(6), 885–893. https://doi.org/10.1002/ca.22362

Jones, K. (2014, January 20). *Fundamental process of heart arrhythmia discovered.* Retrieved May 30, 2019, from https://www.medindia.net/news/fundamental-processof-heart-arrhythmia-discovered-130725-1.htm

Jones, S. A. (2019). *ECG mastery: Improving your ECG interpretation skills* (2nd ed.). F. A. Davis Company.

Mohrman, D. E., & Hellen, L. (2014). Overview of the cardiovascular system. In D. H. Mohrman (Ed.), *Cardiovascular physiology* (8th ed., Ch. 1). McGraw-Hill. Retrieved November 13, 2014, from https://accessmedicine.mhmedical.com/book.aspx?bookID=3346

Mori, S., Spicer, D. E., & Anderson, R. H. (2016). Revisiting the anatomy of the living heart. *Circulation Journal, 80*(1), 24–33. https://doi.org/10.1253/circj.CJ-15-1147

National University Health System. (2017, August 21). Repairing damaged hearts with self-healing heart cells: Researchers discover a new molecule, "Singheart," that may hold the key to triggering the regeneration and repair of damaged heart cells. *ScienceDaily.* Retrieved May 16, 2019, from www.sciencedaily.com/releases/2017/08/170821094253.htm

Newman, T. (2018, January 9). The heart: All you need to know. *Medical News Today.* Retrieved May 30, 2019, from https://www.medicalnewstoday.com/articles/320565.php

Picazo-Angelin, B., Zabala-Argüelles, J. I., Anderson, R. H., & Sánchez-Quintana, D. (2018). Anatomy of the normal fetal heart: The basis for understanding fetal echocardiography. *Annals of Pediatric Cardiology, 11*(2), 164–173. https://doi.org/10.4103/apc.APC_152_17

Spicer, D., Bridgeman, J., Brown, N., Mohun, T., & Anderson, R. (2014). The anatomy and development of the cardiac valves. *Cardiology in the Young, 24*(6), 1008–1022. https://doi.org/10.1017/S1047951114001942

Tkacs, N. C., Herrmann, L. L., & Johnson, R. L. (2021). *Advanced physiology and pathophysiology: Essentials for clinical practice.* Springer Publishing Company.

Zamorano, J. L., González-Gómez, A., & Lancellotti, P. (2014). Mitral valve anatomy: Implications for transcatheter mitral valve interventions. *EuroIntervention, 10*(Suppl U), U106–U111. https://doi.org/10.4244/EIJV10SUA15

Obtaining a rhythm strip

Just the facts

In this chapter, you'll learn:

♦ the importance of ECGs in providing effective patient care

♦ the functions of leads and planes

♦ the types of ECG monitoring systems

♦ proper techniques for applying electrodes, selecting leads, and obtaining rhythm strips

♦ solutions for cardiac monitoring problems.

A look at ECG recordings

The heart's electrical activity produces currents that radiate through the surrounding tissue to the skin. Electrodes attached to the skin sense electrical currents and transmit them to an ECG monitor. The currents are then transformed into waveforms that represent the heart's depolarization–repolarization cycle.

You might remember that myocardial depolarization occurs when an electrical impulse passes through the heart stimulating myocardial contraction. Repolarization is the return to the resting state and results in relaxation.

An ECG shows the precise sequence of electrical events that originate in the cardiac cells and transmit impulses to the myocardium. ECGs allow the health care providers to monitor phases of myocardial contraction and to identify rhythm and conduction disturbances. A series of ECGs can be used as a baseline comparison to assess cardiac function.

An ECG shows the sequence of cardiac events.

Leads and planes

To understand electrocardiography, you need to understand leads and planes. Electrodes placed on the skin measure the direction of electrical current discharged by the heart. This current is then transformed into waveforms.

An ECG records information about those waveforms from different views or perspectives. These perspectives are called *leads* and *planes*.

> Leads and planes offer different views of the heart's electrical activity.

Take the lead

A lead provides a view of the heart's electrical activity between one positive pole and one negative pole. Between the two poles lies an imaginary line representing the *lead's axis*, a term that refers to the direction of the current moving through the heart.

The direction of the current affects the direction in which the waveform points on an ECG. (See *Current direction and wave deflection*) When no electrical activity occurs or the activity is too weak to measure, the waveform looks like a straight line, called an *isoelectric waveform*.

Current direction and wave deflection

The illustration shown depicts the possible directions of electrical current, or depolarization, on a lead. The direction of the electrical current determines the upward or downward deflection of an ECG waveform.

> When current flows perpendicular to the lead, the waveform may be small or go in both directions (biphasic).

> As current travels toward the negative pole, the waveform deflects mostly downward.

> As current travels toward the positive pole, the waveform deflects mostly upward.

Plane and simple

The term *plane* refers to a cross-sectional perspective of the heart's electrical activity. The frontal plane, a vertical cut through the middle of the heart, provides an anterior-to-posterior view of electrical activity. The horizontal plane, a transverse cut through the middle of the heart, provides either a superior or an inferior view.

Types of ECGs

The two types of ECG recordings are the 12-lead ECG and a rhythm strip. Both types give valuable information about heart function.

A dozen views

A 12-lead ECG records information from 12 different views of the heart and provides a complete picture of electrical activity. These 12 views are obtained by placing electrodes on the patient's limbs and chest. The limb leads and the chest, or precordial leads, reflect information from different planes of the heart.

Different leads provide different information. The six limb leads—I, II, III, augmented vector right (aV_R), augmented vector left (aV_L), and augmented vector foot (aV_F)—provide information about the heart's frontal (vertical) plane. Leads I, II, and III require a negative and positive electrode for monitoring, which makes the leads bipolar. The augmented leads record information from one lead and are called *unipolar*.

The six precordial or V leads—V_1, V_2, V_3, V_4, V_5, and V_6—provide information about the heart's horizontal plane. Just like the augmented leads, the precordial leads are also unipolar, requiring only a single electrode. The opposing pole of these leads is the center of the heart as calculated by the ECG.

Just one view

A rhythm strip, which can be used to monitor cardiac status, provides information about the heart's electrical activity from one or more leads simultaneously. Chest electrodes pick up the heart's electrical activity for display on the monitor. The monitor also displays heart rate and other measurements and allows for printing strips of cardiac rhythms.

Commonly monitored leads include the bipolar leads I, II, III, MCL_1, and MCL_6 as well as the unipolar leads V_1 and V_6. The acronym MCL stands for modified chest lead. These leads are similar to the unipolar leads V_1 and V_6 of the 12-lead ECG. MCL_1 and MCL_6, however, are the bipolar leads.

Monitoring ECGs

The type of ECG monitoring system you'll use—hardwire monitoring or telemetry—depends on the patient's condition and the existing equipment. Let's look at each system.

Hardwire basics

With hardwire monitoring, the electrodes are connected directly to the cardiac monitor. Most hardwire monitors are mounted permanently on a shelf or wall near the patient's bed. Some monitors are mounted on an intravenous (IV) pole for portability, and some may include a defibrillator.

The monitor provides a continuous cardiac rhythm display and transmits the ECG tracing to a console at the nurses' station. Both the monitor and the console have alarms and can print rhythm strips. Hardwire monitors can also track pulse oximetry, blood pressure, hemodynamic measurements, and other parameters through various attachments to the patient.

> There are pros and cons with both ECG monitoring systems.

Some drawbacks

Hardwire monitoring is generally used in intensive care units and emergency departments because it permits continuous observation of one or more patients from more than one area in the unit. However, this type of monitoring does have drawbacks, including:

- limited patient mobility because the patient is tethered to a monitor by a cable
- patient discomfort because the electrodes and cables are attached to the chest
- possibility of lead disconnection and loss of cardiac monitoring when the patient moves

Portable points

Telemetry monitoring is generally used in step-down units and medical–surgical units where patients are permitted more physical activity. With telemetry monitoring, the patient carries a small, battery-powered transmitter that sends electrical signals to another location where the signals are displayed on a monitor screen. This type of ECG monitoring frees the patient from cumbersome wires and cables associated with hardwire monitoring.

Telemetry monitoring still requires skin electrodes to be placed on the patient's chest. Each electrode is connected by a thin wire to a small transmitter box carried by the patient in a pocket or pouch. It's especially useful for detecting arrhythmias that occur with activity or stressful situations. Most systems, however, can monitor heart rate and rhythm only.

All about leads

Adjust the leads according to the patient's condition.

Electrode placement is different for each lead, and different leads provide different views of the heart. A lead may be chosen to highlight a particular part of the ECG complex or the electrical events of a specific cardiac cycle.

Although leads II, V_1, and V_6 are among the most commonly used leads for monitoring, you should adjust the leads according to the patient's condition. If your monitoring system has the capability, you may also monitor the patient in more than one lead.

Going to ground

All bipolar leads have a third electrode, known as the *ground*, which is placed on the chest to prevent electrical interference from appearing on the ECG recording.

Here is lead I

Lead I provides a view of the heart that shows current moving from right to left. Because current flows from negative to positive, the positive electrode for this lead is placed on the left arm or on the left side of the chest; the negative electrode is placed on the right arm. Lead I produces a positive deflection on ECG tracings and is helpful in monitoring atrial rhythms and hemiblocks.

Introducing lead II

Lead II produces a positive deflection. This lead is positioned with the positive electrode on the patient's left leg and the negative electrode on the right arm. For continuous monitoring, place the electrodes on the torso for convenience, with the positive electrode below the lowest palpable rib at the left midclavicular line and the negative electrode below the right clavicle. The current travels down and to the left in this lead. Lead II tends to produce a positive, high-voltage deflection, resulting in tall P, R, and T waves. This lead is commonly used for routine monitoring and is useful for detecting sinus node and atrial arrhythmias.

Next up, lead III

Lead III produces a positive deflection. The positive electrode is placed on the left leg, and the negative electrode is placed on the left arm. Along with lead II, this lead is useful for detecting changes associated with an inferior wall myocardial infarction.

Einthoven's triangle

When setting up standard limb leads, you'll place electrodes in positions commonly referred to as *Einthoven's triangle,* shown in the image. The electrodes for leads I, II, and III are about equidistant from the heart and form an equilateral triangle.

Axes

The axis of lead I extends from shoulder to shoulder, with the right arm electrode being the negative electrode and the left arm electrode the positive electrode.

   The axis of lead II runs from the negative right arm electrode to the positive left leg electrode. The axis of lead III extends from the negative left arm electrode to the positive left leg electrode.

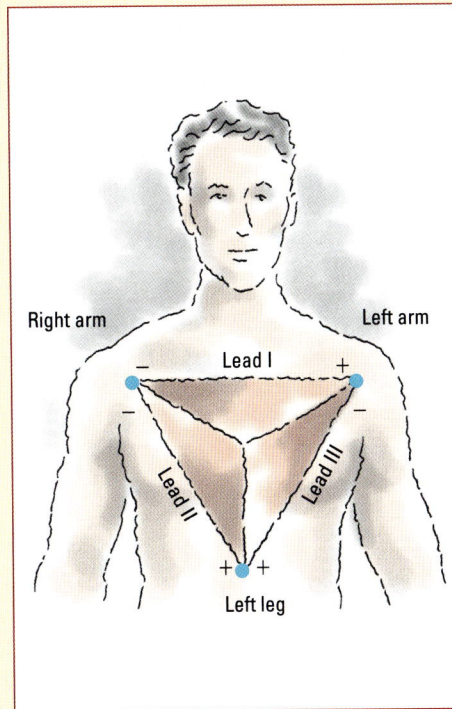

Right arm   Left arm

Lead I

Lead II   Lead III

Left leg

The axes of the three bipolar limb leads—I, II, and III—form a triangle around the heart and provide a frontal plane view of the heart. (See *Einthoven's triangle*)

Placed in sequence across the chest, precordial leads V_1 through V_6 provide a view of the heart's horizontal plane.

The "a" leads

Leads aV_R, aV_L, and aV_F are called *augmented leads* because the small waveforms that normally would appear from these unipolar leads are enhanced by the ECG. (See *Augmented leads*, page 30.) The "a" stands for "augmented," and "R, L, and F" stand for the positive electrode positions of the lead.

   In lead aV_R, the positive electrode is placed on the right arm (hence, the R) and produces a negative deflection because the heart's electrical activity moves away from the lead. In lead aV_L, the positive electrode is on the left arm and produces a positive deflection on the ECG. In lead aV_F, the positive electrode is on the left leg (despite the name aV_F where the F refers to "foot") and produces a positive deflection. These three limb leads also provide a view of the heart's frontal plane.

Augmented leads

Leads aV_R, aV_L, and aV_F are called *augmented leads*. They measure electrical activity between one limb and a single electrode. Lead aV_R provides no specific view of the heart. Lead aV_L shows electrical activity coming from the heart's lateral wall. Lead aV_F shows electrical activity coming from the heart's inferior wall.

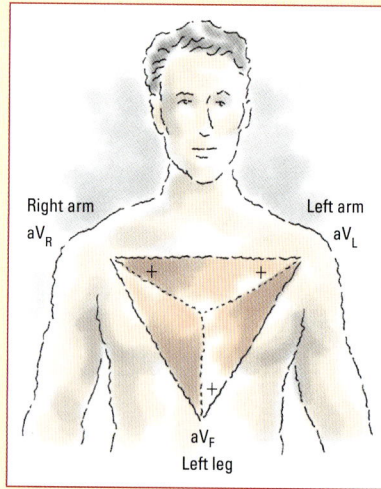

Right arm
aV_R

Left arm
aV_L

aV_F
Left leg

The preeminent precordials

The six unipolar precordial leads are placed in sequence across the chest and provide a view of the heart's horizontal plane. (See *Precordial views*, page 31.) These leads include:

- *Lead V_1:* The precordial lead V_1 electrode is placed on the right side of the sternum at the fourth intercostal rib space. This lead corresponds to the modified chest-lead MCL_1 and shows the P wave, QRS complex, and ST segment particularly well. It helps to distinguish between the right and left ventricular ectopic beats that result from myocardial irritation or other cardiac stimulation outside the normal conduction system. Lead V_1 is also useful in monitoring ventricular arrhythmias, ST-segment changes, and bundle branch blocks.
- *Lead V_2:* Lead V_2 is placed at the left of the sternum at the fourth intercostal rib space.
- *Lead V_3:* Lead V_3 goes between V_2 and V_4. Leads V_1, V_2, and V_3 are biphasic, with both positive and negative deflections. Leads V_2 and V_3 can be used to detect ST-segment elevation.
- *Lead V_4:* Lead V_4 is placed at the fifth intercostal space at the midclavicular line and produces a biphasic waveform.
- *Lead V_5:* Lead V_5 is placed at the fifth intercostal space at the anterior axillary line. It produces a positive deflection on the ECG and, along with V_4, can show changes in the ST segment or T wave.
- *Lead V_6:* Lead V_6, the last of the precordial leads, is placed level with V_4 at the midaxillary line. This lead produces a positive deflection on the ECG.

Precordial views

These illustrations show the different views of the heart obtained from each precordial (chest) lead.

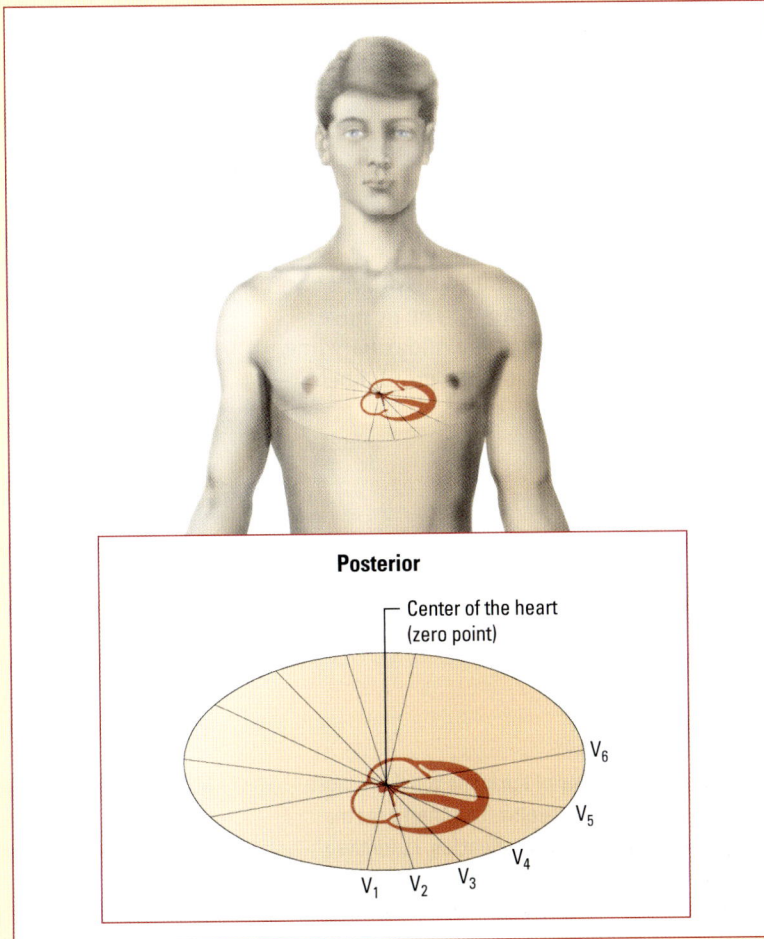

Posterior

Center of the heart
(zero point)

V_6

V_5

V_4

V_1 V_2 V_3

The modest modified lead

MCL$_1$ is similar to lead V$_1$ on the 12-lead ECG and is created by placing the negative electrode on the left upper chest, the positive electrode on the right side of the sternum at the fourth intercostal space, and the ground electrode usually on the right upper chest below the clavicle.

When the positive electrode is on the right side of the heart and the electrical current travels toward the left ventricle, the waveform has a negative deflection. As a result, ectopic or abnormal beats deflect in a positive direction.

You can use this lead to monitor premature ventricular contractions and to distinguish different types of tachycardia, such as ventricular tachycardia and supraventricular tachycardia. Lead MCL_1 can also be used to assess bundle branch defects and P-wave changes and to confirm pacemaker wire placement.

A five-leadwire system allows you to monitor any six MCLs and the standard limb leads. Yippee, Skippy!

A positive option

MCL_6 may be used as an alternative to MCL_1. Just like MCL_1, it monitors ventricular conduction changes. The positive lead in MCL_6 is placed in the same location as its equivalent, lead V_6. The positive electrode is placed at the fifth intercostal space at the midaxillary line, the negative electrode below the left shoulder, and the ground below the right shoulder.

Electrode basics

A three- or five-electrode (or *leadwire*) system may be used for cardiac monitoring. (See *Leadwire systems*) Both systems use a ground electrode to prevent accidental electrical shock to the patient.

These are the electrode positions you'll use most often.

Leadwire systems

This chart shows the correct electrode positions for some of the leads you'll use most often—the five-leadwire, three-leadwire, and telemetry systems. The chart uses the abbreviations RA for the right arm, LA for the left arm, RL for the right leg, LL for the left leg, C for the chest, and G for the ground.

Electrode positions
In the three- and five-leadwire systems, electrode positions for one lead may be identical to those for another lead. When that happens, change the lead selector switch to the setting that corresponds to the lead you want. In some cases, you'll need to reposition the electrodes.

Telemetry
In a telemetry monitoring system, you can create the same leads as the other systems with just two electrodes and a ground wire.

Leadwire systems *(continued)*

Five-leadwire system	Three-leadwire system	Telemetry system

Lead I

Lead II

Lead III

(continued)

Five-leadwire system	Three-leadwire system	Telemetry system

Lead MCL$_1$

Lead MCL$_6$

A three-electrode system consists of one positive electrode, one negative electrode, and a ground.

The popular five-electrode system uses an exploratory chest lead to monitor any six MCLs as well as the standard limb leads. (See *Using a five-leadwire system*) This system uses standardized chest placement. Wires that attach to the electrodes are usually color coded to help you place them correctly on the patient's chest.

Using a five-leadwire system

This illustration shows the correct placement of the leadwires for a five-leadwire system. The chest electrode shown is located in the V_1 position, but you can place it in any of the chest-lead positions. The electrodes are color coded as follows:

White	Black	Green	Red	Brown
Right arm (RA)	Left arm (LA)	Right leg (RL)	Left leg (LL)	Chest (C)

Another application of bedside cardiac monitoring is a reduced lead continuous 12-lead ECG system (EASI* system), which uses an advanced algorithm and only five electrodes uniquely placed on the torso to derive a 12-lead ECG. The system allows all 12 leads to be simultaneously displayed and recorded. (See *Understanding the EASI* system*, page 35.)

Understanding the EASI* system

The five-lead EASI* (reduced lead continuous 12-lead ECG) configuration gives a three-dimensional view of the electrical activity of the heart from the frontal, horizontal, and sagittal planes. This provides 12 leads of information. A mathematical calculation in the electronics of the monitoring system is applied to the information, creating a derived 12-lead ECG.

Placement of the electrodes for the EASI* system includes:

- *E lead:* Lower part of the sternum at the level of the fifth intercostal space
- *A lead:* Left midaxillary line at the level of the fifth intercostal *space*
- *S lead:* Upper part of the sternum
- *I lead:* Right midaxillary line at the level of the fifth intercostal space
- *Ground:* Anywhere on the torso

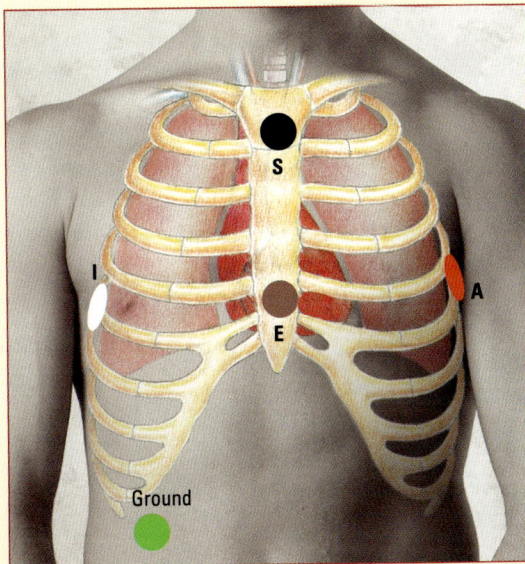

*EASI is a product of Philips Medical Systems, a Division of Philips Healthcare, Andover, MA, 01810-1099.

How to apply electrodes

Before you attach electrodes to your patient, describe the rationale of monitoring their heart rate and rhythm. Explain to the patient that the monitor alarm is a protective feature that notifies nursing staff that the system needs attention; it often means a leadwire has come loose.

Memory jogger

To help you remember where to place electrodes in a five-electrode configuration, think of the phrase "White to the upper right." Then think of snow over trees (white electrode above green electrode) and smoke over fire (black electrode above red electrode). And of course, chocolate (brown electrode) lies close to the heart.

Explain the electrode placement procedure to the patient, provide privacy, and wash your hands. Expose the patient's chest and select electrode sites for the chosen lead. Choose sites over soft tissues or close to bone, not over bony prominences, thick muscles, or skin folds. Those areas can produce ECG artifacts—waveforms not produced by the heart's electrical activity.

Prepare the skin

Next, prepare the patient's skin. To begin, wash the patient's chest with soap and water and then dry it thoroughly. Because body hair may interfere with electrical contact, clip dense hair with clippers or scissors. Then use the special rough patch on the back of the electrode, a dry washcloth, or a gauze pad to rub each site, making sure not to damage or break the skin. Brisk rubbing exfoliates dead skin cells and improves electrical contact.

If the patient has oily skin, clean each site with an alcohol pad and let it air-dry. This ensures proper adhesion and prevents the alcohol from becoming trapped beneath the electrode, which can irritate the skin and cause skin breakdown.

Stick it to me

To apply the electrodes, remove the backing and make sure each pregelled electrode is still moist. If an electrode has become dry, discard it and select another. A dry electrode decreases electrical conductivity, interfering with waveforms.

Apply one electrode to each prepared site using the following method:
- Press one side of the electrode against the patient's skin, pull gently, and then press the opposite side of the electrode against the skin.
- Using two fingers, press the adhesive edge around the outside of the electrode to the patient's chest. This fixes the gel and stabilizes the electrode.
- Repeat this procedure for each electrode.
- Every 24 hours, remove the electrodes, assess the patient's skin, and put new electrodes in place.

Clip, clip, snap, snap

You'll also need to attach leadwires or cable connections to the monitor and attach leadwires to the electrodes. Leadwires may clip on or, more commonly, snap on. (See *Clip-on and snap-on leadwires*) If you're using the snap-on type, attach the electrode to the leadwire just before applying it to the patient's chest. Keep in mind that you may lose electrode contact if you press down to apply the leadwire.

When you use a clip-on leadwire, apply it after the electrode has been secured to the patient's skin. That way, applying the clip won't interfere with the electrode's contact with the skin.

Clip-on and snap-on leadwires

Several kinds of leadwires are available for monitoring. A clip-on leadwire should be attached to the electrode *after* it has been placed on the patient's chest. A snap-on leadwire should be attached to the electrode just *before* it has been placed on the patient's chest. Doing so prevents patient discomfort and disturbance of the contact between the electrode and the skin.

Clip-on leadwire

Leadwire
Electrode

Snap-on leadwire

Electrode

Leadwire

Observing the cardiac rhythm

After the electrodes are in proper position, the monitor is on, and the necessary cables are attached, observe the screen. You should see the patient's ECG waveform. While some monitoring systems allow you to make adjustments by touching the screen, others may require you to manipulate buttons. If the waveform appears too large or too small, change the size by adjusting the gain control. If the waveform appears too high or too low on the screen, adjust the position.

Verify that the monitor detects each heartbeat by comparing the patient's apical rate with the rate displayed on the monitor. Set the upper and lower limits of the heart rate according to your facility's policy and the patient's condition. Heart rate alarms are generally set 10 to 20 beats/min higher and lower than the patient's heart rate.

Monitors with arrhythmia detectors generate a rhythm strip automatically whenever the alarm goes off. You can obtain other views of your patient's cardiac rhythm by selecting different leads. You can select leads with the lead selector button or touch screen.

Printing it out

To get a printout of the patient's cardiac rhythm, press the record control on the monitor. The ECG strip will be printed at the central console. Some systems print the rhythm from a recorder box on the monitor itself.

Most monitor recording systems print the date, time, and the patient's name and identification number; however, if the monitor you're using can't do this, label the rhythm strip with the date, time, patient's name, identification number, and rhythm interpretation. Add any appropriate clinical information to the ECG strip, such as any medication administered, presence of chest pain, or patient activity at the time of the recording.

WOW! Did I really do all of that?!

It's all on paper

Waveforms produced by the heart's electrical current are recorded on graphed ECG paper by a stylus. ECG paper consists of horizontal and vertical lines forming a grid. A piece of ECG paper is called an *ECG strip* or *tracing*. (See *ECG grid*, page 38.)

ECG grid

This ECG grid shows the horizontal axis and vertical axis and their respective measurement values.

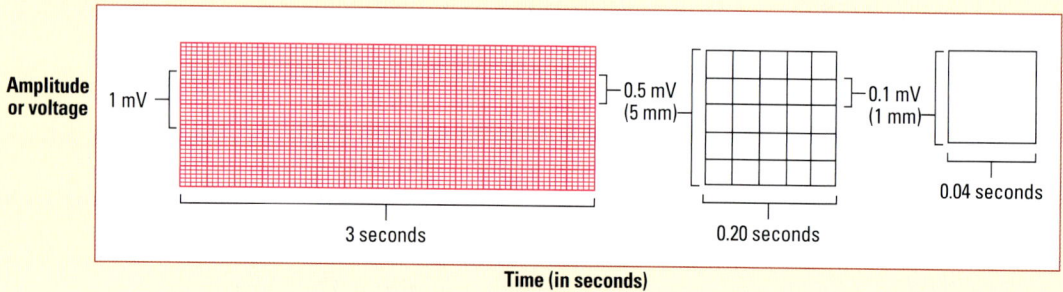

The horizontal axis of the ECG strip represents time. Each small block equals 0.04 seconds, and five small blocks form a large block, which equals 0.2 seconds. This time increment is determined by multiplying 0.04 seconds (for one small block) by 5, the number of small blocks that compose a large block. Five large blocks equal 1 second (5 × 0.2). When measuring or calculating a patient's heart rate, a 6-second strip consisting of 30 large blocks is usually used.

The ECG strip's vertical axis measures amplitude in millimeters (mm) or electrical voltage in millivolts (mV). Each small block represents 1 mm or 0.1 mV and each large block 5 mm or 0.5 mV. To determine the amplitude of a wave, segment, or interval, count the number of small blocks from the baseline to the highest or lowest point of the wave, segment, or interval.

Monitor problems

For optimal cardiac monitoring, you need to anticipate potential problems that can interfere with obtaining a reliable ECG recording. (See *Troubleshooting monitor problems*, page 39.) Causes of interference include artifact from patient movement, and poorly placed, or poorly ill functioning equipment.

Troubleshooting monitor problems

This chart shows several ECG monitoring problems, along with their causes and possible solutions.

What you see	What might cause it	What to do about it	
Artifact (waveform interference)	• Patient experiencing seizures, shaking, chills, or anxiety	• If the patient is having a seizure, notify the practitioner and intervene as ordered. • Keep the patient warm and encourage him or her to relax.	
	• Dirty or corroded connections	• Replace dirty or corroded wires.	
	• Improper electrode application	• Check the electrodes and reapply them if needed. Clean the patient's skin well because skin oils and dead skin cells inhibit conduction.	• Check the electrode gel. If the gel is dry, apply new electrodes.
	• Short circuit in leadwires or cable	• Replace broken equipment.	
	• Static electricity interference from inadequate room humidity	• Make sure all electrical equipment is attached to a common ground. Check all three-pronged plugs to ensure that none of the prongs are loose. Notify the biomedical department.	
	• Electrical interference from other equipment in the room	• Regulate room humidity to 40% if possible.	
False high-rate alarm	• Gain setting too high, particularly with MCL_1 setting	• Reset gain.	

Troubleshooting monitor problems *(continued)*

What you see	What might cause it	What to do about it
Weak signals	• Improper electrode application	• Reapply the electrodes.
	• QRS complex too small to register	• Reset gain so that the height of the complex is greater than 1 mV. • Try monitoring the patient on another lead.
	• Wire or cable failure	• Replace any faulty wires or cables.
Wandering baseline	• Patient is restless.	• Encourage the patient to relax.
	• Chest wall movement during respiration	• Make sure that tension on the cable isn't pulling the electrode away from the patient's body.
	• Improper electrode application; electrode positioned over bone	• Reposition improperly placed electrodes.
Fuzzy baseline (electrical interference)	• Electrical interference from other electrical equipment in the room	• Ensure that all electrical equipment is attached to a common ground. • Check all three-pronged plugs to make sure none of the prongs are loose.
	• Improper grounding of the patient's bed	• Ensure that the bed ground is attached to the room's common ground.
	• Electrode malfunction	• Replace the electrodes.
Baseline (no waveform)	• Improper electrode placement (perpendicular to the axis of heart)	• Reposition improperly placed electrodes.
	• Electrode disconnected	• Check if electrodes are disconnected. Reapply them as necessary.
	• Dry electrode gel	• Check electrode gel. If the gel is dry, apply new electrodes.
	• Wire or cable failure	• Check all wires and cables to see that these are all attached. • Replace faulty wires or cables.

Artifact

Artifact, also called *waveform interference*, may be seen with excessive movement (somatic tremor). The baseline of the ECG appears wavy, bumpy, or tremulous. Dry electrodes may also cause this problem because of poor contact.

Interference

Electrical interference, also called *60-cycle interference*, is caused by electrical power leakage. It may also occur because of interference from other room equipment or improperly grounded equipment. As a result, the lost current pulses at a rate of 60 cycles/sec. This interference appears on the ECG as a thick baseline.

Wandering baseline

A wandering baseline undulates, meaning that all waveforms are present but the baseline isn't stationary. Movement of the chest wall during respiration, poor electrode placement, or poor electrode contact usually causes this problem.

Faulty equipment

Faulty equipment, such as broken leadwires and cables, can also cause monitoring problems. Excessively worn equipment can cause improper grounding, putting the patient at risk for accidental shock.

That's a wrap!

Obtaining a rhythm strip review

Leads and planes

- A *lead* provides a view of the heart's electrical activity between a positive and negative pole.
  - When electrical current travels toward the negative pole, the waveform deflects mostly downward.
  - When the current flows toward the positive pole, the waveform deflects mostly upward.
- A *plane* refers to a cross-sectional view of the electrical activity of the heart.
  - Frontal plane, a vertical cut through the middle of the heart, provides an anterior–posterior view.
  - Horizontal plane, a transverse cut through the middle of the heart, provides a superior or inferior view.

Types of ECGs

- *12-Lead ECG* records electrical activity from 12 views of the heart.
- *Single-lead or dual-lead monitoring* provides continuous cardiac monitoring.

12-lead ECG

- Six limb leads provide information about the heart's frontal (vertical) plane.
- Bipolar leads (leads I, II, and III) require a negative and positive electrode for monitoring.
- Unipolar leads (leads aV_R, aV_L, and aV_F) record information from one lead and require only one electrode.
- The six precordial leads (leads V_1 through V_6) provide information about the heart's horizontal plane and are also unipolar.

Leads I, II, and III

- Leads I, II, and III typically produce positive deflection on ECG tracings.
- Lead I monitors atrial arrhythmias and hemiblocks.
- Lead II commonly aids in routine monitoring and detecting of sinus node and atrial arrhythmias.
- Lead III helps detect changes associated with inferior wall myocardial infarction.

Precordial leads

- Lead V_1
  - Biphasic
  - Distinguishes between the right and left ventricular ectopic beats
  - Monitors ventricular arrhythmias, ST-segment changes, and bundle branch blocks
- Leads V_2 and V_3
  - Produces a biphasic waveform
  - Monitors ST-segment elevation
- Lead V_4
  - Produces a biphasic waveform
  - Monitors ST-segment and T-wave changes
- Lead V_5
  - Produces a positive deflection on the ECG
  - Monitors ST-segment or T-wave changes (when used with lead V_4)
- Lead V_6
  - Produces a positive deflection on the ECG
  - Detects bundle branch blocks

Modified leads

- Lead MCL_1

Obtaining a rhythm strip review (*continued*)

- Similar to V_1
- Assesses QRS-complex arrhythmias, P-wave changes, and bundle branch defects
- Monitors premature ventricular contractions
- Distinguishes different types of tachycardia
- Lead MCL_6
  - Similar to V_6
  - Monitors ventricular conduction changes

Electrode configurations
- Three-electrode system uses one positive electrode, one negative electrode, and a ground.
- *Five-electrode system* uses an exploratory chest lead to monitor modified chest or standard limb leads.

ECG strip
- 1 small horizontal block = 0.04 seconds
- 5 small horizontal blocks = 1 large block = 0.2 seconds
- 5 large horizontal blocks = 1 second
- Normal 6-second strip = 30 large horizontal blocks
- 1 small vertical block = 0.1 mV
- 1 large vertical block = 0.5 mV
- Amplitude (mV) = number of small blocks from baseline to highest or lowest point

Monitoring problems
- *Artifact:* Excessive movement or dry electrode that causes baseline to appear wavy, bumpy, or tremulous
- *Interference:* Electrical power leakage, interference from other equipment, or improper equipment grounding that produces a thick, unreadable baseline
- *Wandering baseline:* Chest wall movement, poor electrode placement, or poor electrode contact that causes an undulating baseline
- *Faulty equipment:* Faulty and worn equipment that causes monitoring problems and places the patient at risk for shock

Worn equipment can cause problems—including a possible shock for the patient.

Be aware that some types of artifact resemble arrhythmias and the monitor will interpret them as such. For example, the monitor may sense a small movement, such as the patient brushing their teeth, as a potentially lethal ventricular tachycardia. Remember to assess the patient and not rely solely on the monitor. The more familiar you become with your unit's monitoring system and with your patient, the more quickly you can recognize and interpret problems and act appropriately.

Quick quiz

1. On ECG graph paper, the horizontal axis measures:
    A. time.
    B. speed.
    C. voltage.
    D. amplitude.

Answer: A. The horizontal axis measures time and is recorded in increments of 0.04 seconds for each small box.

2. On ECG graph paper, the vertical axis measures:
    A. time.
    B. speed.
    C. voltage.
    D. amplitude.

Answer: C. The vertical axis measures voltage by the height of a waveform.

3. A biphasic deflection will occur on an ECG if the electrical current is traveling in a direction:
    A. posterior to the positive electrode.
    B. perpendicular to the positive electrode.
    C. superior to the positive electrode.
    D. anterior to the positive electrode.

Answer: B. A current traveling in a route perpendicular to the positive electrode will generate a biphasic wave, partially above and below the isoelectric line.

4. If a lead comes off the patient's chest, the waveform:
    A. will appear much larger on the monitor.
    B. will appear much smaller on the monitor.
    C. will appear to wander on the monitor.
    D. will be absent on the monitor.

Answer: D. Leadwire disconnection will stop the monitoring process, and the waveform won't be seen on the monitor.

5. To monitor lead II, you would place the:
    A. positive electrode below the lowest palpable rib at the left midclavicular line and the negative electrode below the right clavicle.
    B. positive electrode below the right clavicle at the midline and the negative electrode below the left clavicle at the midline.
    C. positive electrode below the left clavicle and the negative electrode below the right clavicle at the midclavicular line.
    D. positive electrode below the lowest palpable rib at the right midclavicular line and the negative electrode below the left clavicle.

Answer: A. This electrode position is the proper one for monitoring in lead II.

Scoring

☆☆☆ If you answered all five questions correctly, excellent!

☆☆ If you answered four questions correctly, great!

☆ If you answered fewer than four questions correctly, keep at it! A review of the chapter can get your current flowing in the right direction.

Selected references

Bond, M. C., Brady, W., Charlton, N. P., Darby, A. E., Hudson, K., Lipinski, M. J., & Williamson, K. (2021). *Electrocardiogram in clinical medicine.* Wiley Blackwell.

Chen, Y., Kunst, E., Nasrawi, D., Massey, D., Johnston, A. N. B., Keller, K., & Fengzhi Lin, F. (2022). Nurses' competency in electrocardiogram interpretation in acute care settings: A systematic review. *Journal of Advanced Nursing, 78*(5), 1245–1266. https://doi.org/10.1111/jan.15147

Healio. (2019). *ECG reviews and criteria.* https://www.healio.com

Jones, S. A. (2019). *ECG mastery: Improving your ECG interpretation skills* (2nd ed.). F. A. Davis Company.

Klabunde, R. E. (2022). Cardiac function. In *Cardiovascular physiology concepts* (pp. 60–92). Wolters Kluwer.

Philips. (2020). *ECG lead placements.* https://www.philips.com/c-dam/b2bhc/master/Products/Category/supplies/ecg/ecg-lead-placements-poster.pdf

Saitoh, O., Fuse, K., Kasai, T., Tagawa, M., & Chinushi, M. (2022). Incorrect placement of the ground electrode in the 12-lead electrocardiogram: Its clinical implications and a simple identification strategy in healthcare fields. *Ningen Dock International, 10*(1), 92–97. https://doi.org/10.11320/ningendockitn.ND22-021

Sandau, K. E., Funk, M., Auerbach, A., Barsness, G. W., Blum, K., Cvach, M., Lampert, R., May, J. L., McDaniel, G. M., Perez, M. V., Sendelbach, S., Sommargren, C. E., Wang, P. J., & American Heart Association Council on Cardiovascular and Stroke Nursing; Council on Clinical Cardiology; and Council on Cardiovascular Disease in the Young. (2017). Update to practice standards for electrocardiographic monitoring in hospital settings: A scientific statement from the American Heart Association. *Circulation, 136,* e273–e344. https://doi.org/10.1161/CIR.0000000000000527

Tkacs, N. C., Herrmann, L. L., & Johnson, R. L. (2021). *Advanced physiology and pathophysiology: Essentials for clinical practice.* Springer Publishing Company.

Wiegand, D. J. (Ed.). (2017). *AACN procedure manual for high acuity progressive and critical care* (7th ed.). Elsevier.

Interpreting a rhythm strip

Just the facts

In this chapter, you'll learn:

◆ the components of an ECG complex and their significance and variations
◆ the techniques for calculating the rate and rhythm of an ECG recording
◆ the step-by-step approach to ECG interpretation
◆ the properties of normal sinus rhythm.

A look at an ECG complex

An ECG complex represents the electrical events occurring in one cardiac cycle. A complex consists of five waveforms labeled with the letters P, Q, R, S, and T. The middle three letters—Q, R, and S—are referred to as a unit, the QRS complex. ECG tracings represent the conduction of electrical impulses from the atria to the ventricles. (See *Normal ECG*, page 47.)

> ECG tracings represent the conduction of electrical impulses from the atria to the ventricles.

The P wave

The P wave is the first component of a normal ECG waveform. It represents atrial depolarization—conduction of an electrical impulse through the atria. When evaluating a P wave, look closely at its characteristics, especially its location, amplitude, duration, configuration, morphology, and deflection. In a normal ECG, there should be one P wave, which precedes the QRS complex and has the following characteristics:

- Location: Precedes the QRS complex
- Amplitude: Less than 0.25 mV (2.5 mm or 2.5 small squares high)
- Duration: Less than 0.12 seconds (3 small squares in length; each horizontal square equals 0.04 second)
- Configuration: Usually rounded and upright
  ◆ Morphology: Shape has a smooth contour; monophasic in lead II or biphasic in V_1
- Deflection: Positive or upright in leads I, II, aV_F, and V_2 to V_6; usually positive but variable in leads III and aV_L; negative or inverted in lead aV_R

Normal ECG

This strip shows the components of a normal ECG waveform.

If the deflection and configuration of a P wave are normal—for example, if the P wave is upright in lead II and is rounded and smooth—and if one P wave precedes each QRS complex, you can assume that this electrical impulse originated in the sinoatrial (SA) node of the right atrium. Electrical activity of the myocardium precedes muscular contraction. Therefore, the atria contract partway through the P wave and is not recorded on the ECG. Remember, the ECG records only electrical activity and precedes mechanical activity or contraction.

The odd Ps

The configuration, morphology, and amplitude of the P wave are important to note. When a P wave is tall and peaked, with an amplitude of less than 2.5 mm in lead II or less than 1.5 mm in V_1, right atrial enlargement may be indicated. A prolonged P wave that is greater than or equal to 0.12 second in the frontal plane (such as lead II) can suggest left atrial enlargement. Other conditions associated with peaked, notched, or enlarged P waves include chronic obstructive pulmonary disease, pulmonary emboli, valvular disease, or heart failure.

Recall that the SA node, pacemaker of the heart, is located in the right atrium and generates electrical impulses that are relayed to the atrioventricular (AV) node, whereas the AV node is located in the posterior–inferior region of the coronary sinus on the interatrial septum and travel to the ventricles, lower chambers of the heart. Inverted P waves may signify retrograde atrial depolarization or reverse conduction from the AV junction toward the atria. If the P wave has flipped on a repeat ECG, an upright sinus P wave becomes inverted, consider retrograde or reverse conduction as possible conditions.

Varying P waves indicate that the impulse may be generated from different sites, as with a wandering pacemaker rhythm, irritable atrial tissue, or damage near the SA node. Absent P waves may signify conduction by a route other than the SA node, as with a junctional rhythm, such as atrial flutter or fibrillation. In some cases, absent P waves may be caused by hyperkalemia. A flattened baseline with absent or numerous erratic P waves may indicate rapid atrial contraction caused by rhythm disturbances, such as atrial flutter or fibrillation. In atrial flutter, although P waves are not distinct, a saw-toothed flutter wave(s) is apparent on the ECG.

The PR interval

The PR interval is measured on the horizontal axis of the ECG from the beginning of the P wave to the beginning of the adjacent QRS interval. The PR interval tracks the atrial impulse from the atria through the AV node, bundle of His, and right and left bundle branches. When evaluating a PR interval, note duration. Changes in the PR interval indicate an altered impulse formation or a conduction delay, as seen in AV block. Although the amplitude, configuration, and deflection of the PR interval are not measured, it is important to note the following characteristics:
- Location: From the beginning of the P wave to the beginning of the QRS complex
- Duration: 0.12 to 0.20 second (3 to 5 small squares in length; each horizontal square equals 0.04 second).

These characteristics are different for pediatric patients. (See *Pediatric rates and intervals*, page 49.)

Ages and stages

Pediatric rates and intervals

The hearts of infants and children beat faster than those of adults because children have smaller ventricular size and higher metabolic needs. The fast heart rate and small heart size produce short PR intervals and QRS intervals.

Age	Heart rate (beats/min)	PR interval (in seconds)	QRS interval (in seconds)
0–7 days	95–160	0.08–0.12	0.05
1–3 weeks	105–180	0.08–0.12	0.05
1–6 months	110–180	0.08–0.13	0.05
6–12 months	110–170	0.10–0.14	0.05
1–3 years	90–150	0.10–0.14	0.06
4–5 years	65–135	0.11–0.15	0.07
6–8 years	60–130	0.12–0.16	0.07
9–11 years	60–110	0.12–0.17	0.07
12–16 years	60–110	0.12–0.17	0.07

The short and long of it

Short PR intervals (<0.12 second) indicate that the impulse originated somewhere other than the SA node. This variation is associated with young athletes, AV nodal (junctional) arrhythmias and pre-excitation syndromes, such as Wolff–Parkinson–White and Lown–Ganong–Levine syndromes. Prolonged PR intervals (>0.20 second), slowing through the atria or AV junction, represent a conduction delay because of digoxin toxicity, heart block, or myocardial ischemia/infarction associated with heart injury or damaged heart tissue.

The QRS complex

The QRS complex that follows the P wave represents ventricular depolarization and contraction and is also known as ventricular systole. At this time, the atria repolarize and relax. The impulse is transmitted from the AV node to the bundle of His and Purkinje fibers located in the ventricular walls. Ventricular contraction proceeds from the apex of the heart to its base and results in blood being ejected from the ventricles through the semilunar valves (aortic and pulmonary) into the arterial system perfusing the body with oxygenated blood and creating a pulse.

Not necessarily mechanical

The ECG waveform represents only electrical activity of the heart. Remember that electrical conduction of the heart precedes mechanical contraction; however, mechanical contraction does not guarantee successful perfusion. When monitoring the cardiac rhythm, it is important to consider the patient's family and social history, and comorbidities; as well, proper assessment of the patient includes other clinical indicators that determine health and stability. Muscular contraction of the heart can be weak and ineffective, limiting perfusion to the body; this can occur with arrhythmias, such as premature ventricular contractions or pulseless electrical activity. Always check the patient's physiological status (including oxygenation, pulse, blood pressure, and mentation) when performing ECG monitoring.

It's all normal

Pay special attention to the duration and configuration when evaluating a QRS complex. A normal complex has the following characteristics:

- Location: Follows the PR interval
- Amplitude: 5 to 30 mV (1 mm or 6 small squares high) but differs for each lead used
- Duration: 0.06 to 0.12 second (1.5 to 3 small squares in length; each horizontal square equals 0.04 second), or roughly half of the PR interval. Duration is measured from the beginning of the Q wave to the end of the S wave or from the beginning of the R wave if the Q wave is absent.
- Configuration: Consists of the Q wave (the first negative deflection after the P wave), the R wave (the first positive deflection after the P wave or the Q wave), and the S wave (the first negative deflection after the R wave). All three waves may not always be evident on the ECG. The ventricles depolarize quickly, minimizing the contact time between the stylus and the ECG paper, so the QRS complex typically appears thinner than other ECG components. QRS complexes may also appear differently in each lead. (See *QRS waveform variety*, page 51.)
- Deflection: Positive in leads I, II, III, aV_L, aV_F, and V_4 to V_6 and negative in leads aV_R and V_1 to V_3.

Crucial I.D.

Remember that the QRS complex represents intraventricular conduction time. That is why identifying and correctly interpreting this waveform is so crucial. If no P wave appears before the QRS complex, consider that the impulse may have originated in the AV node or bundle of His, such as a junctional rhythm, or the impulse originated in the ventricles, indicating a ventricular arrhythmia. (See *Older adult ECGs*.)

Ages and stages

Older adult ECGs

Always keep the patient's age in mind when interpreting the ECG. ECG changes in the older adult include increased PR, QRS, and QT intervals, decreased amplitude of the QRS complex, and a shift of the QRS axis to the left.

QRS waveform variety

The illustrations below show the various configurations of QRS complexes. When documenting the QRS complex, use uppercase letters to indicate a wave with a normal or high amplitude (>5 mm) and lowercase letters to indicate a wave with a low amplitude (<5 mm). In some instances, a second R wave may appear in a QRS complex. This is called R′.

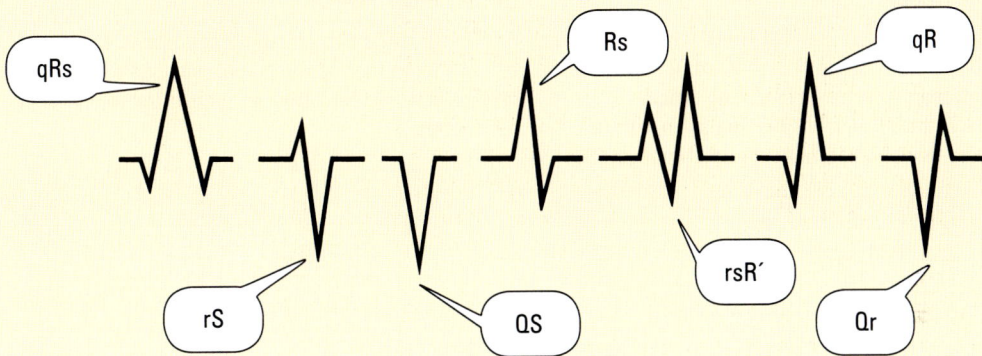

Deep and wide

Deep, wide Q waves may represent myocardial infarction. In this case, the Q-wave amplitude is 25% of the R-wave amplitude, or the duration of the Q wave is 0.04 second. A notched R wave may signify a bundle branch block. A widened QRS complex (>0.12 second) may signify a ventricular conduction delay. Missing QRS complexes may indicate AV block or ventricular standstill.

The ST segment

The ST segment represents the end of ventricular depolarization or conduction and the beginning of ventricular repolarization or recovery. The flat, isoelectric portion of the ECG that occurs at the end of the S wave to the beginning of the T wave is known as the ST segment. The point that marks the end of the QRS complex and the beginning of the ST segment is known as the *J point*. Diffuse J points can be indicative of early repolarization, acute myocardial infarction, left ventricular hypertrophy, or pericarditis, for example.

Normal ST

Pay special attention to the deflection of an ST segment. A normal ST segment has the following characteristics:
- Location: Extends from the S wave to the beginning of the T wave
- Deflection: Usually isoelectric (neither positive or negative); may vary from −0.5 to +1 mm in some precordial leads.

Changes in the ST segment

It is critically important to closely monitor the ST segment on a patient's ECG in order to detect myocardial ischemia or infarction and to limit damage.

ST-segment depression	ST-segment elevation
An ST segment is considered depressed when it is 0.5 mm or more below the baseline. A depressed ST segment may indicate myocardial ischemia or digoxin toxicity. Observe the ST segment for depression, such as upsloping, downsloping, or a horizontal configuration.	An ST segment is considered elevated when it's 1 mm or more above the baseline. An elevated ST segment may indicate myocardial injury, such as from ischemia or pericarditis.

Not so normal ST

A change in the ST segment may indicate myocardial ischemia or infarction. A ST segment may become either elevated or depressed. Observe the ST segment for characteristic patterns of depression changes known as upsloping, downsloping, or horizontal. (See *Changes in the ST segment*.)

The T wave

The T wave represents ventricular repolarization or recovery. When evaluating a T wave, look at the amplitude, configuration, and deflection. Normal T waves have the following characteristics (duration is not measured):

- Location: Follows the S wave
- Amplitude: 0.5 mm in leads I, II, and III and up to 10 mm in the precordial leads
- Configuration: Typically round and smooth
- Deflection: Usually upright in leads I, II, and V_3 to V_6; inverted in lead aV_R; variable in all other leads

Why is that T wave so bumpy?

The T wave may be asymmetrical, and the first slope may appear more gradual than the second one. The T wave's peak represents the relative refractory period of ventricular repolarization, a period during which cells are especially vulnerable to extra stimuli. Bumps or notches in a T wave may indicate that a P wave is hidden within it. If a P wave is hidden, atrial depolarization has occurred, the impulse having originated at a site above the ventricles.

Tall, inverted, or pointy T waves

The amplitude of the T wave typically corresponds to the amplitude of the preceding R wave. T waves may appear taller in leads V_3 and V_4. Tall, peaked, hyperacute, or tented T waves indicate myocardial ischemia or hyperkalemia. Inverted T waves in leads I, II, or V_3 through V_6 may represent myocardial ischemia. Inverted T waves in children may represent a normal variant. Heavily notched or pointed T waves in an adult may suggest pericarditis. Seek to compare prior ECGs in order to evaluate whether or not these represent new findings. New T-wave inversions are an abnormal finding.

> Heavily notched or pointed T waves in an adult may mean pericarditis.

The QT interval

The QT interval measures ventricular depolarization and repolarization. The length of the QT interval varies according to heart rate. The faster the heart rate, the shorter the QT interval. When checking the QT interval, look closely at the duration.

A normal QT interval has the following characteristics (amplitude, configuration, and deflection are not observed):
- Location: Extends from the beginning of the QRS complex to the end of the T wave
- Duration: Varies according to age, sex, and heart rate; usually lasts from 0.36 to 0.44 second; should not be greater than half the distance between consecutive R waves (R to R interval) when the rhythm is regular

The importance of the QT interval

The QT interval shows the time needed for the ventricular depolarization–repolarization cycle. An abnormality in duration may indicate myocardial problems. Prolonged QT intervals indicate that the relative refractory period is longer. A prolonged QT interval increases the risk of a life-threatening ventricular arrhythmia known as *torsades de pointes*.

This variation is also associated with certain medications such as Class IA antiarrhythmics. (See *Drugs that increase the QT interval.*) Prolonged QT syndrome may represent a congenital conduction-system defect. More commonly found, acquired QT prolongation can occur as a result of electrolyte imbalance, such as hypokalemia, hypocalcemia, or hypomagnesemia. Short QT intervals may result from digoxin toxicity, hypercalcemia, or genetic disorders.

Drugs that increase the QT interval

This chart lists the drugs that have been shown to increase the QT interval, which increases the patient's risk of developing torsades de pointes.

Drug class	Drug name	Drug class	Drug name
Antiarrhythmics	Amiodarone (Cordarone or Pacerone) Disopyramide (Norpace) Dofetilide (Tikosyn) Ibutilide fumarate (Corvert) Procainamide (Pronestyl) Propafenone (Rythmol) Quinidine sulfate (Cardioquin or Quinaglute) Sotalol (Betapace)	Antiemetics	Dolasetron (Anzemet)
		Azole antifungals	Fluconazole (Diflucan) Ketoconazole (Nizoral) Metronidazole (Flagyl)
		Antimalarials	Chloroquine (Aralen phosphate) Hydroxychloroquine (Plaquenil)
		Antimigraine medication	Sumatriptan (Imitrex)
Macrolide antibiotics	Azithromycin (Zithromax) Clarithromycin (Biaxin) Erythromycin (Erythrocin)	Antipsychotics/ antiemetics	Chlorpromazine Haloperidol (Haldol) Thioridazine (Mellaril)
Fluoroquinolone antibiotics	Levofloxacin (Levaquin) Moxifloxacin (Avelox)	Opioid antagonists	Methadone (Methadose or Dolophine)
Antidepressants	Amitriptyline (Elavil) Citalopram (Celexa) Desipramine (Norpramin) Fluoxetine (Prozac) Paroxetine (Paxil) Sertraline (Zoloft)	Sedative	Droperidol (Inapsine)

The U wave

The U wave represents the recovery period of the Purkinje or ventricular conduction fibers. It is seen as a small deflection following the T wave, representing the last phase of ventricular depolarization;

however, it is not present on every rhythm strip. The configuration is the most important characteristic of the U wave.

When present, a normal U wave has the following characteristics (amplitude and duration are not measured):

- Location: A small 0.5 mm deflection that immediately follows the T wave; may be seen in anterior leads V_2 and V_3
- Configuration: Typically upright except in aV_R, and rounded
- Deflection: Upright

The U wave may not appear on an ECG. A prominent U wave may be because of hypercalcemia, hypokalemia, or digoxin toxicity.

Eight–step method

Interpreting a rhythm strip is a skill developed through practice. You can use several methods, as long as you employ consistent technique. Rhythm strip analysis requires a sequential and systematic approach, such as the eight steps outlined here.

> What are the keys for reading a rhythm strip? A sequential, systematic approach is the best approach for tackling this task.

Step 1: Determine the rhythm

To determine the heart's atrial and ventricular rhythms, use either the paper-and-pencil method or the caliper method. (See *Methods of measuring rhythm*, page 56.)

For atrial rhythm, measure the P-P intervals—the intervals between consecutive P waves. These intervals should occur regularly, with only small variations associated with respirations. Then compare the P-P intervals in several cycles. Consistently similar P-P intervals indicate regular atrial rhythm; dissimilar P-P intervals indicate irregular atrial rhythm.

To determine the ventricular rhythm, measure the intervals between two consecutive R waves in the QRS complexes. If an R wave is not present, use the Q wave of consecutive QRS complexes. The R-R intervals should occur regularly.

Then compare R-R intervals in several cycles. As with atrial rhythms, consistently similar intervals mean a regular rhythm; dissimilar intervals point to an irregular rhythm.

Ask the question: How irregular is the rhythm? Is it slightly irregular or markedly so? Does the irregularity occur in a pattern (a regularly irregular pattern)? Keep in mind that variations of up to 0.04 second are considered normal.

Methods of measuring rhythm

You can use the paper-and-pen or caliper method to determine atrial or ventricular rhythm.

Paper-and-pen method	Caliper method
Place the ECG strip on a flat surface. Then position the straight edge of a piece of paper along the strip's baseline. Move the paper up slightly so that the straight edge is near the peak of the R wave. With a pen, mark the paper at the R waves of two consecutive QRS complexes, as shown in the image. This is the R-R interval. Next, move the paper across the strip, aligning the two marks with succeeding R-R intervals. If the distance for each R-R interval is the same, the ventricular rhythm is regular. If the distance varies, the rhythm is irregular. Use the same method to measure the distance between the P waves (the P-P interval) and determine whether the atrial rhythm is regular or irregular.	With the ECG on a flat surface, place one point of the caliper on the peak of the first R wave of two consecutive QRS complexes. Then adjust the caliper legs so that the other point is on the peak of the next R wave, as shown in the image. This distance is the R-R interval. Now rotate the first point of the caliper toward the third R wave and note whether it falls on the peak of that wave. Check succeeding R-R intervals in the same way. If the R-R intervals are of the same length, the ventricular rhythm is regular. If the length varies, the ventricular rhythm is irregular. Use the same method to measure the P-P intervals to determine whether the atrial rhythm is regular or irregular.

Step 2: Determine the rate

You can use one of three methods to determine an approximate atrial and ventricular heart rate. Always check a pulse to correlate it with the heart rate on the ECG.

The 10-times method

The simplest way to calculate the heart rate is the 10-times method. Realize that you can use the ECG 6-second rhythm strip to quickly identify the heart rate, which is especially useful when calculating the heart rate for an irregular rhythm. Notice that ECG paper is marked in increments of 3 seconds, or 15 large boxes. To figure the atrial rate, obtain a 6-second strip, count the number of P waves, and multiply these by 10. Ten 6-second strips (10×6) equal 1 minute. Calculate the ventricular rate the same way, using the R waves.

Calculating heart rate

The table can help make the sequencing method of determining heart rate more precise. After counting the number of boxes between the R waves, use the table shown to find the rate.

For example, if you count 20 small blocks or 4 large blocks, the rate would be 75 beats/min. To calculate the atrial rate, use the same method with P waves instead of R waves.

Rapid estimation

This rapid rate calculation is also called the *countdown method.* Using the number of large boxes between R waves and P waves as a guide, you can rapidly estimate ventricular or atrial rates by memorizing the sequence "300, 150, 100, 75, 60, 50."

The 1,500 method

If the heart rhythm is regular, use the 1,500 method—so named because 1,500 small squares represent 1 minute. Count the small squares between identical points on two consecutive P waves and then divide 1,500 by that number to get the atrial rate. To obtain the ventricular rate, use the same method with two consecutive R waves.

Sequence method

The third method of estimating the heart rate is the sequence method, which requires that you memorize a sequence of numbers. (See *Calculating heart rate.*) To get the atrial rate, find a P wave that peaks on a heavy vertical black line on the ECG trace paper and assign the following numbers to the next six heavy vertical black lines: 300, 150, 100, 75, 60, and 50. Then find the next P wave peak and estimate the atrial rate, based on the number assigned to the nearest heavy vertical black line. Estimate the ventricular rate the same way, using the R wave.

Number of small blocks	Heart rate
5 (1 large block)	300
6	250
7	214
8	187
9	166
10 (2 large blocks)	150
11	136
12	125
13	115
14	107
15 (3 large blocks)	100
16	94
17	88
18	83
19	79
20 (4 large blocks)	75
21	71
22	68
23	65
24	63
25 (5 large blocks)	60
26	58
27	56
28	54
29	52
30 (6 large blocks)	50
31	48
32	47
33	45
34	44
35 (7 large blocks)	43
36	42
37	41
38	39
39	38
40 (8 large blocks)	37

Step 3: Evaluate the P wave

When examining a rhythm strip for P waves, ask the question: Are P waves present? Do these P waves all have normal configurations? Do these have a similar size, shape, and location on the ECG? Is there one P wave preceding every QRS complex?

Step 4: Determine the duration of the PR interval

To measure the PR interval, count the small squares between the start of the P wave and the start of the QRS complex; then multiply the number of squares by 0.04 second. Now ask the question: Is the duration a normal 0.12 to 0.20 second? Is the PR interval constant?

Step 5: Determine the duration of the QRS complex

We're up to Step 5!

When determining QRS duration, be sure to measure straight across from the end of the PR interval to the end of the S wave, not just to the peak. Remember, the QRS has no horizontal components. To calculate duration, count the number of small squares between the beginning and end of the QRS complex and multiply this number by 0.04 second. Then ask the question: Is the duration a normal 0.06 to 0.12 second? Are all QRS complexes the same size and shape? (If not, measure each one and describe it individually.) Does a QRS complex appear after every P wave?

Step 6: Evaluate the T waves

Examine the strip for T waves. Then ask the question: Are T waves present? Do they all have a normal shape? Do they all have a normal amplitude? Do they all have the same amplitude? Do the T waves have the same deflection as the QRS complexes?

Step 7: Determine the duration of the QT interval

Count the number of small squares between the beginning of the QRS complex and the end of the T wave, where the T wave returns to the base-line. Multiply this number by 0.04 second. Ask the question: Is the duration a normal 0.36 to 0.44 second? (See *Correcting the QT interval.*)

Step 8: Evaluate any other components

Check for ectopic beats and other abnormalities. Also check the ST segment for abnormalities, and look for the presence of a U wave. Note your findings, and then interpret them by naming the rhythm strip according to one or all of these findings:

- origin of the rhythm (e.g., sinus node, atria, AV node, or ventricles)
- rate characteristics (e.g., bradycardia or tachycardia)
- rhythm abnormalities (e.g., flutter, fibrillation, heart block, escape rhythm, or other arrhythmias)

Correcting the QT interval

The QT interval is affected by the patient's heart rate. As the heart rate increases, the QT interval decreases; as the heart rate decreases, the QT interval increases. For this reason, evaluating the QT interval based on a standard heart rate of 60 is recommended. This corrected QT interval is known as *QTc*. This is particularly important to monitor especially when using antiarrhythmics. The following formula is used to determine the *QTc*:

$$\sqrt{\dfrac{QT\ interval}{R\text{-}R\ interval\ in\ seconds}}$$

The normal QTc for females is less than 0.45 second and for males is less than 0.43 second. When the QTc is longer than 0.50 second in males or females, torsades de pointes is more likely to develop.

Recognizing normal sinus rhythm

Before recognizing an arrhythmia, you must first be able to recognize normal sinus rhythm. Normal sinus rhythm records an impulse that starts in the sinus node and progresses to the ventricles through a normal conduction pathway—from the sinus node to the atria and AV node, through the bundle of His, to the bundle branches, and on to the Purkinje fibers. Normal sinus rhythm is the standard against which all other rhythms are compared. (See *Normal sinus rhythm.*)

Normal sinus rhythm

Normal sinus rhythm, shown in the image, represents normal impulse conduction through the heart.

The atrial and ventricular rhythms are regular.

A P wave precedes each QRS complex.

Each component of the ECG complex is present.

Characteristics of normal sinus rhythm:
- Regular rhythm
- Normal rate
- A P wave for every QRS complex; all P waves similar in size and shape
- All QRS complexes similar in size and shape
- Normal PR and QT intervals
- Normal (upright and round) T waves

What makes for normal?

Using the eight-step method previously described, these are the characteristics of normal sinus rhythm:
- Atrial and ventricular rhythms are regular.
- Atrial and ventricular rates fall between 60 and 100 beats/min, the SA node's normal firing rate, and all impulses are conducted to the ventricles.
- P waves are rounded, smooth, and upright in lead II, signaling that a sinus impulse has reached the atria.

- The PR interval is normal (0.12 to 0.20 second), indicating that the impulse is following normal conduction pathways.
- The QRS complex is of normal duration (<0.12 second), representing normal ventricular impulse conduction and recovery.
- The T wave is upright in lead II, confirming that normal repolarization has taken place.
- The QT interval is within normal limits (0.36 to 0.44 second).
- No ectopic or aberrant beats occur.

That's a wrap!

Rhythm strip interpretation review

Normal P wave
- *Location:* Before the QRS complex
- *Amplitude:* < 0.25 mV high
- *Duration:* < 0.12 second
- *Configuration:* Usually rounded and upright
- *Deflection:* Positive or upright in leads I, II, aV$_F$, and V$_2$ to V$_6$; usually positive but may vary in leads III and aV$_L$; negative or inverted in lead aV$_R$; biphasic or variable in lead V$_1$

Normal PR interval
- *Location:* From the beginning of the P wave to the beginning of the QRS complex
- *Duration:* 0.12 to 0.20 second

Normal QRS complex
- *Location:* Follows the PR interval
- *Amplitude:* > 0.5 mV in at least one standard lead and > 1.0 mV in at least one precordial lead. Upper limit of normal is 2.5 to 3.0 mV.
- *Duration:* 0.06 to 0.12 second, or half the PR interval
- *Configuration:* Consists of the Q wave, the R wave, and the S wave
- *Deflection:* Positive in leads I, II, III, aV$_L$, aV$_F$, and V$_4$ to V$_6$ and negative in leads aV$_R$ and V$_1$ to V$_3$

Normal ST segment
- *Location:* From the S wave to the beginning of the T wave
- *Deflection:* Usually isoelectric; may vary from −0.5 to +1 mm in some precordial leads

Normal T wave
- *Location:* After the S wave
- *Amplitude:* 0.5 mm in leads I, II, and III and up to 10 mm in the precordial leads
- *Configuration:* Typically round and smooth
- *Deflection:* Usually upright in leads I, II, and V$_3$ to V$_6$; inverted in lead aV$_R$; variable in all other leads

Normal QT interval
- *Location:* From the beginning of the QRS complex to the end of the T wave
- *Duration:* Varies; usually lasts from 0.36 to 0.44 second

Normal U wave
- *Location:* Immediately follows the T wave
- *Configuration:* Typically upright and rounded
- *Deflection:* Upright

Rhythm strip interpretation review *(continued)*

Interpreting a rhythm strip: eight-step method

- *Step 1:* Determine the rhythm
- *Step 2:* Determine the rate
- *Step 3:* Evaluate the P wave
- *Step 4:* Measure the PR interval
- *Step 5:* Determine the QRS complex duration
- *Step 6:* Examine the T waves
- *Step 7:* Measure the QT interval duration
- *Step 8:* Check for ectopic beats and other abnormalities

Normal sinus rhythm

Normal sinus rhythm is the standard against which all other rhythms are compared.

Characteristics

- Regular rhythm
- Normal rate
- P wave for every QRS complex; all P waves similar in size and shape
- All QRS complexes similar in size and shape
- Normal PR and QT intervals
- Normal T waves

Quick quiz

1. The P wave represents:
   A. atrial repolarization.
   B. atrial depolarization.
   C. ventricular depolarization.
   D. ventricular repolarization.

Answer: B. The impulse spreading across the atria, or atrial depolarization, generates a P wave.

2. The normal duration of a QRS complex is:
   A. 0.06 to 0.12 seconds.
   B. 0.12 to 0.20 seconds.
   C. 0.24 to 0.28 seconds.
   D. 0.36 to 0.44 seconds.

Answer: A. Normal duration of a QRS complex, which represents ventricular depolarization, is 0.06 to 0.12 seconds.

3. To gather information about impulse conduction from the atria to the ventricles, study the:
   A. P wave.
   B. PR interval.
   C. ST segment.
   D. T wave.

Answer: B. The PR interval measures the interval between atrial depolarization and ventricular depolarization. A normal PR interval is 0.12 to 0.20 second.

4.   The period when myocardial cells are vulnerable to extra stimuli begins with the:

    A.   end of the P wave.
    B.   start of the R wave.
    C.   start of the Q wave.
    D.   peak of the T wave.

Answer: D. The peak of the T wave represents the beginning of the relative, although not the absolute, refractory period, when the cells are vulnerable to stimuli.

5.   Atrial and ventricular rates can be determined by counting the number of small boxes between:

    A.   the end of one P wave and the beginning of another.
    B.   two consecutive P and R waves, respectively.
    C.   the middle of two consecutive T waves.
    D.   the beginning of the P wave and the end of the T wave.

Answer: B. Atrial and ventricular rates can be determined by counting the number of small boxes between two consecutive P or R waves and then dividing that number by 1,500.

Test strips

Now try these test strips. Fill in the blanks with the particular characteristics of the strip.

Strip 1

Atrial rhythm: _____
Ventricular rhythm: _____
Atrial rate: _____
Ventricular rate: _____
P wave: _____
PR interval: _____
QRS complex: _____
T wave: _____
QT interval: _____
Other: _____
Interpretation: _____

Strip 2

Atrial rhythm: _____
Ventricular rhythm: _____
Atrial rate: _____
Ventricular rate: _____
P wave: _____

PR interval: _____

QRS complex: _____

T wave: _____

QT interval: _____

Other: _____

Interpretation: _____

Answers to test strips

1. Rhythm: Atrial and ventricular rhythms are regular.
   Rate: Atrial and ventricular rates are each 79 beats/min.
   P wave: Normal size and configuration
   PR interval: 0.12 second
   QRS complex: 0.08 second; normal size and configuration
   T wave: Normal configuration
   QT interval: 0.44 second
   Other: None
   Interpretation: Normal sinus rhythm

2. Rhythm: Atrial and ventricular rhythms are regular.
   Rate: Atrial and ventricular rates are each 72 beats/min.
   P wave: Normal size and configuration
   PR interval: 0.20 second
   QRS complex: 0.10 second; normal size and configuration
   T wave: Normal configuration
   QT interval: 0.42 second
   Other: None
   Interpretation: Normal sinus rhythm

Scoring

☆☆☆ If you answered all five questions correctly and filled in all the blanks, excellent! You can read rhythm strips with proficiency.

☆☆ If you answered four questions correctly and filled in most of the blanks, very good!

☆ If you answered fewer than four questions correctly and missed most of the blanks, chin up! Review rhythm strips and the chapters and you will be proficient shortly. The trick to learning rhythm strips is repetition.

Selected references

García-Niebla, J. (2009). Comparison of p-wave patterns derived from correct and incorrect placement of V1-V2 electrodes. *Journal of Cardiovascular Nursing, 24*(2), 156–161. https://doi.org/10.1097/JCN.0b013e318197aa73

Katritsis, D. G., Gersch, B. J., & Camm, A. J. (2016). *Clinical cardiology: Current practice guidelines* (2nd ed.). Oxford University Press.

Kligfield, P., Gettes, L. S., Bailey, J. J., Childers, R., Deal, B. J., Hancock, E. W., van Herpen, G., Kors, J. A., Macfarlane, P., Mirvis, D. M., Pahlm, O., Rautaharju, P., Wagner, G. S., Josephson, M., Mason, J. W., Okin, P., Surawicz, B., Wellens, H., American Heart Association Electrocardiography and Arrhythmias Committee, … Heart Rhythm Society. (2007). Recommendations for the standardization and interpretation of the electrocardiogram: Part I: The electrocardiogram and its technology a scientific statement from the American Heart Association Electrocardiography and Arrhythmias Committee, Council on Clinical Cardiology; the American College of Cardiology Foundation; and the Heart Rhythm Society endorsed by the International Society for Computerized Electrocardiology. *Journal of the American College of Cardiology, 49*(10), 1109–1127. https://doi.org/10.1016/j.jacc.2007.01.024

Mann, D. L., Zipes, D. P., Libby, P., & Bonow, R. D. (2015). *Braunwald's heart disease: A textbook of cardiovascular medicine* (10th ed.). Elsevier.

Rasmussen, M. U., Fabricius-Bjerre, A., Kumarathurai, P., Larsen, B. S., Domínguez, H., Kanters, J. K., & Sajadieh, A. (2019). Common source of miscalculation and misclassification of P-wave negativity and P-wave terminal force in lead V1. *Journal of Electrocardiology, 53*, 85–88. https://doi.org/10.1016/j.jelectrocard.2019.01.088

Sandau, K. E., Funk, M., Auerbach, A., Barsness, G. W., Blum, K., Cvach, M., Lampert, R., May, J. L., McDaniel, G. M., Perez, M. V., Sendelbach, S., Sommargren, C. E., & Wang, P. J. (2017). Update to practice standards for electrocardiographic monitoring in hospital settings: A scientific statement from the American Heart Association. *Circulation, 136*(19), e273–e344. https://doi.org/10.1161/CIR.0000000000000527

Shaik, A., Patel, N., Alvarez, C., Panza, G., Baker, W. L., McMahon, S., & Kluger, J. (2023). Erroneous electrocardiographic interpretations and its clinical implications. *Journal of Cardiovascular Electrophysiology, 34*(7), 1515–1522. https://doi.org/10.1111/jce.15943

Strauss, D. G., & Schocken, D. (2021). *Marriott's practical electrocardiography* (13th ed.). Wolters Kluwer.

Urden, L., Stacy, K., & Lough, M. E. (2022). *Critical care nursing* (9th ed.). Elsevier.

Part II

Recognizing arrhythmias

Sinus node arrhythmias

Just the facts

In this chapter, you'll learn:

♦ the proper way to identify the various sinus node arrhythmias

♦ the role of the sinoatrial node in arrhythmia formation

♦ the causes, significance, treatment, and nursing implications of each arrhythmia

♦ assessment findings associated with each arrhythmia

♦ interpretation of sinus node arrhythmias on an electrocardiogram.

A look at the sinus node

When the heart functions normally, the sinoatrial (SA) node, also called the *sinus node*, acts as the primary pacemaker of the heart. The sinus node assumes this role because its automatic firing rate exceeds that of the heart's other pacemakers. In an adult at rest, the sinus node has an inherent firing rate of 60 to 100 times/min.

The SA node is located in the right atrium at the junction of the superior vena cava. The SA node's blood supply comes from either the right coronary artery (60%) or the left circumflex artery (40%). The autonomic nervous system richly innervates the sinus node through the vagus nerve, a parasympathetic nerve, and several sympathetic nerves. The autonomic nervous system regulates the heart rates based on the demands of the body. Stimulation of the vagus nerve decreases the node's firing rate, and stimulation of the sympathetic system increases it.

Sinus arrhythmia

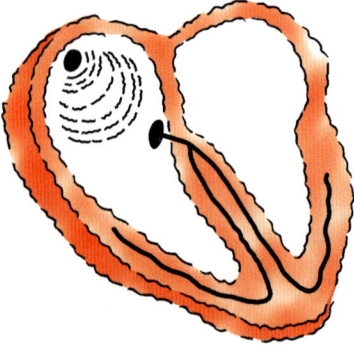

In sinus arrhythmia, the pacemaker cells of the SA node fire irregularly. Sinus arrhythmia is present when there is a sinus rhythm with variability in the cycle lengths between successive P waves, which are usually monoform. The cardiac rate stays within normal limits, but the rate is irregular and corresponds with the respiratory cycle. Sinus arrhythmia is a normal variant occurring commonly in athletes and children, but it rarely occurs in infants. Studies have suggested that the presence of sinus arrhythmia has been an indicator of good cardiovascular health. Studies have also suggested a decrease in sinus arrhythmia occurs among older individuals and in those with comorbidities, such as heart failure and diabetes. Conditions unrelated to respiration may also produce sinus arrhythmia, including inferior wall myocardial infarction (MI), advanced age, use of digoxin (Lanoxin) or morphine, and conditions involving increased intracranial pressure.

How it happens

Sinus arrhythmia, the heart's normal response to respirations, results from an inhibition of reflex vagal activity, or tone. During inspiration, an increase in the flow of blood back to the heart reduces vagal tone, which increases the heart rate. ECG complexes fall closer together, which shortens the P-P interval, the time elapsed between two consecutive P waves.

During expiration, venous return decreases, which, in turn, increases vagal tone, slows the heart rate, and lengthens the P-P interval. (See *Breathing and sinus arrhythmia*, page 71.)

Sick sinus

Sinus arrhythmia is a normal variation of sinus rhythm that does not produce symptoms. Treatment is not needed in its presence. A marked variation in P-P intervals in an older adult, however, may indicate sick sinus syndrome, a related, potentially more serious phenomenon. Sick sinus syndrome results from underlying disease of the conduction system.

Breathing and sinus arrhythmia

When sinus arrhythmia is related to respirations, you'll see an increase in heart rate with inspiration and a decrease with expiration, as shown in the image.

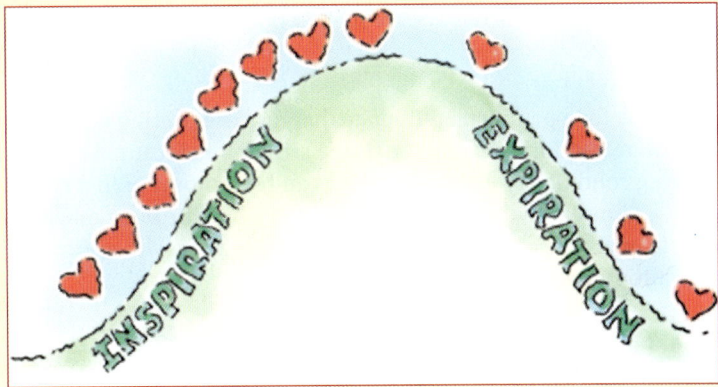

What to look for

When you look for sinus arrhythmia, you'll see that the rate is variable and corresponds to the respiratory cycle. (See *Identifying sinus arrhythmia*.) The difference between the shortest and longest P-P intervals—and the shortest and longest R-R intervals—exceeds 0.12 seconds.

Identifying sinus arrhythmia

This rhythm strip illustrates sinus arrhythmia. Look for the following distinguishing characteristics:

The cyclic irregular rhythm varies with the respiratory cycle.

Expiration   Inspiration   Expiration

- *Rhythm:* Irregular
- *Rate:* Variable, between 60 and 100 beats/min
- *P wave:* Normal
- *PR interval:* 0.16 seconds
- *QRS complex:* 0.06 seconds
- *T wave:* Normal
- *QT interval:* 0.36 seconds
- *Other:* Phasic slowing and quickening

The atrial and ventricular rates are within normal limits (60 to 100 beats/min) and vary with respiration—faster with inspiration, slower with expiration. All other parameters are normal, except for the QT interval, which may vary slightly but remains normal.

It's all in the breath

Look for a peripheral pulse rate that increases during inspiration and decreases during expiration. If the arrhythmia is caused by an underlying condition, you may note signs and symptoms of that condition.

Sinus arrhythmia is easier to detect when the heart rate is slow; it may disappear when the heart rate increases, as with exercise or after atropine administration.

How you intervene

Unless the patient is symptomatic, treatment usually isn't necessary. If sinus arrhythmia is unrelated to respirations, the underlying cause may require treatment.

When caring for a patient with sinus arrhythmia, observe the heart rhythm during respiration to determine whether the arrhythmia coincides with the respiratory cycle. Be sure to check the monitor carefully to avoid an inaccurate interpretation of the waveform. (See *A longer look at sinus arrhythmia*.)

> Notify the practitioner if sinus arrhythmia develops suddenly in a patient taking digoxin.

Mixed signals

A longer look at sinus arrhythmia

Don't mistake sinus arrhythmia for other rhythms. At first glance, it may look like atrial fibrillation, normal sinus rhythm with premature atrial contractions, SA block, or sinus pauses. If the patient is symptomatic with shortness of breath, dyspnea, or edema, there may be an underlying cause other than sinus arrhythmia. Observe the monitor and the patient's respiratory pattern for several minutes to determine the rate and rhythm. As always, check the patient's pulse. Review an ECG and check the patient history, especially of recent fall, head, or neck trauma.

Keep at it

If sinus arrhythmia is induced by drugs, such as morphine sulfate and other sedatives, the practitioner may decide to continue to give the patient those medications. However, if sinus arrhythmia develops suddenly in a patient taking digoxin, notify the practitioner immediately. The patient may be experiencing digoxin toxicity.

Sinus bradycardia

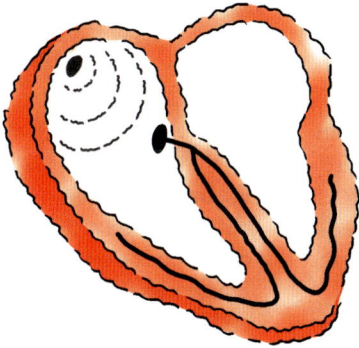

Sinus bradycardia is characterized by a sinus rate below 60 beats/min and a regular rhythm. It may occur normally during sleep or in a person with a well-conditioned heart—an athlete, for example. Many athletes develop sinus bradycardia because their well-conditioned hearts can maintain a normal stroke volume with less than normal effort. Sinus bradycardia also occurs normally during sleep because of decreased metabolic demands.

How it happens

Sinus bradycardia usually occurs as the normal response to a reduced demand for blood flow. In this case, vagal stimulation increases and sympathetic stimulation decreases. (See *Causes of sinus bradycardia.*) As a result, automaticity (the tendency of cells to initiate their own impulses) in the SA node diminishes.

Causes of sinus bradycardia

Sinus bradycardia may be caused by the following:
• noncardiac disorders, such as hyperkalemia, increased intracranial pressure, hypothyroidism, hypothermia, sleep, and glaucoma
• conditions producing excess vagal stimulation or decreased sympathetic stimulation, such as sleep, deep relaxation, Valsalva maneuver, carotid sinus massage, and vomiting

• cardiac diseases, such as SA node disease, cardiomyopathy, myocarditis, and myocardial ischemia, immediately following an inferior wall MI
• certain drugs, especially beta-adrenergic blockers, digoxin (Lanoxin), calcium channel blockers, lithium (Lithobid), and antiarrhythmics, such as sotalol (Betapace), amiodarone (Cordarone), propafenone (Rythmol), dronedarone (Multaq), and quinidine

A tolerable condition?

Sinus bradycardia commonly occurs after an inferior wall MI that involves the right coronary artery, which supplies blood to the SA node. It can also result from numerous other conditions and the use of certain drugs.

The clinical significance of sinus bradycardia depends on how low the rate is and whether the patient is symptomatic. For example, most adults can tolerate a sinus bradycardia of 45 to 59 beats/min but are less tolerant of a rate below 45 beats/min.

No symptoms? No problem?

Usually, sinus bradycardia produces no symptoms and is insignificant. Unless the patient shows symptoms of decreased cardiac output, no treatment is necessary.

Symptoms? Problem!

When sinus bradycardia produces symptoms, however, prompt attention is critical. The heart of a patient with underlying cardiac disease may not be able to compensate for a drop-in rate by increasing its stroke volume. The resulting drop in cardiac output produces signs and symptoms, such as hypotension and dizziness. Bradycardia may also predispose some patients to more serious arrhythmias, such as ventricular tachycardia and ventricular fibrillation.

In a patient with acute inferior wall MI, sinus bradycardia is considered a favorable prognostic sign, unless it's accompanied by hypotension. Because sinus bradycardia rarely affects children, it's considered a poor prognostic sign in children. (See *Bradycardia and tachycardia in children*.)

What to look for

In sinus bradycardia, the atrial and ventricular rhythms are regular, as are their rates, except that they're both less than 60 beats/min. (See *Identifying sinus bradycardia*.) All other characteristics appear normal. You'll see a P wave preceding each QRS complex and a normal PR interval, QRS complex, T wave, and QT interval.

Ages and stages

Bradycardia and tachycardia in children

Evaluate bradycardia and tachycardia in children in context. Bradycardia (<90 beats/min) may occur in a healthy infant during sleep; tachycardia may be a normal response when the child is crying or otherwise upset. Keep in mind that because heart rate varies considerably from the neonate to the adolescent, one definition of bradycardia or tachycardia can't fit all children.

Identifying sinus bradycardia

This rhythm strip illustrates sinus bradycardia. Look for the following distinguishing characteristics:

A normal P wave precedes each QRS complex.

The rhythm is regular with a rate below 60 beats/min.

- *Rhythm:* Regular
- *Rate:* 48 beats/min
- *P wave:* Normal
- *PR interval:* 0.16 seconds
- *QRS complex:* 0.08 seconds
- *T wave:* Normal
- *QT interval:* 0.50 seconds
- *Other:* None

When cardiac output gets low

As long as a patient can compensate for the decreased cardiac output, they are likely to remain asymptomatic. However, if compensatory mechanisms fail, signs and symptoms of declining cardiac output, such as hypotension, dizziness, and fatigue, usually appear.

Palpitations and pulse irregularities may occur if the patient experiences more ectopic beats, such as premature atrial, junctional, or ventricular contractions. Diminished blood flow to the cerebrum may produce signs of decreased level of consciousness (LOC), such as confusion. Bradycardia-induced syncope (Stokes–Adams attack) may also occur.

How you intervene

If the patient is asymptomatic and vital signs are stable, treatment isn't necessary. Continue to observe the heart rhythm, monitoring the progression and duration of the bradycardia. Evaluate the patient's tolerance of the rhythm at rest and with activity. Review and reconcile the patient's medication list. Check with the practitioner about stopping any medications that may be depressing the SA node, such as digoxin, antiarrhythmic drugs, beta-adrenergic blockers, or calcium channel blockers. Before giving those drugs, make sure the heart rate is within a safe range.

Sinus bradycardia in a child is an ominous sign.

Identify and correct

If the patient is symptomatic, treatment aims to identify and correct the underlying cause. Meanwhile, the heart rate must be maintained with transcutaneous pacing. Drugs such as atropine, epinephrine, or dopamine are used while awaiting a temporary or permanent pacemaker or when pacing is ineffective.

Atropine is given as a 0.5-mg dose by rapid injection. The dose may be repeated every 3 to 5 minutes up to a maximum of 3 mg total. If atropine proves ineffective, administer an epinephrine infusion at a rate of 2 to 10 mcg/min. If low blood pressure accompanies bradycardia, administer a dopamine infusion at 2 to 10 mcg/kg/min. Treatment of chronic, symptom-producing sinus bradycardia requires insertion of a permanent pacemaker.

Check the ABCs

If the patient abruptly develops a significant sinus bradycardia, assess the airway, breathing, and circulation (ABCs). If these are adequate, determine whether the patient has an effective cardiac output. If not, the patient will become symptomatic. (See *Clues to symptomatic bradycardia*, page 76.)

Clues to symptomatic bradycardia

If a patient can't tolerate bradycardia, the following signs and symptoms may develop:
- hypotension
- cool, clammy skin
- altered mental status
- dizziness
- blurred vision
- crackles, dyspnea, and an S_3 heart sound, which indicate heart failure
- chest pain
- syncope

When administering atropine, be sure to give the correct dose. Doses lower than 0.5 mg can have a paradoxical effect, slowing the heart rate even further. Keep in mind that a patient with a transplanted heart won't respond to atropine and may require pacing for emergency management.

Sinus tachycardia

If sinus bradycardia is the tortoise of the sinus arrhythmias, sinus tachycardia is the hare. Sinus tachycardia in an adult is characterized by a sinus rate of more than 100 beats/min. The rate rarely exceeds 160 beats/min, except during strenuous exercise; the maximum rate achievable with exercise decreases with age.

How it happens

The clinical significance of sinus tachycardia depends on the underlying cause. (See *Causes of sinus tachycardia*.) The arrhythmia may be the body's response to exercise or high emotional states and may be of no clinical significance. It may also occur with hypovolemia, hemorrhage, fever, or pain. When the stimulus for the tachycardia is removed, the arrhythmia spontaneously resolves.

Causes of sinus tachycardia

Sinus tachycardia may be a normal response to exercise, pain, stress, fever, or strong emotions, such as fear and anxiety. It can also occur during the following conditions:
- in certain cardiac conditions, such as heart failure, cardiogenic shock, and pericarditis
- as a compensatory mechanism in shock, anemia, respiratory distress, pulmonary embolism, sepsis, and hyperthyroidism
- when taking drugs, such as atropine, isoproterenol (Isuprel), aminophylline, dopamine, dobutamine, epinephrine, alcohol, caffeine, nicotine, and amphetamines

Hard on the heart

Sinus tachycardia can also be a significant arrhythmia with dire consequences. Because higher rates increase myocardial demand for oxygen, tachycardia can precipitate an episode of chest pain in patients with coronary artery disease. Sinus tachycardia can also be detrimental for patients with obstructive types of heart conditions, such as aortic stenosis and hypertrophic cardiomyopathy.

Sinus tachycardia occurs in about 30% of patients after acute MI and is considered a poor prognostic sign because it may be associated with massive heart damage. Persistent tachycardia may also signal impending heart failure or cardiogenic shock.

> With sinus tachycardia, look for a pulse rate of more than 100 beats/min but with a regular rhythm.

What to look for

In sinus tachycardia, atrial and ventricular rhythms are regular. (See *Identifying sinus tachycardia.*) Both rates are equal, generally 100 to 160 beats/min. As in sinus bradycardia, the P wave is of normal size and shape and precedes each QRS, but it may increase in amplitude. As the heart rate increases, the P wave may be superimposed on the preceding T wave and difficult to identify the PR interval; QRS complex and T wave are normal. The QT interval normally shortens with tachycardia.

Identifying sinus tachycardia

This rhythm strip illustrates sinus tachycardia. Look for the following distinguishing characteristics:

> A normal P wave precedes each QRS complex.

> The rhythm is regular with a rate above 100 beats/min.

- *Rhythm:* Regular
- *Rate:* 120 beats/min
- *P wave:* Normal
- *PR interval:* 0.14 seconds
- *QRS complex:* 0.06 seconds
- *T wave:* Normal
- *QT interval:* 0.34 seconds
- *Other:* None

Pulse check!

When assessing a patient with sinus tachycardia, look for a pulse rate of more than 100 beats/min but with a regular rhythm. Usually, the patient is asymptomatic. However, if the cardiac output falls and compensatory mechanisms fail, the patient may experience hypotension, syncope, and blurred vision. (See *What happens in tachycardia*.)

What happens in tachycardia

Tachycardia can lower cardiac output by reducing ventricular filling time and the amount of blood pumped by the ventricles during each contraction. Normally, ventricular volume reaches 120 to 130 mL during diastole. In tachycardia, decreased ventricular volume leads to hypotension and decreased peripheral perfusion.

As cardiac output plummets, arterial pressure and peripheral perfusion decrease. Tachycardia worsens myocardial ischemia by increasing the heart's demand for oxygen and reducing the duration of diastole—the period of greatest coronary flow.

Patients may report chest pain and palpitations, commonly described as a pounding chest or a sensation of skipped heartbeats. They may also report a sense of nervousness or anxiety. If heart failure develops, the patient may exhibit crackles, an extra heart sound (S_3), and jugular vein distention.

How you intervene

When treating the asymptomatic patient, focus on determining the cause of the sinus tachycardia. Treatment for a symptomatic patient involves maintaining adequate cardiac output and tissue perfusion and identifying and correcting the underlying cause. For example, if the tachycardia is caused by hemorrhage, treatment includes stopping the bleeding and replacing blood and fluid.

Slow it down

If tachycardia leads to cardiac ischemia, treatment may include medications to slow the heart rate. The most commonly used drugs include beta-adrenergic blockers, such as metoprolol succinate (Toprol XL), metoprolol tartrate (Lopressor), atenolol (Tenormin), and calcium channel blockers, such as diltiazem (Cardizem) or verapamil (Calan).

Getting at the history

Check the patient's medication history and profile. Over-the-counter sympathomimetic agents, which mimic the effects of the sympathetic

Memory jogger

To help you remember how to identify sinus bradycardia from sinus tachycardia, think of the **b** in bradycardia as **b**elow. Sinus bradycardia is **below** 60 beats/min, while sinus tachycardia is **above** 100 beats/min. Both have a normal QRS complex, preceded by a normal P wave.

Advise the patient to avoid caffeine, nicotine, alcohol, and recreational drugs.

nervous system, may contribute to sinus tachycardia. These agents may be contained in nose drops and cold formulas. Also ask about the patient's use of caffeine, nicotine, alcohol, and recreational drugs such as cocaine and amphetamines, any of which can trigger tachycardia. Advise them to avoid these substances.

More steps to take

The following are other steps you should take for the patient with sinus tachycardia:

- Because sinus tachycardia can lead to injury of the heart muscle, check for chest pain or angina. Also assess for signs and symptoms of heart failure, including crackles, an S_3 heart sound, and jugular vein distention.
- Determine the patient's dry weight. Monitor intake and output, as well as daily weight.
- Check the patient's LOC to assess cerebral perfusion.
- Provide the patient with a calm environment. Provide reassurance in an effort to reduce fear and anxiety, which can exacerbate an arrhythmia.
- Educate the patient about procedures and treatments; provide helpful forms of relaxation techniques.
- Be aware that a sudden onset of sinus tachycardia after an MI may signal extension of the infarction. Prompt recognition is vital, so treatment can be started.
- Remember that tachycardia is commonly the first sign of pulmonary embolism. Maintain suspicion, especially if your patient has risk factors for thrombotic emboli.

Sinus arrest

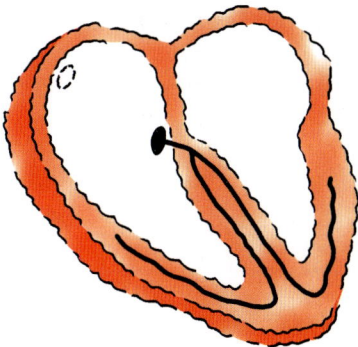

A disorder of impulse formation, sinus arrest is caused by a lack of electrical activity in the atrium, a condition called atrial standstill. (See *Causes of sinus arrest.*) During atrial standstill, the atria aren't stimulated and an entire PQRST complex will be missing from the ECG strip.

Causes of sinus arrest

The following conditions can cause sinus arrest:
- sinus node disease, such as fibrosis and idiopathic degeneration
- increased vagal tone, as occurs with Valsalva maneuver, carotid sinus massage, and vomiting
- digoxin (Lanoxin), quinidine, procainamide, and salicylates, especially if given at toxic levels
- excessive doses of beta-adrenergic blockers, such as metoprolol succinate (Toprol XL), metoprolol tartrate (Lopressor), or propranolol (Inderal)
- cardiac disorders, such as chronic coronary artery disease, acute myocarditis, cardiomyopathy, and hypertensive heart disease
- acute inferior wall MI
- sick sinus syndrome
- acute infection

Except for this missing complex, or pause, the ECG usually remains normal. Atrial standstill is called *sinus pause* when one or two beats are missing and *sinus arrest* when three or more beats are missing.

Sinus arrest closely resembles third-degree SA block, also called *exit block*, on the ECG strip. (See *Understanding SA blocks*.)

Understanding SA blocks

In the SA block, the SA node discharges impulses at regular intervals. Some of those impulses, though, are delayed on their way to the atria. Based on the length of the delay, SA blocks are divided into three categories: first, second, and third degrees. Second-degree atrioventricular blocks are further divided into Mobitz type I (Wenckebach) and Mobitz type II.

First-degree SA block consists of a delay between the firing of the sinus node and the depolarization of the atria. Because the ECG doesn't show sinus node activity, you can't detect first-degree SA block. This is not to be confused with first-degree AV block, which will reveal a prolonged PR interval on an ECG. However, you can detect the other three types of SA block.

Second-degree AV block Mobitz type I (Wenckebach)

In second-degree AV block Mobitz type I, conduction time between the sinus node and the surrounding atrial tissue becomes progressively longer until an entire cycle is dropped. The pause is less than twice the shortest P-P interval.

Eventually, an entire PQRST complex is dropped.

The rhythm is irregular, and the P-P interval gets progressively shorter.

Second-degree AV block type II

In second-degree AV block type II, conduction time between the sinus node and the atrial tissue is normal until an impulse is blocked. The duration of the pause is a multiple of the P-P interval.

Understanding SA blocks (*continued*)

An entire PQRST complex is missing.

The rhythm is regular except for pauses.

Third-degree block

In third-degree AV block, some impulses are blocked, causing long sinus pauses. The pause isn't a multiple of the sinus rhythm. On an ECG, third-degree SA block looks similar to sinus arrest but results from a different cause.

Third-degree SA block is caused by a failure to conduct impulses; sinus arrest results from failure to form impulses. Failure in each case causes atrial activity to stop.

In sinus arrest, the pause commonly ends with a junctional escape beat. In third-degree block, the pause lasts for an indefinite period and ends with a sinus beat.

An entire PQRST complex is missing.

The rhythm is regular except for pauses.

The pause ends with a sinus beat.

SA blocks are divided into three categories based on the length of the delay.

How it happens

Sinus arrest occurs when the SA node fails to generate an impulse. Such failure may result from a number of conditions, including acute infection, heart disease, and vagal stimulation. Sinus arrest may be associated with sick sinus syndrome.

The clinical significance of sinus arrest depends on the patient's symptoms. If the pauses are short and infrequent, the patient will most likely be asymptomatic and won't require treatment. They may have a normal sinus rhythm for days or weeks between episodes of sinus arrest. They may not be able to feel the arrhythmias at all.

Pauses of 2 to 3 seconds normally occur in healthy adults during sleep and occasionally in patients with increased vagal tone or hypersensitive carotid sinus disease.

Too many for too long

If sinus arrest is frequent and prolonged, however, the patient will most likely have symptoms. The arrhythmias can produce syncope or near-syncopal episodes usually within 7 seconds of asystole.

During a prolonged pause, the patient may fall and injure themself. Other situations may be just as serious. For example, a symptom-producing arrhythmia that occurs while the patient is driving a car could result in a fatal accident.

> Sinus arrest can cause accidents. Motor vehicle accidents are of particular concern.

What to look for

When assessing for sinus pause, you'll find that atrial and ventricular rhythms are regular, except for a missing complex at the onset of atrial standstill. (See *Identifying sinus arrest.*) The atrial and ventricular rates are equal and usually within normal limits. The rate may vary, however, as a result of the pauses.

Identifying sinus arrest

This rhythm strip illustrates sinus arrest. Look for the following distinguishing characteristics:

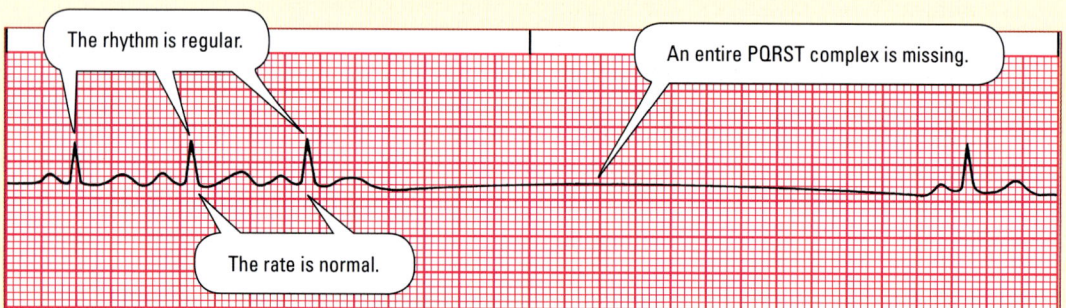

> The rhythm is regular.

> An entire PQRST complex is missing.

> The rate is normal.

- *Rhythm:* Regular, except for the missing PQRST complexes
- *Rate:* 40 beats/min
- *P wave:* Normal; missing during pause

- *PR interval:* 0.20 seconds
- *QRS complex:* 0.08 seconds, absent during pause
- *T wave:* Normal, absent during pause

- *QT interval:* 0.40 seconds, absent during pause
- *Other:* None

Of normal size and shape, a P wave precedes each QRS complex but is absent during a pause. The PR interval is normal and constant when the P wave is present and not measurable when absent. The QRS complex, the T wave, and the QT interval are normal when present and are absent during a pause.

You might see junctional escape beats and premature atrial, junctional, or ventricular contractions. With sinus arrest, the length of the pause isn't a multiple of the previous R-R intervals.

Signs of recurrent pauses

When sinus arrest occurs, a pulse or heartbeat is absent during the pause. Usually, the patient is asymptomatic. However, recurrent pauses may cause signs of decreased cardiac output, such as low blood pressure, altered mental status, syncope or near syncope, and cool, clammy skin. The patient may also complain of lightheadedness, dizziness, or blurred vision.

How you intervene

An asymptomatic patient needs no treatment. For a patient displaying mild symptoms, treatment focuses on maintaining cardiac output and identifying the cause of the sinus arrest. That may involve stopping medications that contribute to SA node suppression, such as digoxin, beta-adrenergic blockers, and calcium channel blockers.

Emergent treatment

A patient who develops signs of circulatory collapse needs immediate treatment. As with sinus bradycardia, emergency treatment includes using a temporary pacemaker and administration of atropine or epinephrine. A permanent pacemaker may be implanted for long-term management.

The goal for the patient with sinus arrest is to maintain adequate cardiac output and perfusion. Be sure to record and document the frequency and duration of pauses. Determine whether a pause is the result of sinus arrest or SA block.

If the patient is dizzy or lightheaded, this may result in syncope or near syncope.

Don't let sleeping pauses lie

Examine the circumstances under which sinus pauses occur. A sinus pause may be insignificant if detected while the patient is sleeping; these are known as nocturnal pauses. If the pauses are recurrent, assess the patient for evidence of decreased cardiac output, such as altered mental status, low blood pressure, and cool, clammy skin.

Ask them whether they feel dizzy or lightheaded or have blurred vision. Does the patient feel like they may pass out? If so, they may be experiencing syncope from a prolonged sinus arrest. (See *Syncope and sinus arrest*, page 84.)

Syncope and sinus arrest

A patient with sinus arrest is at risk for syncope. Ask your patient whether they have ever passed out or nearly passed out.

Also ask about a history of falls and obtain a detailed description of each episode, including where and how the syncope occurred.

Asking questions

If possible, check with friends and family members who witnessed the episodes to find out what happened and how long the patient remained unconscious each time.

The information you gather may help determine whether a vagal mechanism was involved. The presence of syncope or sinus pauses on an electrocardiogram may indicate the need for further electrophysiologic evaluation.

Document the patient's vital signs and how they feel during pauses, as well as any activities that occurred during the episode(s). Activities that increase vagal stimulation, such as Valsalva maneuver or vomiting, increase the likelihood of sinus pauses.

When matters get even worse

Assess for a progression of the arrhythmia. Notify the practitioner immediately if the patient becomes unstable. Lower the head of the bed and administer atropine or epinephrine, as ordered or as your facility's policy directs. Withhold medications that may contribute to sinus pauses and check with the practitioner about whether those drugs should be continued.

If appropriate, be alert for signs of digoxin, quinidine, or procainamide toxicity. Obtain a serum digoxin level and a serum electrolyte level. If a pacemaker is implanted, give the patient discharge instructions about pacemaker care.

Sick sinus syndrome

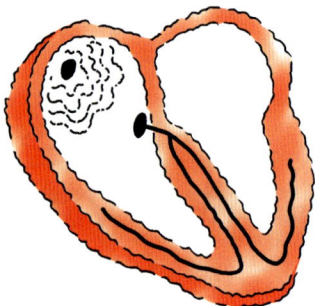

Also called *sinus node disease* or *sinus nodal dysfunction*, sick sinus syndrome refers to a wide spectrum of SA node abnormalities. Sick sinus syndrome is when the SA node is unable to sustain a heart rate that meets the physiological needs of the body. The syndrome is caused by disturbances in the way impulses are generated or the inability to conduct impulses to the atrium.

Causes of sick sinus syndrome

Sick sinus syndrome may result from the following:
• conditions leading to fibrosis of the SA node, such as increased age, atherosclerotic heart disease, hypertension, and cardiomyopathy
• infiltrative diseases, such as sarcoidosis, amyloidosis, or connective tissue diseases
• trauma to the SA node caused by open heart surgery (especially valvular

Sick sinus syndrome usually shows up as bradycardia, with episodes of sinus arrest and SA block interspersed with sudden, brief periods of rapid atrial fibrillation. Patients are also prone to paroxysms of other atrial tachyarrhythmias, such as atrial flutter and ectopic atrial tachycardia, a condition sometimes referred to as *tachycardia–bradycardia syndrome* (or *tachy–brady*) syndrome.

Most patients with sick sinus syndrome are older than age 60, but anyone can develop the arrhythmia. It's rare in children, except after open heart surgery that results in SA node damage. The arrhythmia affects males and females equally. The onset is progressive, insidious, and chronic.

How it happens

Sick sinus syndrome results from a dysfunction of the sinus node's automaticity or abnormal conduction or blockages of impulses coming out of the nodal region. (See *Causes of sick sinus syndrome*, page 84.) These conditions, in turn, stem from a degeneration of the area's autonomic nervous system and partial destruction of the sinus node, as may occur with an interrupted blood supply after an inferior wall MI.

Blocked exits

In addition, certain conditions can affect the atrial wall surrounding the SA node and cause exit blocks. Conditions that cause inflammation or degeneration of atrial tissue can also lead to sick sinus syndrome. In many patients, though, the exact cause of this syndrome is never identified.

Prognosis of the diagnosis

The significance of sick sinus syndrome depends on the patient's age, the presence of other diseases, and the type and duration of the specific arrhythmias that occur. If atrial fibrillation is involved, the prognosis is worse, most likely due to the risk of thromboembolic complications.

If prolonged pauses are involved with sick sinus syndrome, syncope may occur. The length of a pause significant enough to cause syncope varies with the patient's age, posture at the time, and cerebrovascular status. Consider any pause that lasts at least 2 to 3 seconds significant.

Long-term problems

A significant part of the diagnosis is whether the patient experiences symptoms while the disturbance occurs. Because the syndrome is progressive and chronic, a symptomatic patient needs lifelong treatment.

surgery), pericarditis, or rheumatic heart disease
• autonomic disturbances affecting autonomic innervation, such as hypervagotonia and degeneration of the autonomic nervous system
• metabolic and electrolyte disturbances
• cardioactive medications, such as digoxin (Lanoxin), antiarrhythmic drugs, beta-adrenergic blockers, and calcium channel blockers

Prolonged pauses with sick sinus syndrome cause syncope. Consider any pause that lasts 2 to 3 seconds significant.

In addition, thromboembolism may develop as a complication of sick sinus syndrome, possibly resulting in stroke or peripheral embolization.

What to look for

Sick sinus syndrome encompasses several potential rhythm disturbances that may be intermittent or chronic. (See *Identifying sick sinus syndrome*.) Those rhythm disturbances include one or a combination of the following:

Identifying sick sinus syndrome

This rhythm strip illustrates sick sinus syndrome. Look for the following distinguishing characteristics:

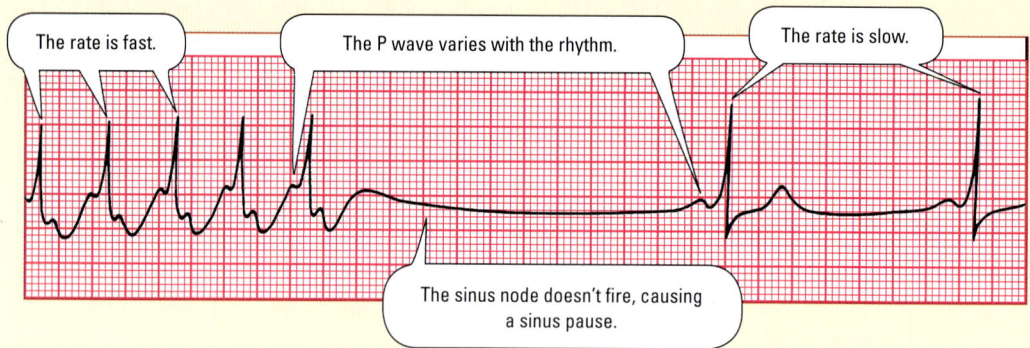

The rate is fast.

The P wave varies with the rhythm.

The rate is slow.

The sinus node doesn't fire, causing a sinus pause.

- *Rhythm:* Irregular
- *Rate:* Atrial—60 beats/min; ventricular—70 beats/min
- *P wave:* Configuration varies
- *PR interval:* Varies with rhythm
- *QRS complex:* 0.10 seconds
- *T wave:* Configuration varies
- *QT interval:* Varies with rhythm changes
- *Other:* None

- sinus bradycardia
- SA block
- sinus arrest
- sinus bradycardia alternating with sinus tachycardia
- episodes of atrial tachyarrhythmias, such as atrial fibrillation and atrial flutter
- failure of the sinus node to increase heart rate with exercise

Check for speed bumps

Also look for an irregular rhythm with sinus pauses and abrupt rate changes. Atrial and ventricular rates may be fast, slow, or alternating periods of fast rates and slow rates interrupted by pauses.

The P wave varies with the rhythm and usually precedes each QRS complex. The PR interval is usually within normal limits but varies with changes in the rhythm. The QRS complex and T wave are usually normal, as is the QT interval, which may vary with rhythm changes.

No set pattern

The patient's pulse rate may be fast, slow, or normal, and the rhythm may be regular or irregular. You can usually detect an irregularity on the monitor or when palpating the pulse, which may feel inappropriately slow, then rapid.

If you monitor the patient's heart rate during exercise or exertion, you may observe an inappropriate response to exercise, such as a failure of the heart rate to increase. You may also detect episodes of brady–tachy syndrome, atrial flutter, atrial fibrillation, SA block, or sinus arrest on the monitor.

Extra sounds

Other assessment findings depend on the patient's condition. For example, they may have crackles in the lungs, an S_3 heart sound, or a dilated and displaced left ventricular apical impulse if they have underlying cardiomyopathy.

The patient may show signs and symptoms of decreased cardiac output, such as hypotension, blurred vision, and syncope, a common experience with this arrhythmia. (See *Check mental status.*)

How you intervene

As with other sinus node arrhythmias, no treatment is necessary if the patient is asymptomatic. If the patient is symptomatic, however, treatment aims to alleviate signs and symptoms and correct the underlying cause of the arrhythmia.

Atropine or epinephrine may be given initially for symptomatic bradycardia. A temporary or permanent pacemaker may be used. Tachyarrhythmias may be treated with antiarrhythmic medications, such as metoprolol and digoxin.

Drugs don't always help

Unfortunately, medications used to suppress tachyarrhythmias may worsen underlying SA node disease and bradyarrhythmias. The patient may need anticoagulants if sudden bursts or paroxysms of atrial fibrillation occur. The anticoagulants help prevent thromboembolism and stroke, a complication of the condition. (See *Recognizing an embolism*, page 88.)

Monitoring heart rate during exercise may show an inappropriate response. Can I stop now?

Ages and stages

Check mental status

Because the older adult with sick sinus syndrome may have mental status changes, be sure to perform a thorough assessment to rule out disorders, such as stroke, delirium, or dementia.

Recognizing an embolism

When caring for a patient with sick sinus syndrome, be alert for signs and symptoms of an embolism, especially if the patient has atrial fibrillation. Any clots that form in the heart can break off and travel through the bloodstream, blocking the blood supply to the lungs, heart, brain, kidneys, intestines, or other organs.

Assess early

Assess the patient for neurologic changes, such as confusion, visual disturbances, weakness, chest pain, dyspnea, tachypnea, tachycardia, and acute onset of pain. Early recognition allows for prompt treatment.

Watch and document

When caring for a patient with sick sinus syndrome, monitor and document all arrhythmias, and signs or symptoms that develop. Assess how the rhythm responds to activity and pain.

Monitor the patient carefully after starting calcium channel blockers, beta-adrenergic blockers, or other antiarrhythmic medications. If treatment includes anticoagulant therapy and the insertion of a pacemaker, ensure that the patient and family receive appropriate instruction.

That's a wrap!

Sinus node arrhythmias review

SA node
- Acts as primary pacemaker
- Inherent firing rate of 60 to 100 times/min in a resting adult
- Supplied by blood from the right coronary artery and left circumflex artery

Sinus arrhythmia
Characteristics
- *Rhythms:* Irregular, corresponding to the respiratory cycle
- *Rates:* Within normal limits, vary with respiration
- *Other parameters:* QT interval variations

Treatment
- No treatment if asymptomatic
- Correction of the underlying cause

Sinus bradycardia
Characteristics
- *Rhythms:* Regular
- *Rates:* Less than 60 beats/min
- *Other parameters:* Normal

Treatment
- No treatment if asymptomatic
- Correction of the underlying cause
- Temporary pacing to increase heart rate
- Atropine or epinephrine to maintain heart rate
- Dopamine for hypotension
- Permanent pacing if necessary

Sinus node arrhythmias review (*continued*)

Sinus tachycardia
Characteristics
- *Rhythms:* Regular
- *Rates:* Both equal, generally 100 to 160 beats/min
- *PR interval:* Normal
- *QRS complex:* Normal
- *T wave:* Normal
- *QT interval:* Shortened

Treatment
- No treatment if asymptomatic
- Correction of the underlying cause
- Beta-adrenergic blockers or calcium channel blockers if symptomatic

Sinus arrest
Characteristics
- *Rhythms:* Regular, except for missing PQRST complex
- *Rates:* Equal and usually within normal limits; may vary as a result of pauses
- *P wave:* Normal and constant when P wave is present; not measurable when P wave is absent
- *QRS complex:* Normal when present; absent during pause
- *T wave:* Normal when present; absent during pause
- *QT interval:* Normal when present; absent during pause

Treatment
- No treatment if asymptomatic
- Correction of the underlying cause
- Atropine or epinephrine to maintain heart rate
- Temporary pacemaker to maintain adequate cardiac output and perfusion
- Permanent pacemaker if necessary

Sick sinus syndrome
Characteristics
- *Rhythms:* Irregular with sinus pauses and abrupt rate changes
- *Rates:* Fast, slow, or combination of both
- *P wave:* Variations with rhythm and usually before QRS complex
- *QRS complex:* Normal
- *T wave:* Normal
- *QT interval:* Normal; variations with rhythm changes

Treatment
- No treatment if asymptomatic
- Correction of the underlying cause
- Atropine or epinephrine for symptomatic bradycardia
- Temporary or permanent pacemaker if necessary
- Antiarrhythmics, such as metoprolol and digoxin, for tachyarrhythmias
- Anticoagulants if atrial fibrillation develops

Quick quiz

1. A patient with symptomatic sinus bradycardia at a rate of 40 beats/min typically experiences:
   - A. high blood pressure.
   - B. hypotension and dyspnea.
   - C. facial flushing and ataxia.
   - D. calf pain and a dry cough.

Answer: B. A patient with symptomatic bradycardia suffers from low cardiac output, which may produce hypotension and dyspnea. The patient may also have chest pain, crackles, an S₃ heart sound, and a sudden onset of confusion.

2. For a patient with symptomatic sinus bradycardia, appropriate nursing interventions include establishing intravenous (IV) access to administer:
      A. atropine.
      B. anticoagulants.
      C. calcium channel blocker.
      D. beta-adrenergic blocker.

Answer: A. Atropine or epinephrine is standard treatment for sinus bradycardia.

3. A monitor shows an irregular rhythm and a rate that increases and decreases in consistent cycles. This rhythm most likely represents:
      A. sinus arrest.
      B. sinus bradycardia.
      C. normal sinus rhythm.
      D. sinus arrhythmia.

Answer: D. In sinus arrhythmia, occurring naturally in athletes and young children, the heart rate varies with the respiratory cycle and is rarely treated.

4. Treatment for symptomatic sick sinus syndrome includes:
      A. beta-adrenergic blockers.
      B. ventilatory support.
      C. pacemaker insertion.
      D. cardioversion.

Answer: C. A temporary or permanent pacemaker is commonly used to maintain a steady heart rate in patients with sick sinus syndrome.

5. Persistent tachycardia in a patient who has had an MI may signal:
      A. chronic sick sinus syndrome.
      B. pulmonary embolism or stroke.
      C. the healing process.
      D. impending heart failure or cardiogenic shock.

Answer: D. Sinus tachycardia occurs in about 30% of patients after acute MI and is considered a poor prognostic sign because it may be associated with massive heart damage.

6. Beta-adrenergic blockers, such as metoprolol and atenolol, and calcium channel blockers, such as diltiazem, may be used to treat:
      A. sinus bradycardia.
      B. sinus tachycardia.
      C. sinus arrest.
      D. sinus arrhythmia.

Answer: B. Beta-adrenergic blockers and calcium channel blockers may be used to treat sinus tachycardia.

Test strips

Try these test strips. Interpret each strip using the eight-step method and fill in the blanks below with the particular characteristics of the strip. Then compare your answers with the answers given.

Strip 1

Atrial rhythm: _____

Ventricular rhythm: _____

Atrial rate: _____

Ventricular rate: _____

P wave: _____

PR interval: _____

QRS complex: _____

T wave: _____

QT interval: _____

Other: _____

Interpretation: _____

Strip 2

Atrial rhythm: _____

Ventricular rhythm: _____

Atrial rate: _____

Ventricular rate: _____

P wave: _____

PR interval: _____

QRS complex: _____

T wave: _____

QT interval: _____

Other: _____

Interpretation: _____

Strip 3

Atrial rhythm: _____

Ventricular rhythm: _____

Atrial rate: _____

Ventricular rate: _____

P wave: _____

PR interval: _____

QRS complex: _____

T wave: _____

QT interval: _____

Other: _____

Interpretation: _____

Answers to test strips

1. Rhythm: Regular except during pause
   Rate: Atrial and ventricular—50 beats/min
   P wave: Normal size and configuration, except when missing during pause
   PR interval: 0.16 seconds
   QRS complex: 0.10 seconds; normal size and configuration except when missing during pause
   T wave: Normal except when missing during pause
   QT interval: 0.42 seconds
   Other: Pause isn't a multiple of a previous sinus rhythm
   Interpretation: Sinus arrest

2. Rhythm: Regular
   Rate: Atrial and ventricular—110 beats/min
   P wave: Normal configuration
   PR interval: 0.14 seconds
   QRS complex: 0.08 seconds; normal size and configuration
   T wave: Normal configuration
   QT interval: 0.36 seconds
   Other: None
   Interpretation: Sinus tachycardia

3. Rhythm: Atrial and ventricular—irregular
   Rate: Atrial and ventricular—90 beats/min
   P wave: Normal
   PR interval: 0.12 seconds
   QRS complex: 0.10 seconds and normal
   T wave: Normal
   QT interval: 0.30 seconds
   Other: None
   Interpretation: Sinus arrhythmia

Scoring

☆☆☆ If you answered all six questions correctly and completed the rhythm strips well, wow!

☆☆ If you answered five questions correctly and correctly completed the rhythm strips, super!

☆ If you answered fewer than five questions correctly and missed most of the blanks, don't worry! A few more lessons will be very useful.

Selected references

De Ponti, R., Marazzato, J., Bagliani, G., Leonelli, F. M., & Padeletti, L. (2018). Sick sinus syndrome. *Cardiac Electrophysiology Clinics, 10*(2), 183–195. https://doi.org/10.1016/j.ccep.2018.02.002

Fadah, K., Yohannan, S., Cartagena, J., Montanez, R., & Roongsritong, C. (2022). Resolution of symptomatic intermittent sinoatrial exit block associated with unstable angina following percutaneous coronary intervention. *Cardiology Research, 13*(3), 172–176. https://doi.org/10.14740/cr1388

Hawks, M. K., Paul, M. L. B., & Malu, O. O. (2021). Sinus node dysfunction. *American Family Physician, 104*(2), 179–185.

Healio. (2019). *ECG reviews and criteria.* https://www.healio.com

Jabbour, F., & Kanmanthareddy, A. (2022). Sinus node dysfunction. In *StatPearls* [Internet]. StatPearls Publishing.

Karki, R., Raina, A., Ezzeddine, F. M., Bois, M. C., & Asorvatham, S. J. (2021). Anatomy and pathology of the cardiac conduction system. *Cardiac Electrophysiology Clinics, 13*(4), 569–584. https://doi.org/10.1016/j.ccep.2021.06.003

Kusumoto, F. M., Schoenfeld, M. H., Barrett, C., Edgerton, J. R., Ellenbogen, K. A., Gold, M. R., Goldschlager, N. F., Hamilton, R. M., Joglar, J. A., Kim, R. J., Lee, R., Marine, J. E., McLeod, C. J., Oken, K. R., Patton, K. K., Pellegrini, C. N., Selzman, K. A., Thompson, A., & Varosky, P. D. (2019). 2018 ACC/AHA/HRS Guideline on the evaluation and management of patients with bradycardia and cardiac conduction delay: A report of the American College of Cardiology/American Heart Association Task Force on Clinical Practice Guidelines and the Heart Rhythm Society. *Journal of the American College of Cardiology, 74*(7), e51–e156. http://www.onlinejacc.org/content/early/2018/10/29/j.jacc.2018.10.044

Manoj, P., Kim, S., Li, T., Sewani, M., Shelu, M. G., & Li, N. (2023). Sinus node dysfunction: Current understanding and future directions. *American Journal of Physiology. Heart and Circulatory Physiology, 324*(3), H259–H278. https://doi.org/10.1152/ajpheart.00618.2022

National Library of Medicine. (2019). *Wolff-Parkinson-White syndrome.* https://ghr.nlm.nih.gov/condition/wolff-parkinson-white-syndrome#

Rogoff, B., & Pride, Y. B. (2022). EKG rhythm. In *StatPearls* [Internet]. StatPearls Publishing.

Sathnur, N., Ebin, E., & Benditt, D. G. (2021). Sinus node dysfunction. *Cardiac Electrophysiology Clinics, 13*(4), 641–659. https://doi.org/10.1016/j.ccep.2021.06.006

Sidhu, S., & Marine, J. E. (2020). Evaluating and managing bradycardia. *Trends in Cardiovascular Medicine, 30*(5), 265–272. https://doi.org/10.1016/j.tcm.2019.07.001

Sole, M. L., Klein, D. G., & Moseley, M. J. (2020). *Introduction to critical care nursing* (8th ed.). Saunders.

Soos, M. P., & McComb, D. (2022). Sinus arrhythmia. In *StatPearls* [Internet]. StatPearls Publishing.

Strauss, D. G., & Schocken, D. D. (2021). *Marriott's practical electrocardiography* (13th ed.). Wolters Kluwer.

Atrial arrhythmias

Just the facts

In this chapter, you'll learn:

◆ the proper way to identify the various atrial arrhythmias

◆ the causes, significance, treatment, and nursing implications of each arrhythmia

◆ assessment findings associated with each arrhythmia

◆ interpretation of atrial arrhythmias on an ECG.

A look at atrial arrhythmias

Atrial arrhythmias, the most common cardiac rhythm disturbances, result from impulses originating in areas outside the sinoatrial (SA) node. These arrhythmias can affect ventricular filling time and diminish the strength of the atrial kick, a contraction that normally provides the ventricles with about 15% to 25% of their blood.

Triple play

Atrial arrhythmias are thought to result from three mechanisms—enhanced automaticity, reentry, and afterdepolarization. Let's look at each cause and review specific atrial arrhythmias:

• Enhanced automaticity: An increase in the automaticity (the ability of cardiac cells to initiate impulses on their own) of the atrial fibers can trigger abnormal impulses. Causes of increased automaticity include extracellular factors, such as hypoxia, acidosis, hypocalcemia, and digoxin toxicity, and conditions in which the function of the heart's normal pacemaker, the SA node, is diminished. For example, increased vagal tone or hypokalemia can increase the refractory period of the SA node and allow atrial fibers to fire impulses.

• Reentry: In reentry, an electrical stimulus is conducted in a circular loop that is large enough to allow the tissue to repolarize and accept a new electrical stimulus. This process continues until something interrupts the continuous cycle. Reentry may occur with coronary artery disease, cardiomyopathy, myocardial infarction (MI), or structural abnormalities of the heart.

- Triggered activity: An injured cell may repolarize only partially. Partial repolarization can lead to a repetitive ectopic firing called *triggered activity*. The depolarization produced by triggered activity is known as *afterdepolarization* and can lead to atrial or ventricular tachycardia. Afterdepolarization can occur with cell injury, digoxin toxicity, and other conditions. Now, let's examine each atrial arrhythmia in detail.

Premature atrial contractions

Premature atrial contractions (PACs) originate outside the SA node and usually result from an irritable focus in the atria that takes over as the pacemaker for one or more beats. Before the SA node can fire an impulse, an irritable atrial focus jumps in, firing its impulse and causing an early beat.

PACs may be conducted through the atrioventricular (AV) node and the rest of the heart, depending on their prematurity and AV and intraventricular conduction system status. Nonconducted or blocked PACs occur when the AV node is recovering and still refractory; therefore, these do not conduct through the AV node or trigger a QRS complex. In this case, a nonsinus P wave is produced and is not followed by a QRS complex.

How it happens

PACs occur in a normal heart and are very common in people who are 50 years or above. PACs can be triggered by alcohol, nicotine, anxiety, fatigue, fever, and infectious diseases. A patient who eliminates or moderates those factors can correct the arrhythmias.

PACs may also be associated with coronary or valvular heart disease, acute respiratory failure, hypoxia, pulmonary disease, digoxin toxicity, and certain electrolyte imbalances.

PACs are rarely dangerous in a patient who has a healthy heart. In fact, they commonly cause no symptoms and can go unrecognized for years. The patient may perceive PACs as normal palpitations or skipped beats.

The nicotine in cigarettes can cause PACs. Yuk!

Early warning sign

However, in patients with heart disease, PACs may lead to more serious arrhythmias, such as atrial fibrillation (AF) and atrial flutter. In a patient with an acute MI, PACs can serve as an early sign of heart failure or an electrolyte imbalance. PACs can also result from the release of the neurohormone catecholamine during episodes of pain or anxiety.

What to look for

The hallmark ECG characteristic of a PAC is a premature (early) P wave with an abnormal shape compared to a sinus P wave. (See *Nonconducted PACs and second-degree AV block*.)

When the PAC is conducted, the QRS complex appears like the underlying QRS complex. PACs are commonly followed by a pause.

The PAC depolarizes the SA node early, causing it to reset itself and disrupt the normal cycle. The next sinus beat occurs sooner than it normally would. This causes a shortening in the P-P interval between two normal beats interrupted by a PAC as compared to a constant P-P interval between three consecutive sinus beats, an occurrence referred to as noncompensatory. (See *Identifying PACs*, page 98.)

Lost in the T

When examining a PAC on an ECG, look for irregular atrial and ventricular rhythms. The underlying rhythm is usually regular. An irregular rhythm results from the PAC and its corresponding pause. The P wave is premature, abnormally shaped, and may be lost in the previous T wave, distorting that waveform's configuration. (The T wave might be bigger or have an extra bump.) Varying configurations of the P wave indicate more than one ectopic site.

The PR interval can be normal, shortened, or slightly prolonged, depending on the origin of the ectopic focus. If no QRS complex follows the premature P wave, then a nonconducted PAC has occurred.

PACs may occur in bigeminy (every other beat is a PAC), trigeminy (every third beat is a PAC), or couplets (two PACs in a row).

The patient will have an irregular peripheral or apical pulse rhythm when the PACs occur. The patient may be asymptomatic or may sense palpitations, skipped beats, or a fluttering sensation in the chest or neck. In a patient with heart disease, signs and symptoms of decreased cardiac output, such as hypotension and syncope, may rarely occur.

Mixed signals

Nonconducted PACs and second-degree AV block

Don't confuse nonconducted PACs with second-degree AV block type II, where the P-P interval is regular and all P waves look identical. A nonconducted PAC, however, is an atrial impulse that arrives early at the AV node, which hasn't yet repolarized.

As a result, the premature P wave fails to be conducted to the ventricle. The rhythm strip below shows an abnormally shaped P wave embedded in the preceding T wave.

Identifying PACs

This rhythm strip illustrates PAC. Look for the following distinguishing characteristics:

The rhythm is irregular when a PAC occurs.

Premature and abnormally shaped P waves occur.

The baseline rhythm is regular.

- *Rhythm:* Irregular
- *Rate:* 90 beats/min
- *P wave:* Abnormal with PAC; some lost in previous T wave

- *PR interval:* 0.20 seconds
- *QRS complex:* 0.08 seconds
- *T wave:* Abnormal with some embedded P waves

- *QT interval:* 0.32 seconds
- *Other:* Noncompensatory pause (as in first PAC)

How you intervene

Most patients who are asymptomatic don't require treatment. In symptomatic patients, however, treatment may focus on eliminating the underlying cause, such as caffeine, alcohol, and nicotine.

When caring for a patient with PACs, assess what may be triggering the ectopic beats. Include in your patient teaching, how to avoid underlying causes, such as eliminating caffeine, nicotine, alcohol; and if appropriate, encourage the patient to use stress reducing techniques that decrease anxiety.

If the patient has ischemic or valvular heart disease, monitor closely for signs and symptoms of heart failure, electrolyte imbalances, and the development of more severe atrial arrhythmias.

PACs may be caused by too much caffeine or alcohol.

Atrial tachycardia

Atrial tachycardia is a supraventricular tachycardia, which means the impulses driving the rapid rhythm originate above the ventricles. Atrial tachycardia has an atrial rate of 100 to 250 beats/min. The rapid rate shortens diastole, reduces cardiac output, and reduces coronary perfusion, potentially causing ischemic myocardial changes.

There are three types of atrial tachycardia: atrial tachycardia with block, multifocal atrial tachycardia (MAT), and paroxysmal atrial tachycardia (PAT).

How it happens

Atrial tachycardia can occur in patients with physiologically normal hearts. In those cases, the condition is commonly related to excessive use of caffeine or other stimulants, marijuana use, electrolyte imbalances, hypoxia, and physical or psychological stress. However, this arrhythmia is usually associated with primary or secondary cardiac problems.

Cardiac conditions that can cause atrial tachycardia include MI, cardiomyopathy, congenital anomalies, Wolff–Parkinson–White syndrome, and valvular heart disease. This rhythm may also be a component of sick sinus syndrome. Other problems resulting in atrial tachycardia include cor pulmonale, hyperthyroidism, systemic hypertension, and digoxin toxicity. (See *Signs of digoxin toxicity*.)

An ominous sign?

In a healthy person, atrial tachycardia is usually benign. However, this rhythm may be a forerunner of a more serious ventricular arrhythmia, especially if it occurs in a patient with an underlying heart condition.

The increased ventricular rate of atrial tachycardia results in a decrease in the time allowed for the ventricles to fill, an increase in myocardial oxygen consumption, and a decrease in oxygen supply. Angina, heart failure, ischemic myocardial changes, and even MI can occur as a result.

What to look for

Atrial tachycardia is characterized by three or more successive ectopic atrial beats at a rate of 100 to 250 beats/min. If the P wave is visible, it will be a different shape than the sinus P, is usually upright, and is followed by a narrow QRS complex.

Signs of digoxin toxicity

With digoxin toxicity, atrial tachycardia isn't the only change you might see in your patient. Patients are at greater risk for digoxin toxicity if the potassium level is low or if they are taking amiodarone (Cordarone); the combination of these can increase digoxin toxicity. Be alert for the following signs and symptoms:
- *Central nervous system (CNS):* Fatigue, general muscle weakness, agitation, hallucinations
- *Eye, ear, nose, and throat (EENT):* Yellow-green halos around visual images, blurred vision
- *Gastrointestinal (GI):* Anorexia, nausea, vomiting
- *Cardiovascular (CV):* Arrhythmias (most commonly, conduction disturbances with or without AV block, premature ventricular contractions, and supraventricular arrhythmias), increased severity of heart failure, hypotension (Digoxin's toxic effects on the heart may be life-threatening and always require immediate attention.)

Keep in mind that atrial beats may be conducted on a 1:1 basis to the ventricles (meaning that each P wave has a QRS complex), so atrial and ventricular rates will be equal. In other cases, atrial beats may be conducted only periodically, meaning the AV node blocks conduction of some of the atrial impulses. The AV node stops the ventricles from receiving every impulse and beating at a very high rate.

Think of the AV node as a gatekeeper. Sometimes, it lets atrial impulses conduct through to the ventricles regularly (every impulse or every other impulse, for instance), and sometimes, it allows them to conduct through irregularly (two impulses might get through, for instance, and then three and then one).

Think of the AV node as a gatekeeper!

Fast but regular

When assessing a rhythm strip for atrial tachycardia, you'll see that atrial rhythm is regular, and ventricular rhythm is regular when the block is constant and irregular when it isn't. (See *Identifying atrial tachycardia*.) The rate consists of three or more successive ectopic atrial beats at a rate of 100 to 250 beats/min. The ventricular rate varies according to the AV conduction ratio.

Identifying atrial tachycardia

This rhythm strip illustrates atrial tachycardia. Look for the following distinguishing characteristics:

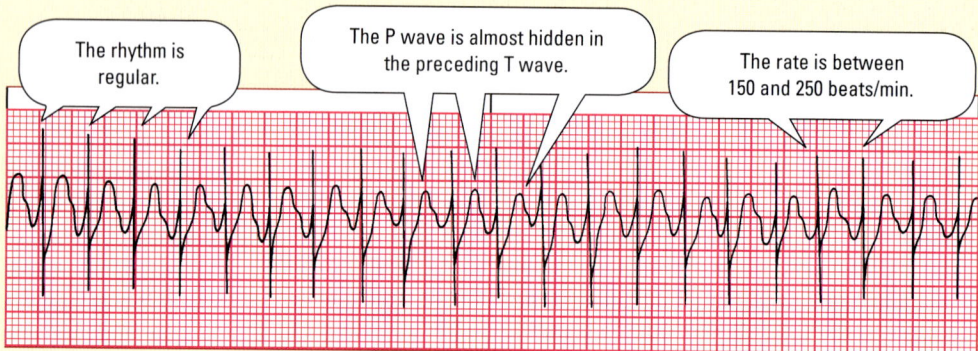

The rhythm is regular.

The P wave is almost hidden in the preceding T wave.

The rate is between 150 and 250 beats/min.

- *Rhythm:* Regular
- *Rate:* 210 beats/min
- *P wave:* Almost hidden in T wave
- *PR interval:* 0.12 seconds
- *QRS complex:* 0.10 seconds
- *T wave:* Distorted by P wave
- *QT interval:* 0.20 seconds
- *Other:* None

The P wave has a 1:1 ratio with the QRS complex unless a block is present. The P wave may not be discernible because of the rapid rate and may be hidden in the previous ST segment or T wave. You may not be able to measure the PR interval if the P wave can't be distinguished from the preceding T wave.

The QRS complex is usually normal unless the impulses are being conducted abnormally through the ventricles. (See *Identifying types of atrial tachycardia*.) The T wave may be normal or inverted if ischemia is present. The QT interval is usually within normal limits but may be shorter because of the rapid rate. ST-segment and T-wave changes may appear if ischemia occurs with a prolonged arrhythmia.

Identifying types of atrial tachycardia

Atrial tachycardia comes in three varieties. Here's a quick rundown of each.

Atrial tachycardia with block

Atrial tachycardia with block is caused by increased automaticity of the atrial tissue. As the atrial rate speeds up and AV conduction becomes impaired, a 2:1 block typically occurs. Occasionally, a second-degree AV block Mobitz type I (Wenckebach) may be seen. Look for the following distinguishing characteristics:

Two P waves occur for each QRS complex.

The ventricular rhythm is regular; the block is constant.

The atrial rhythm is regular.

• *Rhythm:* Atrial—regular; ventricular—regular if block is constant, irregular if block is variable
• *Rate:* Atrial—100 to 250 beats/min, multiples of ventricular rate; ventricular—varies with block

• *P wave:* Slightly abnormal; shape depends on the site of ectopic pacemaker
• *PR interval:* Usually normal
• *QRS complex:* Usually normal
• *T wave:* Usually indistinguishable

• *QT interval:* Possibly indiscernible
• *Other:* More than one P wave for each QRS complex

Identifying types of atrial tachycardia (*continued*)

Multifocal atrial tachycardia

In MAT, atrial tachycardia occurs with numerous atrial foci firing intermittently. MAT produces varying P waves on the strip and occurs most commonly in patients with chronic pulmonary disease. The irregular baseline in this strip is caused by movement of the chest wall. Look for the following distinguishing characteristics:

- *Rhythm:* Atrial and ventricular—irregular
- *Rate:* Atrial—100 to 250 beats/min, usually under 160; ventricular—100 to 250 beats/min
- *P wave:* Configuration varies; must see at least three different P wave shapes
- *PR interval:* Variable
- *QRS complex:* Usually normal; can be aberrant if arrhythmia persists
- *T wave:* Usually distorted
- *QT interval:* Possibly indiscernible
- *Other:* None

Paroxysmal atrial tachycardia

A type of paroxysmal supraventricular tachycardia, PAT features brief periods of tachycardia that alternate with periods of normal sinus rhythm. PAT starts and stops suddenly due to the rapid firing of an ectopic focus. It commonly follows frequent PACs, one of which initiates the tachycardia. Look for the following distinguishing characteristics:

- *Rhythm:* Regular
- *Rate:* 100 to 250 beats/min
- *P wave:* Abnormal, possibly hidden in previous T wave
- *PR interval:* Identical for each cycle
- *QRS complex:* Possibly aberrantly conducted
- *T wave:* Usually distorted
- *QT interval:* Possibly indiscernible
- *Other:* One P wave for each QRS complex

Check out the outward signs

The patient with atrial tachycardia has a rapid apical or peripheral pulse rate. The rhythm may be regular or irregular, depending on the type of atrial tachycardia. A patient with PAT may complain that their heart suddenly starts to beat faster or there are sudden palpitations. Persistent tachycardia and rapid ventricular rate cause decreased cardiac output, which can lead to blurred vision, syncope, and hypotension.

How you intervene

Treatment depends on the type of tachycardia, the width of the QRS complex, and the clinical stability of the patient. Digoxin toxicity is one cause of atrial tachycardia, so assessing the patient for signs and symptoms of toxicity and monitoring serum digoxin levels are important.

Valsalva maneuver or carotid sinus massage may be used to treat atrial tachycardia. (See *No massage for older patients* and *Understanding carotid sinus massage*.) Keep in mind that vagal stimulation can result in bradycardia, ventricular arrhythmias, and asystole. If vagal maneuvers are used, make sure that resuscitative equipment is readily available.

Ages and stages

No massage for older patients

Older adults may have undiagnosed carotid atherosclerosis and carotid bruits may be absent, even with significant disease. As a result, you shouldn't perform cardiac sinus massage in late middle-aged and older patients.

Understanding carotid sinus massage

Carotid sinus massage may be used to diagnose or treat atrial tachycardias. Massaging the carotid sinus stimulates the vagus nerve, which then inhibits the firing of the SA node and slows AV node conduction. As the rate slows down, the atrial arrhythmia can more easily be identified. Sometimes, carotid massage will convert the rhythm back to sinus as the SA node resumes its job as the primary pacemaker. Risks of carotid sinus massage include decreased heart rate, vasodilation, ventricular arrhythmias, stroke, and asystole. Of importance, carotid massage may only be applied to one side of the neck at a time. Direct compression of both carotid arteries simultaneously could cause bradycardia, hypotension, arrythmias, syncope, or anoxia to the brain.

- Internal carotid artery
- External carotid artery
- Vagus nerve
- Carotid sinus

Remember, carotid sinus massage is contraindicated for older patients due to the risk of stroke.

Optimal treatment options

Drug therapy may be used, and initial therapy includes oral beta-blockers or nondihydropyridine calcium channel blockers (i.e., diltiazem or verapamil). If other treatments fail or a recurrence of arrhythmia arises, the patient may be a candidate for a catheter ablation procedure. If clinically unstable, synchronized cardioversion may be used. More aggressive antiarrhythmic drugs can also be considered for patients who fail beta-blockers, diltiazem, and verapamil or are not candidates for ablative procedures. These medications include Class IC (flecainide, propafenone) antiarrhythmic drugs. These drugs can be used in patients without structural or ischemic heart disease. If a patient has significant comorbidities, amiodarone is the preferred drug of choice.

Monitor the strip

When caring for a patient with atrial tachycardia, carefully monitor their rhythm. Doing so may provide information about the cause of atrial tachycardia, which can facilitate treatment. In addition, monitor the patient for chest pain, indications of decreased cardiac output, hypotension, and signs and symptoms of heart failure or myocardial ischemia.

Atrial flutter

Atrial flutter, a supraventricular tachycardia, is characterized by an atrial rate of 250 to 350 beats/min, although it's generally around 300 beats/min. Originating in a single atrial focus, this rhythm results from reentry and, possibly, increased automaticity.

On an ECG, the P waves lose their distinction because of the rapid atrial rate. The waves blend in a saw-toothed appearance and are called *flutter waves*. These waves are the hallmark of atrial flutter. The distance from one R wave to the next is regular in atrial flutter.

Atrial flutter is commonly associated with AV nodal block.

How it happens

Atrial flutter is commonly associated with AV nodal block. The AV node prevents the conduction of every impulse to the ventricles. As a result, the ventricular rate is slower than the atrial rate. This protects the ventricles from excessive rates.

Atrial flutter may be caused by conditions that enlarge atrial tissue and elevate atrial pressures. It's commonly found in patients with heart failure, severe mitral valve disease, hyperthyroidism, alcoholism, pericardial disease, obesity, obstructive sleep apnea, and primary myocardial disease. The rhythm is also sometimes encountered in patients after cardiac surgery or in patients with acute MI, chronic obstructive pulmonary disease (COPD), pulmonary embolus, and systemic arterial hypoxia. Atrial flutter rarely occurs in healthy people. When it does, it may indicate intrinsic cardiac disease.

> Saw-toothed flutter waves are the hallmark of atrial flutter.

Rating the ratio

The clinical significance of atrial flutter is determined by the number of impulses conducted through the node—expressed as a conduction ratio, for example, 2:1 or 4:1—and the resulting ventricular rate. If the ventricular rate is too slow (<40 beats/min) or too fast (>150 beats/min), cardiac output can be seriously compromised.

Usually, the faster the ventricular rate, the more dangerous the arrhythmia. The rapid rate reduces ventricular filling time and coronary perfusion, which can cause angina, heart failure, pulmonary edema, hypotension, and syncope.

What to look for

Atrial flutter is characterized by abnormal P waves that produce a saw-toothed appearance, the hallmark flutter-wave appearance. (See *Identifying atrial flutter*.) Varying degrees of AV block produce ventricular rates one half to one fourth of the atrial rate.

Identifying atrial flutter

This rhythm strip illustrates atrial flutter. Look for the following distinguishing characteristics:

> Classic, saw-toothed flutter waves occur.

> The ventricular rate is less than the atrial rate.

- *Rhythm:* Atrial—regular; ventricular—irregular
- *Rate:* Atrial—280 beats/min; ventricular—60 beats/min
- *P wave:* Classic saw-toothed appearance
- *PR interval:* Unmeasurable
- *QRS complex:* 0.08 seconds
- *T wave:* Unidentifiable
- *QT interval:* Unidentifiable
- *Other:* None

The AV node usually won't accept more than 180 impulses/min and allows every second, third, or fourth impulse to be conducted, the ratio of which determines the ventricular rate.

The most common ventricular rate is 150 beats/min. With an atrial rate of 300, that rhythm is referred to as a 2:1 block. (See *Atrial flutter and sinus tachycardia.*)

The QRS complex is usually normal but may be widened if flutter waves are buried in the complex. You won't be able to identify a T wave, nor will you be able to measure the QT interval.

The atrial rhythm may vary between fibrillatory waves and flutter waves, an arrhythmia commonly referred to as *atrial fibrillation and flutter.*

Misleading pulses

When caring for a patient with atrial flutter, you may note that their peripheral or apical pulse is normal in rate and rhythm. That is because the pulse reflects the number of ventricular contractions, not the number of atrial impulses.

If the ventricular rate is normal, the patient may be asymptomatic. However, if the ventricular rate is rapid, the patient may exhibit signs and symptoms of reduced cardiac output and cardiac decompensation.

How you intervene

If the patient is hemodynamically unstable, synchronized electrical cardioversion should be administered immediately. Cardioversion delivers transthoracic electrical current to the heart (applied to the anterior chest) in order to correct an arrhythmia. The electrical energy is synchronized to discharge at the peak of the R wave. Synchronizing the energy to be delivered on the R wave ensures that the current will avoid the vulnerable T wave, which could induce ventricular tachycardia or ventricular fibrillation. Procedural sedation is administered prior to cardioversion to reduce the discomfort for the patient.

Control and convert operation

The focus of treatment for hemodynamically stable patients includes controlling the rate and converting the rhythm. For patients in an atrial flutter with normal cardiac function and duration, synchronized cardioversion may be considered; for a duration greater than 48 hours, synchronized cardioversion would not be considered because it increases the risk of thromboembolism unless the patient has been adequately anticoagulated (anticoagulation should be uninterrupted for 3 to 4 weeks preceding direct current cardioversion).

Mixed signals

Atrial flutter and sinus tachycardia

Whenever you see sinus tachycardia with a consistent rate of 150 beats/min, take another look. That rate is a common one for atrial flutter with 2:1 conduction. Look closely for flutter waves; these may be hidden in the QRS complex. You may need to check another lead for these to be clearly discernable. Another hint: If you turn the rhythm strip upside down, you may be able to see the flutter waves more easily.

Due to the high recurrence rate of atrial flutter, radiofrequency catheter ablation is the preferred treatment for most patients. Radiofrequency catheter ablation for atrial flutter is a highly successful and more definitive treatment. It is less preferable for patients to be converted with antiarrhythmic drugs because of the side effects. If it is necessary, ibutilide, through intravenous (IV) administration, is the drug of choice.

If synchronized cardioversion or catheter ablation is not indicated, medications may be used. Rate control medications can be used, including a nondihydropyridine calcium channel blocker or a beta-blocker. Amiodarone may also be used for rate control, in acutely ill patients, but it is not generally used long term due to the risk of potential side effects.

Stay alert

Because atrial flutter may indicate intrinsic cardiac disease, monitor the patient closely for signs and symptoms of low cardiac output. If cardioversion is necessary, prepare the patient for IV administration of a sedative or anesthetic as ordered. Keep resuscitative equipment at the bedside. Also be alert for bradycardia because cardioversion can decrease the heart rate.

Atrial fibrillation

Atrial fibrillation, sometimes called *A-fib*, is defined as chaotic, asynchronous electrical activity in atrial tissue. It's the most common arrhythmia, affecting at least three to six million people in the United States. AF stems from the firing of fast and irregular impulses across multiple reentry pathways. As with atrial flutter, AF results in a loss of atrial kick. The ectopic impulses may fire at a rate of 400 to 600 times/min, causing the atria to quiver instead of contract.

The ventricles respond only to those impulses that make it through the AV node. On an ECG, atrial activity is no longer represented by P waves but by erratic baseline waves called *fibrillatory waves*, or *f waves*. This rhythm may be either paroxysmal (occurring usually less than 24 hours and can last up to a week), persistent (lasting more than a week), long-standing persistent (lasting more than a year), or permanent AF (at which point, the patient and physician decide to stop attempts to restore or maintain sinus rhythm).

The irregular conduction of impulses through the AV node produces a characteristic irregular ventricular response. If you see no P waves and a ventricular rhythm that is irregularly irregular, suspect AF.

How it happens

AF occurs more commonly than atrial flutter or atrial tachycardia. AF can occur following cardiac surgery, or it can be caused by long-standing hypertension, diabetes, obesity, obstructive sleep apnea, smoking, pulmonary embolism, COPD, electrolyte imbalances, mitral insufficiency, mitral stenosis, hyperthyroidism, infection, coronary artery disease, acute MI, pericarditis, hypoxia, congenital heart disease, and atrial septal defects.

The rhythm may also occur in a healthy person who has a familial predisposition or who uses coffee, excessive alcohol consumption, high-fat intake, or nicotine in excess or who's fatigued and under stress. Catecholamine release during exercise may also trigger the arrhythmia.

Where have all the atrial kicks gone?

As with other atrial arrhythmias, AF eliminates atrial kick. That loss, combined with the decreased filling times associated with rapid rates, can lead to clinically significant problems. If the ventricular response is greater than 100 beats/min—a condition called *atrial fibrillation with rapid ventricular response* (RVR)—the patient may develop hypotension, heart failure, angina, or syncope.

Patients with preexisting cardiac disease, such as hypertrophic obstructive cardiomyopathy, mitral stenosis, rheumatic heart disease, and mitral prosthetic valves, tend to tolerate AF poorly and may develop shock and severe heart failure.

Left untreated, AF can lead to CV collapse, atrial thrombus formation, and systemic arterial or pulmonary embolism. AF is a common cause of stroke. (See *Risk of restoring sinus rhythm.*)

What to look for

AF is distinguished by the absence of P waves and an irregular ventricular response. When several ectopic sites in the atria fire impulses, depolarization can't spread in an organized manner. (See *Identifying AF*, page 109.)

Risk of restoring sinus rhythm

A patient with AF is at increased risk for developing atrial thrombus and systemic arterial embolism. Because the atria don't contract, blood may pool on the atrial wall and thrombi can form.

If normal sinus rhythm is restored and the atria contract normally, clots can break away and travel through the pulmonary or systemic circulation with potentially disastrous results.

Identifying AF

This rhythm strip illustrates AF. Look for the following distinguishing characteristics:

> The sinus P wave is replaced by erratic fibrillatory waves.

> The rhythm is irregularly irregular.

- *Rhythm:* Irregularly irregular
- *Rate:* Atrial—indiscernible; ventricular—130 beats/min
- *P wave:* Absent; replaced by fine fibrillatory waves
- *PR interval:* Indiscernible
- *QRS complex:* 0.08 seconds
- *T wave:* Indiscernible
- *QT interval:* Unmeasurable
- *Other:* None

Small sections of the atria are activated individually, which results in the atrial muscle quivering instead of contracting. On an ECG, you'll see uneven baseline and f waves rather than clearly distinguishable P waves.

That fabulous filter

The AV node protects the ventricles from the 400 to 600 erratic atrial impulses that occur each minute by acting as a filter and blocking some of the impulses. The AV node itself, however, doesn't receive all the impulses. If muscle tissue around the AV node is in a refractory state, impulses from other areas of the atria can't reach the AV node, which further reduces the number of atrial impulses conducted through to the ventricles.

Those two factors help explain the characteristic wide variation in R-R intervals in AF.

Barely measurable

The atrial rate is indiscernible but is usually greater than 400 impulses/min. It is important to note that with AF, atrial response is chaotic without any organized atrial contraction. The ventricular rate usually varies from 100 to 150 beats/min but can be lower or higher.

AF is called *coarse* if the P waves are pronounced and *fine* if they aren't. AF and flutter may also occur. Look for a configuration that varies between fibrillatory waves and flutter waves.

How you intervene

The major therapeutic goal in treating AF is early rhythm control in patients with AF that has not become long-standing. Early rhythm control can help prevent irreversible atrial remodeling. It can also prevent heart failure, stroke, and AF-related death. There has been a shift from favoring rhythm control over rate control for patients with new-onset AF. Rhythm control can be accomplished by using antiarrhythmic medications, cardioversion, or catheter ablation. In patients with permanent AF and symptomatic, rate control medications are recommended. In patients who continue to be symptomatic with rate control medications, AV node ablation with a pacemaker is an option.

Timing is everything

Electrical cardioversion is most successful if used within the first 48 hours of treatment and less successful if the rhythm has existed for a long time. If the patient shows signs of more severe angina or a decreased cardiac output, emergency measures are necessary.

Cardioversion

A symptomatic patient needs immediate synchronized cardioversion. The patient should receive appropriate anticoagulation therapy first because cardioversion can cause emboli to be released from the atrial wall, especially in a patient with chronic or paroxysmal AF.

A conversion to normal sinus rhythm will cause forceful atrial contractions to resume abruptly. If a thrombus forms in the atria, the resumption of contractions can result in systemic emboli. (See *How synchronized cardioversion works*.)

> Immediate synchronized cardioversion can reestablish normal sinus rhythm in a symptomatic patient.

How synchronized cardioversion works

A patient whose arrhythmia causes low cardiac output and hypotension may be a candidate for synchronized cardioversion. This may be an elective or emergency procedure. For instance, it may be used to make a person with AF more comfortable or to save the life of a patient with ventricular tachycardia.

Synchronize the energy

Synchronized cardioversion is like defibrillation, except that cardioversion generally requires lower energy levels. In synchronized cardioversion, the R wave on the patient's ECG is synchronized with the cardioverter (defibrillator). After the firing buttons have been pressed, the defibrillator discharges energy when it senses the next R wave.

How synchronized cardioversion works (*continued*)

When the stimulus hits

To stop atrial depolarization and reestablish normal sinus rhythm, electrical stimulation must occur during the R wave. Stimulation that hits a T wave increases the risk of fatal arrhythmias. Keep in mind that there's a slight delay between the time the firing button is pressed and the moment the energy is actually discharged. Call "All clear," and observe that no one is touching the patient until the energy is actually discharged.

Digoxin toxicity warning

Be aware that synchronized cardioversion carries the risk of lethal arrhythmias when used in patients with digoxin toxicity.

Reestablishing its role

Drugs such as amiodarone, dofetilide, dronedarone, flecainide, propafenone, and sotalol are antiarrhythmic drugs that are used for restoration and/or maintenance of sinus rhythm. Regarding dronedarone, studies have shown that this drug is effective in maintaining sinus rhythm and has a better safety profile than amiodarone, thus making it a first-line treatment option for rhythm management. Pharmacological rate control strategies can be used prior to or after a cardioversion, and they include beta-blockers (metoprolol), nondihydropyridine calcium channel blockers, digoxin, and amiodarone.

Symptomatic AF that does not respond to routine treatment may be treated with radiofrequency catheter ablation therapy (pulmonary vein isolation) or, rarely, an AV node ablation and permanent pacemaker.

When assessing a patient with AF, assess both the peripheral and apical pulses. If the patient isn't on a cardiac monitor, be alert for an irregular pulse and differences in the apical and radial pulse rates.

Assess for symptoms of decreased cardiac output and heart failure. If drug therapy is used, monitor ECG changes (QTc), liver function levels, and thyroid levels (in amiodarone use), and observe the patient for evidence of toxicity. Tell the patient to report pulse rate changes, syncope or dizziness, chest pain, or signs of heart failure, such as increasing dyspnea and peripheral edema.

Meds to the rescue! Drugs can help maintain normal sinus rhythm after cardioversion.

Wandering pacemaker

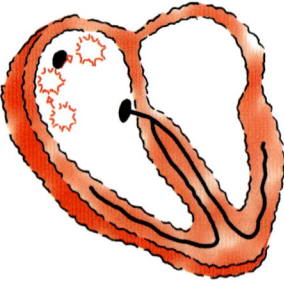

A wandering pacemaker (also termed "multifocal atrial rhythm") is an atrial arrhythmia when the electrical impulses causing the atrial activity are moving or wandering. Due to the different locations of stimulation, the P-wave morphology changes. In a wandering pacemaker ECG, three different shaped P waves need to be observed. A dominant P wave cannot be identified. The rate is less than 100 beats/min usually. The PR interval can or cannot be affected. The rhythm on an ECG strip will look slightly irregular because the sites of impulse initiation vary.

How it happens

Wandering pacemaker may be caused by:
- sleep apnea
- asthma
- chronic bronchitis
- emphysema
- COPD

The arrhythmia can be seen in very young or very old people and can be common in athletes. It rarely causes symptoms and rarely requires treatment.

Identifying wandering pacemaker

This rhythm strip illustrates wandering pacemaker. Look for the following distinguishing characteristics:

The rhythm is irregular.

The QRS complex is normal.

The P waves change in appearance.

- *Rhythm:* Atrial and ventricular—irregular
- *Rate:* Atrial and ventricular—50 beats/min
- *P wave:* Changes in size and shape; first P wave inverted, second upright
- *PR interval:* Variable
- *QRS complex:* 0.08 seconds
- *T wave:* Normal
- *QT interval:* 0.44 seconds
- *Other:* None

How you intervene

Usually, no treatment is needed for a wandering pacemaker, but monitor the rhythm and keep a close eye on the patient.

That's a wrap!

Atrial arrhythmias review

Premature atrial contractions
Characteristics
- *Rhythms:* Irregular as a result of PACs
- *P wave:* Premature with an abnormal configuration; may be buried in the previous T wave
- *PR interval:* Usually normal; may be slightly shortened or prolonged
- *QRS complex:* Similar to the underlying QRS complex when PAC is conducted; may not follow the premature P wave when a nonconducted PAC occurs

Treatment
- No treatment if asymptomatic
- Correction of the underlying cause

Atrial tachycardia
Characteristics
- *Rhythms:* Atrial—regular, irregular in MAT; ventricular—regular when the block is constant and irregular when it isn't
- *Rates:* Atrial—three or more successive ectopic atrial beats at a rate of 100 to 250 beats/min; ventricular—varies
- *P wave:* A 1:1 ratio with QRS complex (unless a block is present); may not be discernible; may be hidden in previous ST segment or T wave; in MAT, at least three different P waves seen
- *PR interval:* Sometimes not measurable; varies in MAT
- *QRS complex:* Usually normal
- *T wave:* Normal or inverted
- *QT interval:* Usually within normal limits; may be shorter

- *ST-segment and T-wave changes:* Sometimes with ischemia

Treatment
- Correction of underlying cause
- Monitoring of blood digoxin levels for toxicity
- Valsalva maneuver or carotid sinus massage
- Calcium channel blocker, beta-adrenergic blocker, or digoxin; synchronized cardioversion
- Atrial overdrive pacing to stop arrhythmia

Atrial flutter
Characteristics
- *Rhythms:* Atrial—regular; ventricular—depends on the AV conduction pattern
- *Rates:* Atrial—250 to 350; ventricular—less than atrial
- *P waves:* Abnormal with saw-toothed appearance
- *QRS complex:* Usually normal; may be widened if flutter waves are buried in complex
- *T wave:* Unidentifiable
- *QT interval:* Unmeasurable

Treatment
- Anticoagulation therapy before converting rhythm if flutter is present for more than 48 hours
- Diltiazem, verapamil or digoxin, or amiodarone to control rate if heart function is impaired; synchronized cardioversion or amiodarone to convert rhythm if less than 48 hours

Atrial arrhythmias review (*continued*)

Atrial fibrillation
Characteristics
- *Rhythms:* Irregularly irregular
- *Rates:* Atrial—greater than 400 impulses/min, unable to measure; ventricular—varies from 100 to 150 beats/min but can be lower or higher
- *P waves:* Absent
- *f waves:* Seen as uneven baseline on ECG rather than distinguishable P waves
- *R-R intervals:* Irregularly irregular

Treatment
- Rhythm control with catheter ablation, cardioversion, and/or antiarrhythmic medications, or rate control

Wandering pacemaker
Characteristics
- *Rhythms:* Irregular
- *Rates:* Usually normal or below 60 beats/min
- *P wave:* At least three P waves of different size and shape
- *PR interval:* Varies; always less than 0.20 seconds
- *QRS complex:* Usually normal; less than 0.12 seconds
- *QT interval:* Sometimes varies

Treatment
- No treatment if asymptomatic
- Correction of the underlying cause

Quick quiz

1. The hallmark of a PAC is:
   A. regular atrial rhythm.
   B. premature, abnormally shaped P wave.
   C. P wave followed by an aberrantly conducted QRS complex.
   D. regular ventricular rhythm.

Answer: B. Because PACs originate outside the SA node, the P wave comes earlier in the cycle and has a different configuration than the sinus P wave.

2. In atrial flutter, the key consideration in determining treatment is the:
   A. atrial rate.
   B. ventricular rate.
   C. configuration of the flutter waves.
   D. QT interval.

Answer: B. If the ventricular rate is too fast or too slow, cardiac output will be compromised. A rapid ventricular rate may require immediate cardioversion.

3. In AF with RVR, the ventricular response rate is:
   A. less than 60 beats/min.
   B. less than or equal to 80 beats/min.
   C. greater than 100 beats/min.
   D. greater than 120 beats/min.

Answer: C. AF with a ventricular response of greater than 100, which is considered AF with RVR and may cause symptoms and require cardioversion or other treatment.

4. Carotid sinus massage is used to:
   A. prevent the continued development of PACs.
   B. increase the ventricular rate in AV block.
   C. convert atrial tachycardia to sinus rhythm.
   D. suppress the development of flutter waves.

Answer: C. Carotid sinus massage slows the atrial rate by inhibiting firing of the SA node and slowing AV conduction. This allows the SA node to reestablish itself as the primary pacemaker. In atrial flutter, the technique may increase the block and slow the ventricular rate but won't convert the rhythm.

5. For AF, electrical cardioversion is most successful if used:
   A. during the first 48 hours after the onset of the arrhythmia.
   B. during the first 2 weeks of treatment for the arrhythmia.
   C. during the first 4 months after the onset of the arrhythmia.
   D. anytime during the first year after the onset of the arrhythmia.

Answer: A. Electrical cardioversion is most successful if used within the first 48 hours of treatment and less successful if the rhythm has existed for a long time.

6. In a patient with wandering pacemaker, the ECG strip will show:
   A. an early beat causing irregularity.
   B. a regular rhythm of 40 beats/min.
   C. slight irregularity because the sites of impulse initiation vary.
   D. a regular rhythm and a rate of 60 to 100 beats/min.

Answer: C. Wandering pacemaker is an irregular rhythm that results when the heart's pacemaker changes its focus from the SA node to another area above the ventricles. So, the rhythm on the ECG strip will look slightly irregular because of the variation of the impulse sites.

Test strips

Try these test strips. Interpret each strip using the eight-step method and fill in the blanks below with the particular characteristics of the strip. Then compare your answers with the answers given.

Strip 1

Atrial rhythm: _____

Ventricular rhythm: _____

Atrial rate: _____

Ventricular rate: _____

P wave: _____

PR interval: _____

QRS complex: _____

T wave: _____

QT interval: _____

Other: _____

Interpretation: _____

Strip 2

Atrial rhythm: _____

Ventricular rhythm: _____

Atrial rate: _____

Ventricular rate: _____

P wave: _____

PR interval: _____

QRS complex: _____

T wave: _____

QT interval: _____

Other: _____

Interpretation: _____

Strip 3

Atrial rhythm: _____

Ventricular rhythm: _____

Atrial rate: _____

Ventricular rate: _____

P wave: _____

PR interval: _____

QRS complex: _____

T wave: _____

QT interval: _____

Other: _____

Interpretation: _____

Answers to test strips

1. Rhythm: Regular
Rate: Atrial—310 beats/min; ventricular—80 beats/min
P wave: Saw toothed
PR interval: Unmeasurable
QRS complex: 0.08 seconds
T wave: Normal configuration
QT interval: Unmeasurable
Other: None
Interpretation: Atrial flutter

2. Rhythm: Irregular
Rate: Atrial and ventricular—80 beats/min
P wave: Normal configuration, early P's look different than the
sinus P's
PR interval: 0.14 seconds
QRS complex: 0.08 seconds
T wave: Normal configuration
QT interval: 0.36 seconds
Other: Every other beat is a PAC
Interpretation: Normal sinus rhythm with bigeminal PACs

3. Rhythm: Irregular
Rate: Atrial—undetermined; ventricular—60 beats/min
P wave: Absent; coarse fibrillatory waves present
PR interval: Indiscernible
QRS complex: 0.12 seconds
T wave: Indiscernible
QT interval: Unmeasurable
Other: None
Interpretation: Atrial fibrillation

Scoring

☆☆☆ If you answered all six questions correctly and filled in all the blanks close to what we did, outstanding! You're the MVP of the Atrial World Series.

☆☆ If you answered five questions correctly and filled in most of the blanks, terrific! You're an up-and-coming power hitter, destined for the Atrial Hall of Fame.

☆ If you answered fewer than five questions correctly and missed most of the blanks, hang in there. With a bit of batting practice, you'll be smacking home runs outta Atrial Park in no time.

Selected References

Brundel, B. J. J. M., Ai, X., Hills, M. T., Kuipers, M. F., Lip, G. Y. H., & de Groot, N. M. S. (2022, April 7). Atrial fibrillation. *Nature News*. Retrieved April 22, 2023, from https://www.nature.com/articles/s41572-022-00347-9

Camm, A. J., Naccarelli, G. V., Mittal, S., Crijns, H. J. G. M., Hohnloser, S. H., Ma, C. S., Natale, A., Turakhia, M. P., & Kirchhof, P. (2022). The increasing role of rhythm control in patients with atrial fibrillation: JACC state-of-the-art review. *Journal of the American College of Cardiology, 79*(19), 1932–1948. https://doi.org/10.1016/j.jacc.2022.03.337

January, C. T., Wann, L. S., Calkins, H., Chen, L. Y., Cigarroa J. E., Cleveland, J. C., Jr, Ellinor, P. T., Ezekowitz, M. D., Field, M. E., Furie, K. L., Heidenreich, P. A., Murray, K. T., Shea, J. B., Tracy, C. M., & Yancy, C. W. (2019). 2019 AHA/ACC/HRS focused update of the 2014 AHA/ACC/HRS Guideline for the management of patients with atrial fibrillation: A report of the American College of Cardiology/American Heart Association Task Force on practice guidelines and the Heart Rhythm Society in collaboration with the Society of Thoracic Surgeons. *Circulation, 140*(2), e125–e151. https://doi.org/10.1161/CIR.0000000000000665

Kistler, P. (2022, June 30). Focal atrial tachycardia. *UpToDate*. https://www.uptodate.com/contents/focal-atrial-tachycardia?search=atrial%20tachycardia&sectionRank=1&usage_type=default&anchor=H4348457&source=machineLearning&selectedTitle=1~150&display_rank=1#H4348457

Kornej, J., Borschel, C. S., Benjamin, E. J., & Schnabel, R. B. (2020). Epidemiology of atrial fibrillation in the 21st century. *Circulation Research, 127*, 4–20. https://doi.org/10.1161/CIRCRESAHA.120.316340

Kumar, K., Zimetbaum, P. J., & Parikh, N. (2023, March 22). Atrial fibrillation: Overview and management of new-onset atrial fibrillation. *UpToDate*. Retrieved April 20, 2023, from https://www.uptodate.com/contents/atrial-fibrillation-overview-and-management-of-new-onset-atrial-fibrillation?search=atrial+fibrillation+treatment&source=search_result&selectedTitle=1~150&usage_type=default&display_rank=1#H3067512081

Liwanag, M., & Willoughby, C. (2022, June 27). Atrial tachycardia. In *StatPearls* [Internet]. National Center for Biotechnology Information. https://www.ncbi.nlm.nih.gov/books/NBK542235/

O'Brien, T. (2022, June 15). *Wandering atrial pacemaker—EKG lesson #312*. Retrieved April 26, 2023, from https://ekg.academy/lesson/5/wandering-atrial-pacemaker

Phang, R., & Prutkin, J. M. (2022, June 16). Overview of atrial flutter. *UpToDate*. https://www.uptodate.com/contents/overview-of-atrial-flutter#H28361313

Podrid, P. J., Gersh, B. J., & Yeon, S. B. (2023, February 3). Reentry and the development of cardiac arrhythmias. *UpToDate*. Retrieved April 20, 2023, from https://www.uptodate.com/contents/reentry-and-the-development-of-cardiac-arrhythmias/print

Prutkin, J. M., Goldberger, A. L., & Yeon, S. B. (2022, June 30). ECG tutorial: Atrial and atrioventricular nodal (supraventricular) arrhythmias. *UpToDate*. Retrieved

April 26, 2023, from https://www.uptodate.com/contents/ecg-tutorial-atrial-and-atrioventricular-nodal-supraventricular-arrhythmias?search=wandering+pacemaker&source=search_result&selectedTitle=1~7&usage_type=default&display_rank=1#H4

U.S. Department of Health and Human Services. (2022, November 30). Atrial fibrillation: Diagnosis. National Heart Lung and Blood Institute. Retrieved April 25, 2023, from https://www.nhlbi.nih.gov/health/atrial-fibrillation/diagnosis

Junctional arrhythmias

Just the facts

In this chapter, you'll learn:

♦ the proper way to identify various junctional arrhythmias

♦ the causes, significance, treatment, and nursing implications of each arrhythmia

♦ assessment findings associated with each arrhythmia interpretation of junctional arrhythmias on an ECG.

A look at junctional arrhythmias

Junctional arrhythmias originate in the atrioventricular (AV) junction—the area around the AV node and the bundle of His. The arrhythmias occur when the sinoatrial (SA) node, a higher pacemaker, is suppressed and fails to conduct impulses, or when a block occurs in conduction. If this occurs, electrical impulses may then be initiated by pacemaker cells in the AV junction. Junctional rhythms can also occur when there is an irritable focus in the AV junction that causes those cells to depolarize early, ahead of the heart's normal pacemaker in the SA node.

Normal impulses keep the blood pumping.

Just your normal impulse

In normal impulse conduction, the AV node slightly slows transmission of the impulse from the atria to the ventricles, giving the atria time to contract and pump as much blood as they can into the ventricles before the ventricles contract. However, impulses aren't always conducted normally.

Which way did the impulse go?

Because the AV junction is located in the lower part of the right atrium near the tricuspid valve, impulses generated in this area cause the heart to be depolarized in an abnormal way. The impulse moves upward and causes backward, or *retrograde*, depolarization of the atria. P waves might not be seen on the rhythm strip. However, if P waves are present, these may be inverted in leads II, III, and aV$_F$, leads in which you would normally see upright P waves. (See *Finding the P wave*.)

Mixed signals

Finding the P wave

When the pacemaker fires in the AV junction, the impulse may reach either the atria or the ventricles first. Therefore, the inverted P wave and the following QRS complex won't have a consistent relationship. These rhythm strips show the various positions the P wave can take in junctional rhythms.

Atria first
If the atria are depolarized first, the P wave will occur before the QRS complex.

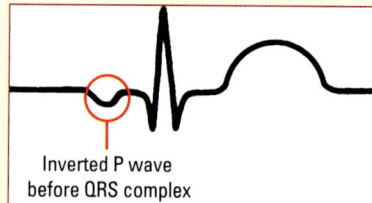

Inverted P wave
before QRS complex

Ventricles first
If the ventricles are depolarized first, the inverted P wave will follow the QRS complex.

Inverted P wave
after QRS complex

Simultaneous
If the ventricles and atria are depolarized simultaneously, the P wave will be hidden in the QRS complex and will not be seen.

Inverted P wave hidden
in QRS complex

Junctional mimic

Atrial arrhythmias are sometimes mistaken for junctional arrhythmias because impulses are generated so low in the atria that they cause retrograde depolarization and inverted P waves. Looking at the PR interval will help you determine whether an arrhythmia is atrial or junctional.

An arrhythmia with an inverted P wave before the QRS complex and a normal PR interval (0.12 to 0.20 seconds) originated in the atria. An arrhythmia with an inverted P wave before the QRS complex and a PR interval less than 0.12 seconds originated in the AV junction.

Premature junctional contraction

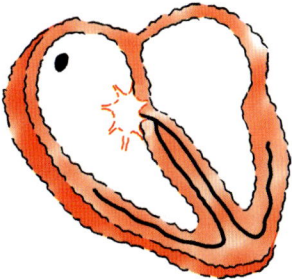

A premature junctional contraction (PJC) is a beat that occurs as a normal beat and causes an irregular rhythm. This ectopic beat occurs when an irritable location within the AV junction acts as a pacemaker and fires either prematurely or out of sequence.

As with all beats produced by the AV junction, the atria are depolarized in a retrograde manner, causing an inverted P wave. This P wave can occur before, during, or after the QRS. The ventricles are depolarized normally.

How it happens

PJCs may be caused medications, excessive caffeine intake, myocardial infarction (MI) (usually the inferior wall), electrolyte imbalances, hypothyroidism, rheumatic heart disease, valvular disease, hypoxia, heart failure, smoking, alcohol, edema of the AV junction after heart surgery, or other causes of inflammation or ischemia. One example of medication-induced PJCs is toxic levels of digoxin (Lanoxin) (level greater than 2.5 mg/mL).

Memory jogger

To help you remember what a PJC is, think of "early" for premature, "originated in the AV junction" for junctional, and "beat" for contraction. A PJC is an "early beat originating in the AV junction."

The beat goes on

Although PJCs themselves usually aren't dangerous, you'll need to monitor the patient carefully and assess for other signs of intrinsic pacemaker failure.

> There's an early beat on the waveform with a PJC. I prefer it when the beat goes on ... the beat goes on...

What to look for

A PJC appears on a rhythm strip as an early beat and causes an irregularity. The rest of the strip will show the patient's underlying rhythm, which can be regular or irregular atrial and ventricular rhythms.

P–wave inversion

Look for an inverted P wave in leads II, III, and aV_F. Depending on when the impulse occurs, the P wave may fall before, during, or after the QRS complex. (See *Identifying a PJC.*) If it falls during the QRS complex, it's hidden. If it comes before the QRS complex, the PR interval is less than 0.12 seconds.

Identifying a PJC

This rhythm strip illustrates PJCs. Look for the following distinguishing characteristics:

The rhythm is irregular.

The P wave is inverted with PR interval less than 0.12 seconds.

PJC

PJC

- *Rhythm:* Irregular atrial and ventricular rhythms
- *Rate:* 100 beats/min
- *P wave:* Inverted and precedes the QRS complex with PJC; otherwise,

normal configuration as expected with underlying sinus rhythm
- *PR interval:* 0.14 seconds for the underlying rhythm and 0.06 seconds for the PJC

- *QRS complex:* 0.06 seconds
- *T wave:* Normal configuration
- *QT interval:* 0.36 seconds
- *Other:* Pause after PJC

Because the ventricles are usually depolarized normally, the QRS complex has a normal configuration and a normal duration of less than 0.12 seconds. The T wave and the QT interval are also usually normal.

That quickening feeling

The patient may be asymptomatic or may complain of palpitations or a feeling of quickening in the chest. You may be able to palpate an irregular pulse. If the PJCs are frequent enough, the patient may experience hypotension from a transient decrease in cardiac output.

How you intervene

In addition to monitoring the ECG, evaluation includes vital signs, identifying underlying causes, and assessing the patient's medication list. PJCs usually only require treatment when symptoms arise. In those cases, the underlying cause should be treated. If digoxin toxicity is the culprit, the medication should be discontinued and serum digoxin levels should be monitored.

You should also monitor the patient for hemodynamic instability. If ectopic beats are frequent, the patient should decrease or eliminate their caffeine intake if it is excessive.

Junctional escape rhythm

A junctional escape rhythm is a string of beats that occur after a conduction delay from the atria. The normal intrinsic firing rate for cells in the AV junction is 40 to 60 beats/min.

Remember that myocardial cells have automaticity, and the AV junction can take over as the heart's pacemaker if higher pacemaker sites slow down or fail to fire or conduct. The junctional escape beat is an example of this compensatory mechanism. Junctional escape beats prevent ventricular standstill and should never be suppressed.

Backward and upside down

In a junctional escape rhythm, as in all junctional arrhythmias, the atria are depolarized by means of retrograde conduction. The P waves are inverted, and impulse conduction through the ventricles is normal. (See *Check age and lifestyle.*)

How it happens

A junctional escape rhythm can be caused by any condition that disturbs SA node function or disrupts conduction through the AV node. Common causes of the arrhythmia include the following:

- sick sinus syndrome
- vagal stimulation
- electrolyte imbalances
- medications (including, but not limited to, digoxin, beta-adrenergic blockers, calcium channel blockers, sotalol, amiodarone, adenosine, and lithium)
- myocardial ischemia or MI
- rheumatic heart disease
- Lyme disease
- chest trauma
- intracranial hemorrhage.

The great escape

Whether junctional escape rhythm harms the patient depends on how well the patient's heart tolerates a decreased heart rate and decreased cardiac output. The less tolerant the heart is, the more significant the effects of the arrhythmia.

What to look for

A junctional escape rhythm shows a regular rhythm of 40 to 60 beats/min on an ECG strip. Look for inverted P waves in leads II, III, and aV$_F$.

The P waves occur before, after, or hidden within the QRS complex. The PR interval is less than 0.12 seconds and is measurable only if the P wave comes before the QRS complex. (See *Identifying junctional escape rhythm*, page 127.)

The rest of the ECG waveform—including the QRS complex, T wave, and QT interval—should appear normal because impulses through the ventricles are usually conducted normally.

Identifying junctional escape rhythm

This rhythm strip illustrates junctional escape rhythm. Look for the following distinguishing characteristics:

The rhythm is regular with a rate of 40 to 60 beats/min.

The P wave is inverted.

- *Rhythm:* Regular
- *Rate:* 60 beats/min
- *P wave:* Inverted and preceding each QRS complex
- *PR interval:* 0.10 seconds
- *QRS complex:* 0.10 seconds
- *T wave:* Normal
- *QT interval:* 0.44 seconds
- *Other:* None

It may be slow, but at least it's regular

A patient with a junctional escape rhythm has a slow, regular pulse rate of 40 to 60 beats/min. The patient may be asymptomatic. However, pulse rates less than 60 beats/min may lead to inadequate cardiac output causing hypotension, syncope, or decreased urine output—among other signs and symptoms of inadequate perfusion.

How you intervene

Treatment for a junctional escape rhythm involves correcting the underlying cause—for example, digoxin may be withheld, electrolyte imbalances may be restored, Lyme disease may be treated with antibiotics, or myocardial ischemia may be reversed. Atropine may be given to stimulate the sympathetic nervous system and increase the heart rate, or a temporary or permanent pacemaker may be inserted if the patient remains symptomatic.

Nursing care includes monitoring the patient's serum digoxin and electrolyte levels and watching for signs of decreased cardiac output. If the patient is hypotensive, lower the head of the bed as far as tolerated and keep atropine at the bedside. Discontinue digoxin if indicated.

Accelerated junctional rhythm

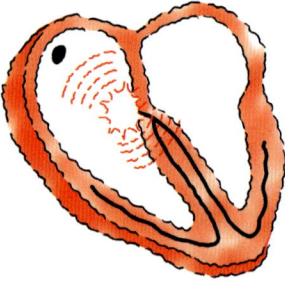

An accelerated junctional rhythm is caused by an irritable focus in the AV junction, and if this stimulus triggers an impulse at a rate faster than the rate of the SA node, then the AV junction takes over as the heart's pacemaker. The atria are depolarized by means of retrograde conduction, and the ventricles are depolarized normally. The accelerated rate is usually between 60 and 100 beats/min.

How it happens

Conditions that affect SA node or AV node automaticity can cause accelerated junctional rhythm. These conditions include:

- digoxin toxicity
- electrolyte imbalances (e.g., hypokalemia, hypercalcemia)
- MI
- rheumatic heart disease
- valvular heart disease.

Getting a kick out of it

This arrhythmia is significant if the patient has symptoms of decreased cardiac output—hypotension, syncope, and decreased urine output. These symptoms can occur if the atria are depolarized after the QRS complex, which prevents blood ejection from the atria into the ventricles, or atrial kick.

What to look for

With an accelerated junctional rhythm, look for a regular rhythm and a rate of 60 to 100 beats/min. (See *Identifying accelerated junctional rhythm*, page 129.) If the P wave is present, it will be inverted in leads II, III, and aV$_F$ and will occur before or after the QRS complex or be hidden in it. If the P wave comes before the

---

Ages and stages

Escape rate higher in young children

Up to age 3, the AV nodal escape rhythm is 50 to 80 beats/min. Consequently, a junctional rhythm is considered accelerated in infants and toddlers only when greater than 80 beats/min.

QRS complex, the PR interval will be less than 0.12 seconds. The QRS complex, T wave, and QT interval all appear normal. (See *Escape rate higher in young children*, page 128.)

Identifying accelerated junctional rhythm

This rhythm strip illustrates accelerated junctional rhythm. Look for the following distinguishing characteristics:

The P wave is absent.

The rhythm is regular with a rate between 60 and 100 beats/min.

- *Rhythm:* Regular
- *Rate:* 80 beats/min
- *P wave:* Hidden in T wave
- *PR interval:* Unmeasurable
- *QRS complex:* 0.10 seconds
- *T wave:* Distorted by P wave
- *QT interval:* 0.32 seconds
- *Other:* None

Low-down, dizzy, and confused

The patient may be asymptomatic because accelerated junctional rhythm has the same rate as sinus rhythm. However, the atria may be unable to empty sufficiently into the ventricles, thereby lowering the cardiac output. Due to decreased cardiac output, the patient may become lightheaded, hypotensive, and confused.

Look for a regular rhythm.

How you intervene

Treatment for accelerated junctional arrhythmia involves correcting the underlying cause. Nursing interventions include observing the patient to see how well the rhythm is tolerated, monitoring the serum digoxin level, and withholding the digoxin dose.

Serum potassium and other electrolyte levels should be assessed and supplements administered as needed. Monitoring vital signs for hemodynamic instability and observing for signs of decreased cardiac output are useful. Temporary or permanent pacing may be necessary if the patient remains symptomatic.

Junctional tachycardia

In junctional tachycardia, three or more PJCs occur in a row. This supraventricular tachycardia occurs when an irritable focus from the AV junction has enhanced automaticity, overriding the SA node to function as the heart's pacemaker.

In this arrhythmia, the atria are depolarized by means of retrograde conduction, and conduction through the ventricles is normal. The rate is usually 100 to 200 beats/min, although this can vary by age. (See *Identifying junctional tachycardia*.)

Identifying junctional tachycardia

This rhythm strip illustrates junctional tachycardia. Look for the following distinguishing characteristics:

The rhythm is regular with a rate of 100 to 200 beats/min.

The P wave is inverted.

- *Rhythm:* Atrial and ventricular—regular
- *Rate:* Atrial and ventricular—115 beats/min

- *P wave:* Inverted; follows QRS complex
- *PR interval:* Unmeasurable
- *QRS complex:* 0.08 seconds

- *T wave:* Normal
- *QT interval:* 0.36 seconds
- *Other:* None

How it happens

Possible causes of junctional tachycardia include:

- digoxin toxicity (most common cause), which can be enhanced by hypokalemia
- MI or myocardial ischemia
- autonomic or metabolic disturbance
- congenital heart disease in children
- irritation and edema of the AV junction after heart surgery (or atrioventricular nodal reentrant tachycardia [AVNRT] ablation).

Compromising rhythm

The significance of junctional tachycardia depends on the rate, underlying cause, and severity of the accompanying cardiac disease. At higher ventricular rates, junctional tachycardia may compromise cardiac output by decreasing atrial kick or the amount of blood filling the ventricles prior to each ventricular contraction.

What to look for

When assessing a rhythm strip for junctional tachycardia, look for a rate of 100 to 200 beats/min. The P wave is inverted in leads II, III, and aV_F and can occur before, during (hidden P wave), or after the QRS complex.

Measurement of the PR interval depends on whether the P wave falls before, in, or after the QRS complex. If it comes before the QRS complex, the only time the PR interval can be measured it will always be less than 0.12 seconds.

The QRS complexes look normal, as does the T wave, unless a P wave occurs in it, or the rate is so fast that the T wave is unable to be detected. (See *Junctional and supraventricular tachycardia.*)

Mixed signals

Junctional and supraventricular tachycardia

If a tachycardia has a narrow QRS complex, you may have trouble deciding whether its source is junctional or atrial. When the rate approaches 150 beats/min, a formerly visible P wave is hidden in the previous T wave, and the origin of the P wave cannot be determined.

In these cases, call the rhythm *supraventricular* tachycardia, a general term that refers to the origin as being above the ventricles. Examples of supraventricular tachycardia include atrial flutter, multifocal atrial tachycardia, and junctional tachycardia.

Rapid rate = instability

Patients with rapid heart rates may have decreased cardiac output and hemodynamic instability. The pulse will be rapid, and lightheadedness, low blood pressure, and other signs of decreased cardiac output may be present.

How you intervene

The underlying cause should be treated. If the cause is digoxin toxicity, the digoxin should be discontinued. Vagal maneuvers and medications such as intravenous (IV) adenosine may slow the heart rate for the symptomatic patient. Diltiazem, beta-blockers, and amiodarone can also treat junctional tachycardia. (See *Comparing junctional rates.*)

Comparing junctional rates

The names given to junctional rhythms vary according to rate. The following illustration shows how each rhythm's name and rate are correlated.

If the patient recently had an MI or heart surgery, they may need a temporary pacemaker to reset the heart's rhythm until the inflammation or irritation resolves and the heart tissue returns to normal. A child with a permanent arrhythmia may be resistant to drug therapy and require surgery. The patient with recurrent junctional tachycardia may be treated with ablation therapy, followed by possible permanent pacemaker insertion.

Monitor patients with junctional tachycardia for signs of decreased cardiac output. You should also check serum digoxin and potassium

That's a wrap!

Junctional arrhythmias review

Overview of junctional arrhythmias
- Originate in the AV junction
- Occur when the SA node is suppressed, conduction is blocked, or there is an irritable focus in the AV junction
- Impulses cause retrograde atrial depolarization and inverted P waves in leads II, III, and aV_F (delta wave).

Premature junctional contraction
Characteristics
- *Rhythms:* Irregular with PJC appearance
- *Rates:* Vary with underlying rhythm
- *P wave:* Inverted; occurs before, during, or after QRS complex; may be absent; other P waves consistent with the underlying rhythm
- *PR interval:* Less than 0.12 seconds or unmeasurable
- *QRS complex:* Usually normal
- *T wave:* Usually normal
- *QT interval:* Usually normal
- *Other:* Sometimes a compensatory pause after PJC

Treatment
- No treatment if asymptomatic
- Correction of the underlying cause
- Discontinuation of digoxin if indicated
- Reduction or elimination of caffeine intake

Junctional escape rhythm
Characteristics
- *Rhythms:* Regular. If the escape rhythm is intermittent, it will begin after a pause in the underlying rhythm
- *Rates:* 40 to 60 beats/min
- *P wave:* Inverted in leads II, III, and aV_F; can occur before, during, or after QRS complex
- *PR interval:* Less than 0.12 seconds if P wave comes before QRS complex
- *QRS complex:* Normal; less than 0.12 seconds
- *T wave:* Normal
- *QT interval:* Normal

Treatment
- Correction of the underlying cause
- Atropine for symptomatic bradycardia

- Temporary or permanent pacemaker insertion if arrhythmia refractory to drugs
- Discontinuation of digoxin if indicated

Accelerated junctional rhythm
Characteristics
- *Rhythms:* Regular
- *Rates:* 60 to 100 beats/min
- *P wave:* Inverted in leads II, III, and aV_F (if present); occurs before, during, or after QRS complex
- *PR interval:* Measurable only with P wave that comes before QRS complex; 0.12 seconds or less
- *QRS complex:* Normal
- *T wave:* Normal
- *QT interval:* Normal

Treatment
- Correction of the underlying cause
- Discontinuation of digoxin if indicated
- Temporary or permanent pacemaker insertion if symptomatic
- Antiarrhythmic medications generally are not indicated.

Junctional tachycardia
Characteristics
- *Rhythms:* Regular
- *Rates:* 100 to 200 beats/min
- *P wave:* Inverted in leads II, III, and aV_F; before, during, or after QRS complex
- *PR interval:* Shortened at less than 0.12 seconds or unmeasurable
- *QRS complex:* Normal
- *T wave:* Usually normal; may contain P wave
- *QT interval:* Usually normal

Treatment
- Correction of the underlying cause
- Discontinuation of digoxin if indicated
- Temporary or permanent pacemaker insertion if symptomatic
- Vagal maneuvers or drugs such as adenosine to slow heart rate if symptomatic

levels. Administer potassium supplements and hold digoxin as ordered. If symptoms are severe and digoxin is the culprit, the practitioner may order digoxin immune fab, a digoxin-binding drug.

Quick quiz

1. In a junctional escape rhythm, the P wave can occur:
    A. within the T wave.
    B. on top of the preceding Q wave.
    C. before, during, or after the QRS complex.
    D. earlier than expected.

Answer: C. In all junctional arrhythmias, the P wave is inverted in leads II, III, and aV$_F$ and may appear before, during, or after the QRS complex.

2. In an accelerated junctional rhythm, the QRS complex appears:
    A. narrowed.
    B. widened.
    C. damped.
    D. normal.

Answer: D. Because the ventricles are usually depolarized normally in this rhythm, the QRS complex has a normal configuration and a normal duration of less than 0.12 seconds.

3. The normal slowing of impulses as they pass through the AV node allows the atria to:
    A. fill completely with blood from the venae cavae.
    B. pump the maximum amount of blood possible into the ventricles.
    C. remain insensitive to ectopic impulse formation outside the sinus node.
    D. contract simultaneously.

Answer: B. In normal impulse conduction, the AV node slows impulse transmission from the atria to the ventricles and allows the atria to pump as much blood as possible into the ventricles before the ventricles contract.

4. If the ventricles are depolarized first in a junctional rhythm, the P wave will:
    A. appear before the QRS complex.
    B. appear within the QRS complex.
    C. appear after the QRS complex.
    D. not be apparent.

Answer: C. If the ventricles are depolarized first, the P wave will come after the QRS complex.

Test strips

Try these test strips. Interpret each strip using the eight-step method and fill in the blanks below with the particular characteristics of the strip. Then compare your answers with the answers given.

Strip 1

Atrial rhythm: _____

Ventricular rhythm: _____

Atrial rate: _____

Ventricular rate: _____

P wave: _____

PR interval: _____

QRS complex: _____

T wave: _____

QT interval: _____

Other: _____

Interpretation: _____

Strip 2

Atrial rhythm: _____

Ventricular rhythm: _____

Atrial rate: _____

Ventricular rate: _____

P wave: _____

PR interval: _____

QRS complex: _____

T wave: _____

QT interval: _____

Other: _____

Interpretation: _____

Answers to test strips

1. Rhythm: Regular
    Rate: 47 beats/min
    P wave: Inverted
    PR interval: 0.08 seconds
    QRS complex: 0.06 seconds
    T wave: Normal configuration
    QT interval: 0.42 seconds
    Other: None
    Interpretation: Junctional escape rhythm

2. Rhythm: Regular
    Rate: 75 beats/min
    P wave: Abnormal within T wave
    PR interval: Unmeasurable
    QRS complex: 0.08 seconds
    T wave: Distorted by P wave
    QT interval: Unmeasurable
    Other: None
    Interpretation: Accelerated junctional rhythm

Scoring

☆☆☆ If you answered all four questions correctly and correctly filled in all the blanks, that is impressive!

☆☆ If you answered three questions correctly and correctly filled in most of the blanks, wow!

☆ If you answered fewer than three questions correctly and missed most of the blanks, keep reviewing.

Recommended References

Alasti, M., Mirzaee, S., Machado, C., Healy, S., Bittinger, L., Adam, D., Kotschet, E., Krafchek, J., & Alison, J. (2020, July 27). Junctional ectopic tachycardia. *Journal of Arrhythmia, 36*(5), 837–844. https://doi.org/10.1002/joa3.12410

Beinart, S. C. (2018, November 27). *Junctional rhythm treatment and management.* Medscape. https://emedicine.medscape.com/article/155146-treatment

Hafeez, Y., & Grossman, S. (2019). *Junctional rhythm.* STATPearls. https://www.ncbi.nlm.nih.gov/books/NBK507715/

Healio. (2019). *ECG reviews and criteria.* https://www.healio.com/cardiology/learn-the-heart/ecg-review/ecg-topic-reviews-and-criteria

Kusumoto, F. M., Schoenfeld, M. H., Barrett, C., Edgerton, J. R., Ellenbogen, K. A., Gold, M. R., Goldschlager, N. F., Hamilton, R. M., Joglar, J. A., Kim, R. J., Lee, R., Marine, L. E., McLeod, C. J., Oken, K. R., Patton, K. K., Pellegrini, C. N., Selzman, K. A., Thompson, A., & Varosy, P. D. (2019). 2018 ACC/AHA/HRS Guideline on the evaluation and management of patients with bradycardia and cardiac conduction delay: A report of the American College of Cardiology/American Heart Association Task Force on Clinical Practice Guidelines and the Heart Rhythm Society. *Circulation, 140*(8), e382–e482. https://doi.org/10.1161/CIR.0000000000000628

Ventricular arrhythmias

Just the facts

In this chapter, you'll learn:

♦ the proper way to identify various ventricular arrhythmias (aka, dysrhythmias)

♦ the role of the ventricles in arrhythmia formation

♦ the causes, significance, treatment, and nursing implications of each arrhythmia

♦ assessment findings associated with each arrhythmia

♦ interpretation of ventricular arrhythmias on an ECG.

A look at ventricular arrhythmias

Ventricular arrhythmias originate in the ventricles below the bundle of His. These occur when electrical impulses depolarize the myocardium using a different pathway from normal impulses.

Ventricular arrhythmias appear on an ECG in characteristic ways. The QRS complex is wider than normal (>0.10) because of the prolonged conduction time through the ventricles. The T wave and the QRS complex deflect in opposite directions because of the difference in the action potential during ventricular depolarization and repolarization. Also, the P wave is absent because atrial depolarization doesn't occur.

No atrial kick

When electrical impulses are generated from the ventricles instead of the atria, atrial kick is lost and cardiac output decreases by as much as 30%. Patients with ventricular arrhythmias may show signs and symptoms of cardiac decompensation, including hypotension, angina, syncope, and respiratory distress.

Potential to kill

Ventricular arrhythmias may be benign or potentially lethal based on the frequency, type, and duration of the arrhythmia since the ventricles are ultimately responsible for cardiac output. Rapid recognition and treatment of ventricular arrhythmias increase the chance for successful resuscitation.

Premature ventricular contraction

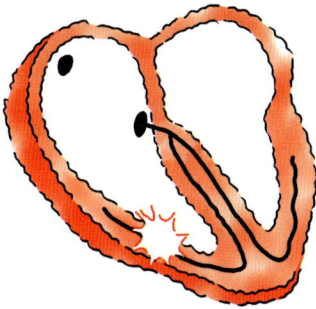

A premature ventricular contraction (PVC) is an ectopic beat that may occur in healthy people without causing problems. PVCs may occur singly, in clusters of two or more, or in repeating patterns, such as bigeminy or trigeminy. (See *Identifying PVCs*, page 140.) When PVCs occur in patients with underlying heart disease, they may indicate impending lethal ventricular arrhythmias, especially if it is a change from baseline.

Memory jogger

To help you remember the characteristics of PVCs, think of **1, 2, 3.** *PVCs may occur singly (***1***), in clusters of two or more (***2a***), or in repeating patterns, such as bigeminy (***2b***) (bi— means 2 or every other beat) and trigeminy (***3***) (tri—means 3 or every third beat).*

How it happens

PVCs are usually caused by electrical irritability in the ventricular conduction system or muscle tissue. This irritability may be provoked by anything that disrupts normal electrolyte shifts during cell depolarization and repolarization. Conditions that can disrupt electrolyte shifts include:

- electrolyte imbalances, such as hypokalemia, hyperkalemia, hypomagnesemia, and hypocalcemia
- metabolic acidosis
- hypoxia
- myocardial ischemia and infarction
- drug intoxication, particularly cocaine, amphetamines, and tricyclic antidepressants
- enlargement of the ventricular chambers
- increased sympathetic stimulation
- myocarditis
- caffeine or alcohol ingestion
- proarrhythmic effects of some antiarrhythmic
- tobacco (vaping, smoking, chew) use.

Identifying PVCs

This rhythm strip illustrates PVCs on beats 1, 6, and 11. Look for these distinguishing characteristics:

Premature QRS complex appears wide and bizarre.

The rhythm is irregular.

- *Rhythm:* Irregular
- *Rate:* 120 beats/min
- *P wave:* Absent with PVC, but present with other QRS complexes
- *PR interval:* 0.12 to 0.20 (normal) seconds in underlying rhythm

- *QRS complex:* Early with bizarre configuration and duration of greater than 0.10 seconds in PVC; less than 1.0 seconds in underlying rhythm; note the configuration of these ectopic beats is similar or unifocal, which will be discussed shortly.

- *T wave:* Normal; opposite direction from QRS complex with PVC
- *QT interval:* 0.28 seconds with underlying rhythm
- *Other:* Full compensatory pause after PVC

This could get serious

PVCs are significant for two reasons. First, these arrhythmias can lead to more serious ones, such as ventricular tachycardia or ventricular fibrillation. The risk of developing a more serious arrhythmia increases in patients with ischemic or damaged hearts.

PVCs also decrease cardiac output, especially if the ectopic beats are frequent or sustained. Decreased cardiac output is caused by reduced ventricular diastolic filling time and a loss of atrial kick. The clinical impact of PVCs hinges on how well perfusion is maintained and how long the abnormal rhythm lasts.

People with damaged hearts are more likely to develop serious arrhythmias.

What to look for

On the ECG strip, PVCs look wide and bizarre and appear as early beats causing atrial and ventricular irregularity. The rate follows the underlying rhythm, which is usually regular.

The P wave is usually absent. Retrograde P waves may be stimulated by the PVC and cause distortion of the ST segment. The PR interval and QT interval aren't measurable on a premature beat, only on the normal beats.

Complex configuration

The QRS complex occurs early. Configuration of the QRS complex is usually normal in the underlying rhythm. The duration of the QRS complex in the premature beat exceeds 0.10 seconds. The T wave in the premature beat has a deflection opposite that of the QRS complex.

When a PVC strikes on the downslope of the preceding normal T wave—the R-on-T phenomenon—it can trigger more serious rhythm disturbances (torsades de pointes).

The pause that compensates

A horizontal baseline called a full *compensatory pause* may follow the T wave of the PVC. This pause occurs because the ventricle is refractory and unable to respond to the next regularly timed P wave from the sinus node. When a compensatory pause doesn't occur, the PVC is referred to as interpolated. A compensatory pause is also helpful in determining the underlying rhythm, a regular or irregular rhythm, such as in an atrial arrhythmia. (See *Compensatory pause.*)

PVCs all in a row

PVCs that look alike are called *uniform or unifocal* and may originate from the same ectopic focus. These beats, also known as monomorphic, are usually benign in nature but may progress to more lethal arrhythmias. (See *When PVCs spell danger.*)

Compensatory pause

You can determine if a compensatory pause exists by using calipers to mark off two normal P-P intervals. Place one leg of the calipers on the sinus P wave that comes just before the PVC. If the pause is compensatory, the other leg of the calipers will fall precisely on the P wave that comes after the pause. Note that this does not apply to patients who are in an atrial arrhythmia.

When PVCs spell danger

Here are some examples of patterns of dangerous PVCs.

Paired PVCs

Two PVCs in a row is called a pair or *couplet* (see highlighted areas). A pair can produce ventricular tachycardia because the second depolarization usually meets refractory tissue. Three or more PVCs in a row is ventricular tachycardia. If the patient spontaneously converts to an underlying rhythm, it is called a run of nonsustained V-tach (NSVT). Measure the rate and count the number of beats of the V-tach, for example, a run of 20 beats at a rate of 300/min. This would be very clinically significant. Not all V-tach is the same.

When PVCs spell danger

Multiform or multifocal PVCs

PVCs that look different from one another arise from different sites or from the same site with abnormal conduction (see highlighted areas). Multiform/multifocal also known as polymorphic PVCs may indicate increased ventricular irritability. Review patients' baseline to confirm this is new for the patient. With increasing age, some patients have PVCs as part of their baseline rhythm. It should be assessed and determined to be benign.

Bigeminy and trigeminy

PVCs that occur every other beat (bigeminy) or every third beat (trigeminy) may indicate increased ventricular irritability (see highlighted areas on the rhythm strip).

R-on-T phenomenon

In R-on-T phenomenon, the PVC occurs so early that it falls on the T wave of the preceding beat (see highlighted area) and can lead to lethal arrhythmias. Since the cells haven't fully repolarized, ventricular tachycardia, ventricular fibrillation, or torsades de pointes can result.

Ruling out trouble

To help determine the seriousness of PVCs, ask yourself these questions:

- How often do they occur? In patients with chronic PVCs, an increase in frequency or a change in the pattern of PVCs from the baseline rhythm may signal a more serious condition.
- What pattern do they occur in? If the ECG shows a dangerous pattern—such as paired PVCs, PVCs with more than one morphology (shape), bigeminy, or R-on-T phenomenon—the patient may require immediate treatment.
- Are they really PVCs? Make sure the complex you see is a PVC, not another, less dangerous arrhythmia. (See *Deciphering PVCs*, page 143.) Early assessment and treatment are important. If patient is symptomatic and unstable, treatment must be immediate.

Outward signs tell a story

The patient with PVCs will have a much weaker pulse wave after the premature beat and a longer-than-normal pause between pulse waves. At times, you won't be able to palpate any pulse after the PVC. If the carotid pulse is visible, however, you may see a weaker pulse wave after the premature beat. When auscultating for heart sounds, you'll hear an abnormally early heart sound and a diminished amplitude with each premature beat.

Patients with frequent PVCs may complain of their heart racing or thumping (palpitations) and may also experience hypotension or syncope.

How you intervene

Sporadic PVCs are a normal part of the heart's conduction system. Frequent PVCs, whether the patient is symptomatic or not, may require further investigation and treatment. If the patient has symptoms or a dangerous form of PVCs, the type of treatment depends on the cause of the problem.

Intravenous (IV) potassium chloride may be given IV or orally to correct hypokalemia, and magnesium sulfate IV may be given to correct hypomagnesemia. Other treatments may be aimed at adjusting drug therapy or correcting acidosis, hypothermia, or hypoxia. See Chapter 10 for pharmacologic treatments of ventricular arrhythmia, if warranted.

Stat assessment

Patients who have recently developed PVCs need prompt assessment, especially if they have underlying heart disease or complex medical problems. Those with chronic PVCs should be observed closely for

Mixed signals

Deciphering PVCs

To determine whether the rhythm you're assessing is a PVC or some other beat, ask yourself these questions:
- Are you seeing ventricular escape beats rather than PVCs? Escape beats act as a safety mechanism to protect the heart from ventricular standstill. The ventricular escape beat will be late, rather than premature.
- Are you seeing normal beats with aberrant ventricular conduction? Some supraventricular impulses may take an abnormal pathway through the ventricular conduction system, causing the QRS complex to appear abnormal. This aberrantly conducted beat will have a P wave, whereas a PVC doesn't.

the development of more frequent PVCs or more dangerous PVC patterns.

Until effective treatment is begun, a patient with frequent PVCs accompanied by serious symptoms should have continuous ECG monitoring and ambulate only with assistance. If the patient is discharged from the health care facility on antiarrhythmic drugs, family members should know how to contact the emergency medical service (EMS) and know how to perform cardiopulmonary resuscitation (CPR).

Further investigation

Other causes of PVCs include the following:
- Dehydration
- Ischemic heart disease/coronary artery disease (CAD)
- Advanced age
- Medications, such as diuretics
- Alcohol, drugs, or stimulants, such as caffeine
- Cardiomyopathy

Idioventricular rhythms

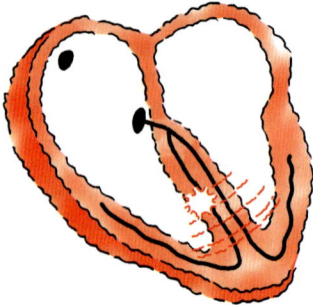

Called the *rhythms of last resort*, idioventricular rhythms act as safety mechanisms to prevent ventricular standstill when no impulses are conducted to the ventricles from above the bundle of His. The cells of the His–Purkinje system take over and act as the heart's pacemaker to generate electrical impulses.

Idioventricular rhythms can occur as ventricular escape beats, idioventricular rhythm, or accelerated idioventricular rhythm.

How it happens

Idioventricular rhythms occur when all of the heart's other pacemakers have failed to function or when supraventricular impulses are unable to reach the ventricles because of a block in the conduction system. The arrhythmias may accompany third-degree heart block or be caused by:
- myocardial ischemia
- myocardial infarction (MI)
- digoxin toxicity
- beta-adrenergic blockers
- pacemaker failure
- metabolic imbalances.

The slow ventricular rate of these arrhythmias combined with the loss of atrial kick markedly reduce cardiac output. Patients require close observation because this problem can progress to more lethal arrhythmias. Idioventricular arrhythmias also commonly occur in dying patients.

Carefully monitor patients who have idioventricular rhythms.

What to look for

If just one idioventricular beat is generated, it's called a *ventricular escape beat*. (See *Identifying idioventricular rhythm*.) The beat appears late in the conduction cycle, when the rate drops to 40 beats/min.

Don't skip this strip

Identifying idioventricular rhythm

This rhythm strip illustrates idioventricular rhythm. Look for these distinguishing characteristics:

The rate is below 40 beats/min.

The QRS complex is wide and bizarre.

- *Rhythm:* Regular
- *Rate:* Unable to determine atrial rate; ventricular rate of 35 beats/min
- *P wave:* Absent
- *PR interval:* Unmeasurable
- *QRS complex:* Wide and bizarre
- *T wave:* Deflection opposite QRS complex
- *QT interval:* 0.60 seconds
- *Other:* None

Consecutive ventricular beats on the ECG strip make up idioventricular rhythm. When this arrhythmia occurs, atrial rhythm and rate can't be determined. The ventricular rhythm is usually regular at 20 to 40 beats/min, the inherent rate of the ventricles. If the rate is faster, it's called an *accelerated idioventricular rhythm*. (See *Accelerated idioventricular rhythm*, page 146.)

Accelerated idioventricular rhythm

An accelerated idioventricular rhythm has the same characteristics as an idioventricular rhythm except that it's faster. The rate shown here varies between 40 and 100 beats/min.

The rate is between 40 and 100 beats/min.

The QRS complex is wide and bizarre.

A telltale arrhythmia

Distinguishing characteristics of idioventricular rhythm include an absent P wave or one that can't conduct through to the ventricles. This makes the PR interval unmeasurable.

Because of abnormal ventricular depolarization, the QRS complex has a duration of longer than 0.10 seconds, with a wide and bizarre configuration. The T-wave deflection will be opposite the QRS complex. The QT interval is usually prolonged, indicating delayed depolarization and repolarization.

The patient may complain of palpitations, dizziness, or lightheadedness, or may have a syncopal episode. If the arrhythmia persists, hypotension, weak peripheral pulses, decreased urine output, or confusion can occur.

How you intervene

If the patient is symptomatic, treatment should be initiated immediately to increase the heart rate, improve cardiac output, and establish a normal rhythm. Atropine may be prescribed to increase the heart rate by increasing sinus node automaticity. However, atropine will not work to increase ventricular rate if the normal conduction system is not intact because vagus nerve intervention is at the level of the bundle. Atropine antagonizes the effects of acetylcholine.

If atropine isn't effective or if the patient develops hypotension or other signs of instability, a pacemaker may be needed to reestablish a heart rate that provides enough cardiac output to perfuse organs properly. A transcutaneous pacemaker may be used in an emergency until a temporary or permanent transvenous pacemaker can be inserted. Also, direct-acting catecholamine drips may be used to increase heart rate. These include dopamine or epinephrine drips. (See *Transcutaneous pacemaker*.)

I can't waste time

Transcutaneous pacemaker

In life-threatening situations in which time is critical, a transcutaneous pacemaker may be used to regulate heart rate. This device sends an electrical impulse from the pulse generator to the heart by way of two electrodes placed on the patient's chest and back, as shown.

The electrodes are placed at heart level, on either side of the heart, so the electrical stimulus has only a short distance to travel to the heart. Transcutaneous pacing is quick and effective but will be painful. It's used as an interim measure until transvenous pacing/epinephrine or dopamine drip can be initiated.

Anterior pacing electrode

Posterior pacing electrode

Remember: The goal of treatment doesn't include suppressing the idioventricular rhythm because it acts as a safety mechanism to protect the heart from standstill. *Idioventricular rhythm should never be treated with lidocaine or other antiarrhythmic that would suppress that safety mechanism.*

Continuous monitoring needed

Patients with idioventricular rhythms need continuous ECG monitoring and constant assessment until treatment restores hemodynamic stability. Keep pacemaker equipment at the bedside and have atropine readily available. Enforce bed rest until a permanent system is in place for maintaining an effective heart rate.

Be sure to tell the patient and their family about the serious nature of this arrhythmia and all aspects of treatment. If a permanent pacemaker is inserted, teach the patient and their family how it works, how to recognize problems, when to contact the practitioner, and how pacemaker function will be monitored.

Ventricular tachycardia

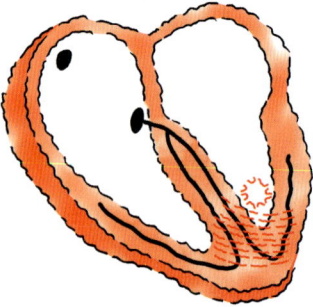

In ventricular tachycardia, commonly called *V-tach*, three or more PVCs occur in a row and the ventricular rate exceeds 100 beats/min. This arrhythmia may precede ventricular fibrillation and sudden cardiac death, especially if the patient isn't in a health care facility.

Ventricular tachycardia is an extremely unstable rhythm. It can occur in short, paroxysmal bursts lasting fewer than 30 seconds and causing few or no symptoms. Alternatively, it can be sustained, requiring immediate treatment to prevent death; even in patients initially able to maintain adequate cardiac output, 30% to 50% will have no pulse.

V-tach may be unstable and can occur in short paroxysmal bursts.

How it happens

Ventricular tachycardia usually results from increased myocardial irritability, which may be triggered by enhanced automaticity or reentry within the Purkinje system or by PVCs initiating the R-on-T phenomenon. Conditions that can cause ventricular tachycardia (note these are similar to causes of PVCs) include the following:

- myocardial ischemia
- MI
- CAD
- valvular heart disease
- heart failure
- cardiomyopathy
- electrolyte imbalances, such as hypokalemia
- drug intoxication from digoxin (Lanoxin), procainamide, quinidine, cocaine, or meta-amphetamines
- proarrhythmic effects of some antiarrhythmic.

Unpredictable V-tach

Ventricular tachycardia is significant because of its unpredictability and potential to cause death. A patient may be stable with a normal pulse and adequate hemodynamics or unstable with hypotension and no detectable pulse. Because of reduced ventricular filling time and the drop in cardiac output, the patient's condition can quickly deteriorate to ventricular fibrillation and complete cardiac collapse.

What to look for

On the ECG strip, the atrial rhythm and rate can't be determined. The ventricular rhythm is usually regular but may be slightly irregular. The ventricular rate is usually rapid—100 to 250 beats/min.

The P wave is usually absent but may be obscured by the QRS complex. Retrograde P waves may be present. Because the P wave can't be seen in most cases, you can't measure the PR interval. The QRS complex is wide and bizarre, usually with an increased amplitude and a duration of longer than 0.12 seconds.

All about uniformity

QRS complexes in monomorphic ventricular tachycardia have a uniform shape. In polymorphic ventricular tachycardia, the shape of the QRS complex constantly changes. If the T wave is visible, it occurs opposite the QRS complex. The QT interval isn't measurable. (See *Identifying ventricular tachycardia*.)

Torsades de pointes is a special variation of polymorphic ventricular tachycardia. (See *Torsades de pointes* and *Pediatric torsades de pointes*, page 150.)

Don't skip this strip

Identifying ventricular tachycardia

This rhythm strip illustrates ventricular tachycardia. Look for these distinguishing characteristics:

The QRS complex is wide and bizarre.

The ventricular rate is 100 to 250 beats/min.

- *Rhythm:* Regular
- *Rate:* 187 beats/min
- *P wave:* Absent
- *PR interval:* Unmeasurable
- *QRS complex:* 0.16 seconds; wide and bizarre
- *T wave:* Opposite direction of QRS complex
- *QT interval:* Unmeasurable
- *Other:* None

Torsades de pointes

Torsades de pointes, which means "twisting about the points," is a special form of polymorphic ventricular tachycardia. The hallmark characteristics of this rhythm, shown later, are QRS complexes that rotate about the baseline, deflecting downward and upward for several beats.

The rate is 150 to 250 beats/min, usually with an irregular rhythm, and the QRS complexes are wide with changing amplitude. The P wave is usually absent.

Paroxysmal rhythm

This arrhythmia may be paroxysmal, starting and stopping suddenly, and may deteriorate into ventricular fibrillation. It should be considered when ventricular tachycardia doesn't respond to antiarrhythmic therapy or other treatments.

Reversible causes

The cause of this form of ventricular tachycardia is usually reversible. The most common causes are drugs that lengthen the QT interval, such as amiodarone, ibutilide, erythromycin, haloperidol, droperidol, and sotalol. Other causes include myocardial ischemia and electrolyte abnormalities, such as hypokalemia, hypomagnesemia, and hypocalcemia.

Going into overdrive

Torsades de pointes is treated by correcting the underlying cause, especially if the cause is related to specific drug therapy. The practitioner may order mechanical overdrive pacing, which overrides the ventricular rate and breaks the triggered mechanism for the arrhythmia. This type of treatment may not be readily available and the patient must be monitored closely. Magnesium sulfate IV may also be effective. Electrical cardioversion may be used when torsades de pointes doesn't respond to other treatment or defibrillation if the patient has no pulse.

Ages and stages

Pediatric torsades de pointes

Torsades de pointes at an early age usually originates from congenital long QT syndrome. Ask the parents about a family history of sudden cardiac death or sudden infant death syndrome.

The ventricular rate is 150 to 250 beats/min.

The QRS complexes are wide, with phasic variation that seems to twist around the baseline.

Quick work prevents collapse

Although some patients have only minor symptoms at first, they still need rapid intervention and treatment to prevent cardiac collapse. Most patients with ventricular tachycardia have weak or absent pulses. Low cardiac output will cause hypotension and a decreased level of consciousness (LOC) leading to unresponsiveness. Because of the significant increase in cardiac oxygen demand, ventricular tachycardia may precipitate angina, heart failure, or a substantial decrease in organ perfusion.

How you intervene

Treatment depends on whether the patient's pulse is detectable or un-detectable. A patient with pulseless ventricular tachycardia receives the same treatment as one with ventricular fibrillation and requires CPR and immediate defibrillation. Treatment for the patient with a detect-able pulse depends on whether their condition is stable or unstable and whether the QRS complexes are monomorphic or polymorphic.

Patients who are unstable generally have heart rates greater than 150 beats/min. They may also have hypotension, shortness of breath, an altered LOC, heart failure, angina, or MI—conditions that indicate cardiac decompensation. These patients are treated immediately with direct-current synchronized cardioversion.

Typical tachycardia complex

A hemodynamically stable patient with monomorphic ventricular tachycardia is treated differently. First, consider adenosine—to help slow down the rhythm for better diagnosis—and then consider antiarrhythmic drugs. If need be, administer amiodarone following advanced cardiac life support (ACLS) protocols to correct the rhythm disturbance. If the drug doesn't correct the disturbance or if the patient at any time becomes unstable, prepare the patient for synchronized cardioversion.

If the patient has polymorphic ventricular tachycardia with a nor-mal QT interval, correct ischemia and electrolyte imbalances. Then administer amiodarone, lidocaine, beta-adrenergic blockers, follow-ing ACLS protocol. Again, if drug therapy is unsuccessful or if the patient at any time becomes unstable, synchronized cardioversion is performed.

Correct electrolyte abnormalities in the patient with polymorphic ventricular tachycardia with a prolonged QT interval and administer magnesium IV. If the rhythm persists, prepare the patient for overdrive pacing.

Patients with chronic, recurrent episodes of ventricular tachycardia who are unresponsive to drug therapy may have an implantable cardioverter defibrillator (ICD) implanted. This device is a more permanent solution to recurrent episodes of ventricular tachycardia. (For more information about the ICD, see Chapter 9.)

Always assume the worst

Any wide QRS complex tachycardia should be treated as ventricular tachycardia until definitive evidence is found to establish another diagnosis, such as supraventricular tachycardia with abnormal ventricular conduction. *Always assume that the patient has ventricular tachycardia and treat them accordingly. Rapid intervention will prevent cardiac decompensation or the onset of more lethal arrhythmias.*

Teacher, teacher

Be sure to teach the patient and family about the serious nature of this arrhythmia and the need for prompt treatment. If the patient is undergoing cardioversion, explain the role of an analgesia or a sedative in preventing discomfort.

If a patient will be discharged with an ICD or a prescription for long-term antiarrhythmic drugs, teach the family how to contact the EMS and how to perform CPR. Also, teach the family the ICD cannot cause harm to any family member if the ICD discharges while touching the patient.

Ventricular fibrillation

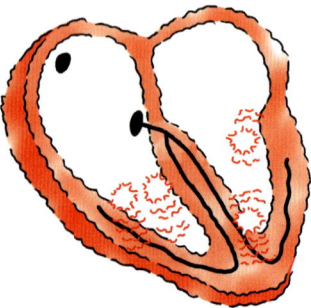

Ventricular fibrillation, commonly called *V-fib*, is a chaotic pattern of electrical activity in the ventricles in which electrical impulses arise from many different foci. It produces no effective muscular contraction and no cardiac output. Untreated ventricular fibrillation causes most cases of sudden cardiac death in people outside of a hospital.

How it happens

Causes of ventricular fibrillation include:
- myocardial ischemia
- MI
- untreated ventricular tachycardia
- underlying heart disease

- acid–base imbalance
- electrical shock
- severe hypothermia
- electrolyte imbalances, such as hypokalemia, hyperkalemia, and hypercalcemia
- drug toxicity, including digoxin
- inherited cardiac arrhythmias
- cardiomyopathy
- certain infiltrative diseases such as amyloidosis and sarcoidosis
- congenital heart disease
- severe hypoxia.

Quivering ventricles

With ventricular fibrillation, the ventricles quiver instead of contract, so cardiac output falls to zero. If ventricular fibrillation continues, it leads to ventricular standstill and death.

What to look for

On the ECG strip, ventricular activity appears as fibrillatory waves with no recognizable pattern. Atrial rate and rhythm can't be determined, nor can ventricular rhythm because no pattern or regularity occurs.

As a result, the ventricular rate, P wave, PR interval, QRS complex, T wave, and QT interval can't be determined. Larger, or coarse, fibrillatory waves are easier to convert to a normal rhythm than are smaller waves because larger waves indicate a greater degree of electrical activity in the heart. (See *Identifying ventricular fibrillation*, page 154.)

Extreme urgency

The patient in ventricular fibrillation is in full cardiac arrest, unresponsive, and without a detectable blood pressure or carotid or femoral pulse. Whenever you see a pattern resembling ventricular fibrillation, check the patient immediately by palpating for a carotid pulse and start treatment.

Be aware that other factors can mimic ventricular fibrillation on an ECG strip. Interference from an electric razor is one such mimic, as is muscle movement from shivering.

With V-fib, the ventricles quiver instead of contract, so no pattern or regularity can be detected on the ECG strip.

How you intervene

Defibrillation is the most effective treatment for ventricular fibrillation. (See https://cpr.heart.org/en/resuscitation-science/cpr-and-ecc-guidelines/algorithms for the ACLS algorithms.) CPR must be

Identifying ventricular fibrillation

The following rhythm strips illustrate coarse ventricular fibrillation (first strip) and fine ventricular fibrillation (second strip). Look for these distinguishing characteristics:

> The presence of large fibrillatory waves indicates coarse ventricular fibrillation.

> The presence of small fibrillatory waves indicates fine ventricular fibrillation.

- *Rhythm:* Chaotic
- *Rate:* Undetermined
- *P wave:* Absent

- *PR interval:* Unmeasurable
- *QRS complex:* Indiscernible
- *T wave:* Indiscernible

- *QT interval:* Not applicable
- *Other:* Waveform is a wavy line.

performed until the defibrillator arrives to preserve oxygen supply to the brain, heart, and other vital organs. Assist with endotracheal intubation. Such drugs as epinephrine may help the heart respond better to defibrillation. Drugs such as amiodarone, lidocaine, and magnesium sulfate may also be given.

A shock for life

During defibrillation, hands-free patches or paddles direct an electrical current through the patient's heart. The current causes the myocardium to depolarize, which, in turn, encourages the sinoatrial node to resume normal control of the heart's electrical activity.

One paddle is placed to the right of the upper sternum, and the other is placed over the fifth or sixth intercostal space at the left anterior axillary line. A hands-free methodology places large patches in the location where paddles were placed. These patches can be used to monitor the patient's rhythm, defibrillate, and even transcutaneously pace the patient (three-lead ECG required for pacing). During cardiac surgery, internal paddles are placed directly on the myocardium.

Automated external defibrillators are increasingly being used to provide early defibrillation. In this method, electrode pads are placed on the patient's chest and a microcomputer in the unit interprets the cardiac rhythm, providing the caregiver with step-by-step instructions on how to proceed. These defibrillators can be used by people without medical experience.

Speed is the key

For the patient with ventricular fibrillation, successful resuscitation requires rapid recognition of the problem and prompt defibrillation (<2 minutes per American Heart Association [AHA]). Many health care facilities and EMS providers have established protocols based on ACLS algorithms to help health care workers initiate prompt treatment. Make sure you know where your facility keeps its emergency equipment, be proficient in its use, and know how to recognize and deal with lethal arrhythmias. Every minute significantly decreases risk of survival.

You'll also need to teach the patient and their family how to contact the EMS. Family members need instruction in CPR. Teach them about long-term therapies that prevent recurrent episodes of ventricular fibrillation, including chronic antiarrhythmic drugs and implantation of an ICD.

Asystole

Asystole is ventricular standstill. The patient is completely unresponsive, with no electrical activity in the heart and no cardiac output. This arrhythmia results most commonly from a prolonged period of cardiac arrest without effective resuscitation. It's extremely important to distinguish asystole from fine ventricular fibrillation, which is managed differently. Therefore, asystole must be confirmed in more than one ECG lead.

Asystole has been called the *arrhythmia of death*. The patient is in cardiopulmonary arrest. Without rapid initiation of CPR and appropriate treatment, the situation quickly becomes irreversible.

How it happens

Anything that causes inadequate blood flow to the heart may lead to asystole, including:

- MI
- severe electrolyte disturbances, such as hyperkalemia
- massive pulmonary embolism
- prolonged hypoxemia
- severe, uncorrected acid–base disturbances
- electrical shock
- drug intoxication such as cocaine overdose
- cardiac tamponade
- hypothermia.

What to look for

On the ECG strip, asystole looks like a nearly flat line (except for changes caused by chest compressions during CPR). No electrical activity is evident, except possibly P waves for a time. Atrial and ventricular activity is at a standstill, so no intervals can be measured. (See *Identifying asystole.*)

Don't skip this strip

Identifying asystole

This rhythm strip illustrates asystole, the absence of electrical activity in the ventricles. Except for a few P waves or pacer spikes, nothing appears on the waveform and the line is almost flat.

> The absence of electrical activity in the ventricles results in a nearly flat line.

In the patient with a pacemaker, pacer spikes may be evident on the strip, but no P wave or QRS complex occurs in response to the stimulus.

The patient will be unresponsive, without any discernible pulse or blood pressure.

How you intervene

The immediate treatment for asystole is CPR. Start CPR as soon as you determine that the patient has no pulse.

Give repeated doses of epinephrine and atropine, as ordered. Transcutaneous pacing should be initiated as soon as possible. Subsequent treatment for asystole focuses on identifying and either treating or removing the underlying cause.

Quick recognition

Your job is to recognize this life-threatening arrhythmia and start resuscitation right away. Unfortunately, most patients with asystole can't be resuscitated, especially after a prolonged period of cardiac arrest.

Be aware that pulseless electrical activity can lead to asystole. Know how to recognize this problem and treat it. (See *Pulseless electrical activity*.)

> Arrhythmias can be life-threatening. If asystole occurs, start CPR immediately.

I can't waste time

Pulseless electrical activity

In pulseless electrical activity, the heart muscle loses its ability to contract even though electrical activity is preserved. As a result, the patient goes into cardiac arrest.

On an electrocardiogram, you'll see evidence of organized electrical activity, but you won't be able to palpate a pulse or measure the blood pressure.

Causes
This condition requires rapid identification and treatment. Causes include hypovolemia, hypoxia, acidosis, tension pneumothorax, cardiac tamponade, massive pulmonary embolism, hypothermia, hyperkalemia, massive acute MI, and an overdose of drugs such as tricyclic antidepressants.

Treatment
CPR is the immediate treatment, along with epinephrine. Atropine may be given to patients with bradycardia. Subsequent treatment focuses on identifying and correcting the underlying cause.

That's a wrap!

Ventricular arrhythmias review

Overview of ventricular arrhythmias
- Originate in the ventricles, below the bundle of His
- Loss of atrial kick, decreasing cardiac output
- Potentially fatal without treatment or resuscitation

Characteristics
- QRS complex—wider than normal
- T wave and QRS complex deflect in opposite directions.
- P wave is absent.

Premature ventricular contraction
Characteristics
- *Rhythms:* Irregular during PVC; underlying rhythm may be regular.
- *Rates:* Patterned after underlying rhythm
- *P wave:* Absent
- *PR interval:* Unmeasurable
- *QRS complex:* Wide and bizarre
- *T wave:* Opposite direction from QRS complex
- *QT interval:* Unmeasurable
- *Other:* Possible compensatory pause

Treatment
- Correction of the underlying cause
- Discontinuation of drug that may be causing toxicity
- Correction of electrolyte imbalances
- Amiodarone or lidocaine if warranted

Idioventricular rhythms
- Act as a safety mechanism to prevent ventricular standstill
- Occur as escape beats, idioventricular rhythm, or accelerated idioventricular rhythm

Characteristics
- *Rhythms:* Atrial—undetermined; ventricular—usually regular

- *Rates:* Atrial—unmeasurable; ventricular—20 to 40 beats/min
- *P wave:* Absent
- *PR interval:* Unmeasurable
- *QRS complex:* Wide and bizarre
- *T wave:* Deflection opposite that of QRS complex
- *QT interval:* Greater than 0.44 seconds

Treatment
- Atropine to increase heart rate, dopamine or epinephrine drips to increase heart rate
- Temporary or permanent pacemaker if arrhythmia is refractory to drugs
- Avoidance of drugs that suppress the idioventricular rhythm, such as lidocaine and other antiarrhythmics

Ventricular tachycardia
Characteristics
- *Rhythms:* Atrial—can't be determined; ventricular—regular or slightly irregular
- *Rates:* Atrial—can't be determined; ventricular—100 to 250 beats/min
- *P wave:* Absent or hidden by QRS complex
- *PR interval:* Unmeasurable
- *QRS complex:* Wide and bizarre, with increased amplitude; duration greater than 0.12 seconds
- *T wave:* Opposite direction of QRS complex
- *Other:* Possible torsades de pointes

Treatment
ACLS protocols:
- Amiodarone; if patient is stable with monomorphic QRS complexes and drugs are unsuccessful, cardioversion
- Beta-adrenergic blockers, lidocaine, amiodarone, if patient's ECG shows polymorphic QRS complexes and normal QT interval; cardioversion if unsuccessful

Ventricular arrhythmias review (continued)

- Magnesium sulfate IV if patient shows polymorphic QRS and QT interval is prolonged, then overdrive pacing if rhythm persists (possibly also isoproterenol)
- Defibrillation; CPR, endotracheal intubation, and epinephrine, if patient is pulseless (possibly also consider amiodarone, lidocaine, or magnesium sulfate)
- Cardioverter-defibrillator possibly implanted for recurrent ventricular tachycardia

Torsades de pointes
- A form of polymorphic ventricular tachycardia
- Sometimes deteriorates into ventricular fibrillation

Characteristics
- *Rhythms:* Ventricular—irregular
- *Rates:* 150 to 250 beats/min
- *P wave:* Usually absent
- *PR interval:* Unmeasurable
- *QRS complex:* Wide; rotates around the baseline; deflection downward and upward for several beats

Treatment
- Correction of the underlying cause
- Discontinuation of offending drug (usually one that lengthens the QT interval)
- Overdrive pacing
- Magnesium sulfate (per ACLS)
- Cardioversion if unresponsive to other treatment

Ventricular fibrillation
- Electrical impulses arise from many different foci in the ventricles.
- Produces no effective muscular contraction and no cardiac output
- If untreated, it causes most cases of sudden cardiac death out of hospital.

Characteristics
- *Rhythms:* Can't be determined
- *Rates:* Can't be determined
- *P wave:* Can't be determined
- *PR interval:* Can't be determined
- *QRS complex:* Can't be determined
- *T wave:* Can't be determined
- *QT interval:* Isn't applicable
- *Other:* Variations in size of fibrillatory waves

Treatment
ACLS protocols for VF/pulseless VT:
- Initiation of CPR
- Give oxygen
- If rhythm is shockable, defibrillate
- Continue CPR for 2 minutes
- IV/Intraosseous access
- If rhythm is shockable, defibrillate
- Continue CPR for 2 minutes
- Drug therapy: Administer epinephrine every 3-5 minutes
- Consider advanced airway
- If rhythm is shockable, defibrillate
- Continue CPR for 2 minutes
- Drug therapy: Administer amiodarone or lidocaine
- Treat reversible causes
Implantation of cardioverter-defibrillator if patient is at risk for recurrent ventricular fibrillation

Asystole
- Characterized by ventricular standstill and cardiac arrest
- Fatal without prompt CPR and treatment

Characteristics
- Lack of electrical activity seen on ECG as a nearly flat line

Ventricular arrhythmias review (*continued*)

Pulseless electrical activity

Characteristics

- Electrical activity is present on ECG but heart muscle can't contract.
- Result is no palpable pulse or blood pressure and cardiac arrest.

Treatment

ACLS protocols for Asystole/Pulseless electrical activity (PEA)

- Initiation of CPR
- Give oxygen
- Rhythm is determined not shockable

- Drug therapy: Administer epinephrine immediately
- Continue CPR for 2 minutes
- Obtain IV/Intraosseous access
- Drug therapy: Administer epinephrine every 3-5 minutes
- Consider advanced airway
- If rhythm is not shockable, continue CPR for 2 minutes
- Treat reversible causes
- If rhythm is not shockable, continue CPR, repeat epinephrine administration
- Consider appropriateness of continuing resuscitation protocol

Quick quiz

1. PVCs are most dangerous if they:
    A. are multiformed and increase in frequency.
    B. appear wide and bizarre.
    C. occur after the T wave.
    D. are uniform and wide.

Answer: A. PVCs that have different shapes (multiformed) and increase in frequency may signal increased ventricular irritability and progress to a lethal arrhythmia.

2. The treatment of choice for a patient with ventricular fibrillation is:
    A. defibrillation.
    B. transesophageal pacing.
    C. synchronized cardioversion.
    D. administration of epinephrine.

Answer: A. Patients with ventricular fibrillation are in cardiac arrest and require defibrillation.

3. Patients with a slow idioventricular rhythm that doesn't respond to atropine should receive:
    A. lidocaine.
    B. dobutamine.
    C. synchronized cardioversion.
    D. transcutaneous pacing.

Answer: D. Transcutaneous pacing is a temporary way to increase the rate and ensure adequate cardiac output.

4. A compensatory pause occurs after a PVC because the:
   A. atria conduct a retrograde impulse.
   B. ventricle is refractory at that point.
   C. bundle of His blocks sinus impulses to the ventricles.
   D. atria are refractory and can't respond.

Answer: B. A compensatory pause occurs because the ventricle is refractory and can't respond to the next regularly timed P wave from the sinus node.

5. The term *pulseless electrical activity* refers to a condition in which there's:
   A. an extremely slow heart rate but no pulse.
   B. asystole on a monitor or rhythm strip.
   C. electrical activity in the heart but no actual contraction.
   D. asystole and a palpable pulse and blood pressure.

Answer: C. Pulseless electrical activity is electrical activity without mechanical contraction. The patient is in cardiac arrest, with no blood pressure or pulse.

Test strips

Ready for a few test strips? Interpret the two strips using the eight-step method. Fill in the blanks with the characteristics of the strip and then check your answers with ours.

Strip 1

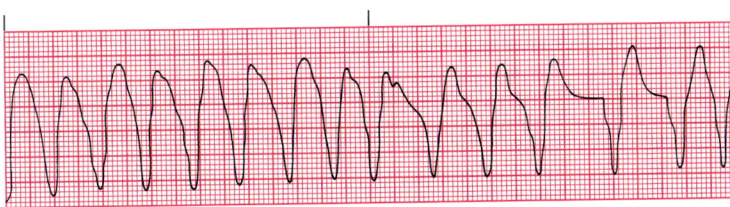

Atrial rhythm: _____

Ventricular rhythm: _____

Atrial rate: _____

Ventricular rate: _____

P wave: _____

PR interval: _____

QRS complex: _____

T wave: _____

QT interval: _____

Other: _____

Interpretation: _____

Strip 2

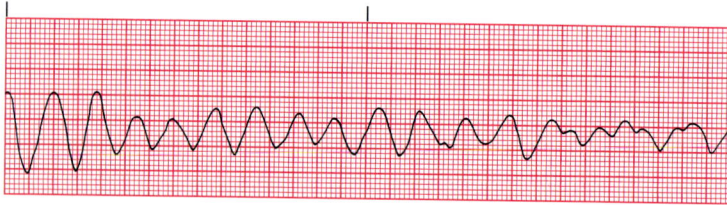

Atrial rhythm: _____

Ventricular rhythm: _____

Atrial rate: _____

Ventricular rate: _____

P wave: _____

PR interval: _____

QRS complex: _____

T wave: _____

QT interval: _____

Other: _____

Interpretation: _____

Answers to test strips

1. Rhythm: Irregular ventricular rhythm
   Rate: Ventricular rate is 130 beats/min.
   P wave: Absent
   PR interval: Unmeasurable
   QRS complex: Wide and bizarre with varying duration
   T wave: Opposite QRS complex
   QT interval: Unmeasurable
   Other: None
   Interpretation: Ventricular tachycardia

2. Rhythm: Chaotic ventricular rhythm
   Rate: Can't be determined
   P wave: Indiscernible
   PR interval: Indiscernible
   QRS complex: Indiscernible
   T wave: Indiscernible
   QT interval: Indiscernible
   Other: None
   Interpretation: Ventricular fibrillation

> Keep going ... you're halfway through this book!

Scoring

☆☆☆ If you answered all five questions correctly and filled in all the blanks as we did, sensational! You're simply the best.

☆☆ If you answered four questions correctly and filled in most of the blanks pretty much as we did, super! You've got a great eye for those tricky ventricular rhythms.

☆ If you answered fewer than four questions correctly and missed most of the blanks, that's okay. Read this chapter again and you'll get de pointes.

Selected references

Al-Khatib, S. M., Stevenson, W. G., Ackerman, M. J., Bryant, W. J., Callans, D. J., Curtis, A. B., Deal, B. J., Dickfeld, T., Field, M. E., Fonarow, G. C., Gillis, A. M., Granger, C. B., Hammill, S. C., Hlatky, M. A., Joglar, J. A., Kay, G. N., Matlock, D. D., Myerburg, R. J., & Page, R. L. (2018). 2017 AHA/ACC/HRS Guideline for Management of Patients With Ventricular Arrhythmias and the Prevention of Sudden Cardiac Death: Executive Summary: A Report of the American College of Cardiology/American Heart Association Task Force on Clinical Practice Guidelines and the Heart Rhythm Society. *Journal of the American College of Cardiology (JACC), 72*(14), 1677–1749. https://doi-org.proxy.library.nyu.edu/10.1016/j.jacc.2017.10.053

American Heart Association. (2020). 2020 American Heart Association guidelines for cardiopulmonary resuscitation and emergency cardiovascular care. *Circulation, 142*(16_Suppl_2), S571–S620.

Chiampo, A., & Di Salvo, A. (2018). *ECG mastery: The simplest way to learn the ECG.* CreateSpace Independent Publishing Platform.

Fuster, V., Harrington, R. A., Narula, J., & Eapen, Z. J. (Eds.). (2017). *Hurst's the heart* (14th ed., 2 Volume set). McGraw-Hill Education.

Kuntz, K. J., & Humphrey, M. (2018). *Electrocardiography for healthcare professionals.* Jones & Bartlett Learning.

Lyon, R. M., Richardson, S. E., Hay, A. W., Andrews, L. P., Mpotos, N., & Robertson, L. (2018). Advanced life support for out-of-hospital cardiac arrest due to ventricular tachycardia or ventricular fibrillation: A systematic review and meta-analysis. *Resuscitation, 126,* 69–81.

Mann, D. L., Bonow, R. O., & Braunwald, E. (Eds.). (2019). *Braunwald's heart disease: A textbook of cardiovascular medicine* (11th ed.). Elsevier.

Okada, D. R., Smith, J., Derakhshan, A., Gowani, Z., Misra, S., Berger, R. D., Calkins, H., Tandri, H., & Chrispin, J. (2018). Ventricular arrhythmias in cardiac sarcoidosis. *Circulation, 138*(12), 1253–1264. https://doi.org/10.1161/CIRCULATIONAHA.118.034687

Perman, S. M., Elmer, J., Maciel, C. B., Uzendu, A., May, T., Mumma, B. E., Bartos, J. A., Rodriguez, A. J., Kurz, M. C., Panchal, A. R., Rittenberger, J. C., & American Heart Association. (2024). 2023 American Heart Association focused update on adult advanced cardiovascular life support: An update to the American Heart Association guidelines for cardiopulmonary resuscitation and emergency cardiovascular care. *Circulation, 149*(5), e254–e273. https://doi.org/10.1161/CIR.0000000000001194

Stouffer, G., Runge, M. S., Patterson, C., & Rossi, J. S. (Eds.). (2018). *Netter's cardiology* (3rd ed.). Elsevier.

Thaler, M. S. (2018). *The only EKG book you'll ever need.* Lippincott Williams & Wilkins.

Atrioventricular blocks

Just the facts

In this chapter, you'll learn:

♦ the proper way to identify the various forms of atrioventricular (AV) block and interpret their rhythms

♦ the reason that AV block is a significant arrhythmia

♦ patients who are at risk for developing AV block

♦ signs and symptoms of AV block

♦ nursing care for patients with AV block.

A look at atrioventricular block

Atrioventricular (AV) heart block results from an interruption in the conduction of impulses between the atria and the ventricles. AV block can be total or partial, or it may delay conduction. The block can occur at the AV node, the bundle of His, or the bundle branches.

The heart's electrical impulses normally originate in the sinoatrial (SA) node, so when those impulses are blocked at the AV node, atrial rates are commonly normal (60 to 100 beats/min). The clinical effect of the block depends on how many impulses are completely blocked, how slow the ventricular rate is as a result, and how the block ultimately affects the heart. A slow ventricular rate can decrease cardiac output, possibly causing lightheadedness, hypotension, and confusion.

In AV block, the transmission of impulses between the atria and the ventricles is delayed, or partially or completely interrupted.

The cause before the block

Various factors can lead to AV block, including underlying heart conditions, use of certain drugs, congenital anomalies, and conditions that disrupt the cardiac conduction system. (See *Causes of AV block*, page 166.)

Causes of AV block

AV blocks can be temporary or permanent. Here's a look at the causes of each kind of AV block.

Causes of temporary block
- Myocardial infarction (MI), usually inferior wall MI
- Digoxin (Lanoxin) toxicity
- Acute myocarditis
- Calcium channel blockers
- Beta-adrenergic blockers
- Cardiac surgery

Causes of permanent block
- Changes associated with aging
- Congenital abnormalities
- MI, usually anteroseptal MI
- Cardiomyopathy
- Cardiac surgery
- Myocarditis, such as Lyme carditis

Typical examples include:
- myocardial ischemia, which impairs cellular function so cells repolarize more slowly or incompletely. The injured cells, in turn, may conduct impulses slowly or inconsistently. Relief of the ischemia can restore normal function to the AV node.
- MI, in which cell death occurs. If the necrotic cells are part of the conduction system, they no longer conduct impulses and a permanent AV block occurs.
- excessive dosage of, or an exaggerated response to, a drug that can cause AV block or increase the likelihood that a block will develop. Although many antiarrhythmic medications can have this effect, the drugs more commonly known to cause or exacerbate AV blocks include digoxin, beta-adrenergic blockers, and calcium channel blockers.
- congenital anomalies such as congenital ventricular septal defect that involve cardiac structures and affect the conduction system. Anomalies of the conduction system, such as an AV node that doesn't conduct impulses, can also occur in the absence of structural defects. (See *AV block in elderly patients*.)

Under the knife

AV block may also be caused by inadvertent damage to the heart's conduction system during cardiac surgery. Damage is most likely to occur in surgery involving the mitral or tricuspid valve or in the closure of a ventricular septal defect. If the injury involves tissues adjacent to the surgical site and the conduction system isn't physically disrupted, the block may be only temporary. If a portion of the conduction system itself is severed, a permanent block results.

Ages and stages

AV block in elderly patients

In elderly patients, AV block may be because of fibrosis of the conduction system. Other causes include the use of digoxin and the presence of aortic valve calcification.

Radio blackout

Similar disruption of the conduction system can occur from a procedure called *radiofrequency ablation.* In this invasive procedure, a transvenous catheter is used to locate the area within the heart that participates in initiating or perpetuating certain tachyarrhythmias.

Radiofrequency energy is then delivered to the myocardium through this catheter to produce a small area of necrosis. The damaged tissue can no longer cause or participate in the tachyarrhythmia. If the energy is delivered close to the AV node, bundle of His, or bundle branches, block can occur.

Degrees of block

AV blocks are classified according to their severity, not their location. That severity is measured according to how well the node conducts impulses and is separated by degrees—first, second, and third. Let's take a look at them one at a time.

First-degree AV block

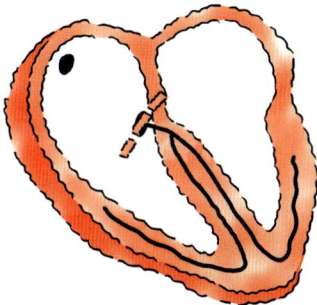

First-degree AV block occurs when impulses from the atria are consistently delayed during conduction through the AV node. All atrial impulses reach the ventricle; however, the conduction delay occurs within the AV node. Conduction eventually occurs; it just takes longer than normal. It's as if people are walking in a line through a doorway, but each person hesitates before crossing the threshold.

How it happens

First-degree AV block may appear normally in a healthy person or result from myocardial ischemia or MI, myocarditis, or degenerative changes in the heart. The condition may also be caused by medications, such as digoxin, calcium channel blockers, and beta-adrenergic blockers.

First-degree AV block may be temporary, particularly if it stems from medications or ischemia early in the course of an MI. The presence of first-degree block, the least dangerous type of AV block, indicates some kind of problem in the conduction system. Usually, this block does not cause any symptoms.

Because first-degree AV block can progress to a more severe block, it should be monitored for changes.

What to look for

In general, a rhythm strip with this block looks like normal sinus rhythm, except that the PR interval is longer than normal. (See *Identifying first-degree AV block*.) The rhythm will be regular, with one normal P wave for every QRS complex.

Identifying first-degree AV block

This rhythm strip illustrates first-degree AV block. Look for these distinguishing characteristics:

The PR interval is greater than 0.20 second.

The rhythm is regular.

- *Rhythm:* Regular
- *Rate:* 75 beats/min
- *P wave:* Normal
- *PR interval:* 0.32 seconds
- *QRS complex:* 0.08 seconds
- *T wave:* Normal
- *QT interval:* 0.40 seconds
- *Other:* PR interval prolonged but constant

The PR interval will be greater than 0.20 seconds and will be consistent for each beat. The QRS complex is usually normal, although sometimes a bundle branch block may occur along with first-degree AV block and cause a widening of the QRS complex.

No signs of block

Most patients with first-degree AV block show no symptoms of the block because cardiac output isn't significantly affected. If the PR interval is extremely long, a longer interval between S_1 and S_2 may be noted on cardiac auscultation.

How you intervene

Usually, just the underlying cause will be treated, not the conduction disturbance itself. For example, if a medication is causing the block, the dosage may be reduced or the medication may be discontinued.

Close monitoring helps to detect the progression of first-degree AV block to a more serious form of block.

When caring for a patient with first-degree AV block, evaluate any underlying causes that can be corrected, such as medications or ischemia. Observe the ECG for progression of the block to a more severe form of block. Administer digoxin, calcium channel blockers, or beta-adrenergic blockers cautiously.

Second-degree AV block type I

Also called *Mobitz type I block* or *Wenckebach*, second-degree AV block type I occurs when each successive impulse from the SA node is delayed slightly longer than the previous impulse. That pattern continues until an impulse fails to be conducted to the ventricles, and the cycle then repeats. The block generally will occur at the AV node but can also occur in the bundle of His or the Purkinje system. It's similar to a line of people trying to get through a revolving doorway, each one taking longer and longer until finally one can't get through.

How it happens

Causes of second-degree AV block type I include coronary artery disease, inferior wall MI, rheumatic fever, and cardiac surgery. It may also be because of antiarrhythmic agents, cardiac medication toxicity (AV nodal blockers), such as beta-adrenergic blockers, digoxin, and calcium channel blockers, hyperkalemia, cardiomyopathy, and myocarditis (Lyme disease). Increased vagal stimulation can also cause this type of block.

Second-degree AV block type I may occur normally in an otherwise healthy person. Almost always temporary, this type of block resolves when the underlying condition is corrected. Although an asymptomatic patient with this block has a good prognosis, the block may progress to a more serious form, especially if it occurs early during an MI.

What to look for

When monitoring a patient with second-degree AV block type I, since the SA node isn't affected by this lower block, it continues its normal activity. As a result, the atrial rhythm is normal. (See *Identifying type I second-degree AV block*, page 170.)

Identifying second-degree AV block type I

This rhythm strip illustrates second-degree AV block type I. Look for these distinguishing characteristics:

The PR interval gets progressively longer...

...until a QRS complex is dropped.

- *Rhythm:* Atrial—regular; ventricular—irregular
- *Rate:* Atrial—80 beats/min; ventricular—50 beats/min
- *P wave:* Normal

- *PR interval:* Progressively prolonged
- *QRS complex:* 0.08 seconds
- *T wave:* Inverted
- *QT interval:* 0.46 seconds

- *Other:* Wenckebach pattern of grouped beats; PR interval appearing progressively longer until QRS complex drops

The PR interval gets gradually longer with each successive beat until finally a P wave drops, representing failure to conduct through to the ventricles. This makes the ventricular rhythm irregular, with a repeating pattern of groups of QRS complexes followed by a dropped beat whereby the P wave isn't followed by a QRS complex.

Famous footprints

The pattern of grouped beating is sometimes referred to as the *footprints of Wenckebach*. (Karel Frederik Wenckebach was a Dutch internist who, at the turn of the century and long before the introduction of the ECG, described the two forms of what is now known as *second-degree AV block* by analyzing waves in the jugular venous pulse. Following the introduction of the ECG, German internist Woldemar Mobitz differentiated Wenckebach's findings as type I and type II.)

As you've probably noticed by now, rhythm strips have distinctive patterns. (See *Rhythm strip patterns,* page 171.)

Memory jogger

To help you identify second-degree AV block type I, think of the phrase "longer, longer, drop," which describes the progressively prolonged PR intervals and the missing QRS complex. (The QRS complexes, by the way, are usually normal because the delays occur in the AV node.)

Rhythm strip patterns

The more you look at rhythm strips, the more you'll notice patterns. The symbols in the image represent some of the patterns you might see as you study rhythm strips.

Normal, regular (as in normal sinus rhythm)	♥ ♥ ♥ ♥ ♥ ♥
Slow, regular (as in sinus bradycardia)	♥ ♥ ♥
Fast, regular (as in sinus tachycardia)	♥ ♥ ♥ ♥ ♥ ♥ ♥ ♥ ♥ ♥
Premature (as in a premature ventricular contraction)	♥ ♥ ♥ ♥ ♥ ♥
Grouped (as in second-degree AV block type I)	♥ ♥ ♥ ♥ ♥ ♥ ♥ ♥ ♥
Irregularly irregular (as in atrial fibrillation)	♥ ♥♥ ♥ ♥ ♥ ♥ ♥ ♥
Paroxysm or burst (as in paroxysmal atrial tachycardia)	♥ ♥ ♥ ♥ ♥ ♥ ♥ ♥ ♥♥♥

Lonely Ps, lightheaded patients

Usually asymptomatic, a patient with second-degree AV block type I may show signs and symptoms of decreased cardiac output, such as lightheadedness or hypotension. Symptoms may be especially pronounced if the ventricular rate is slow.

How you intervene

No treatment is needed if the patient is asymptomatic. For a symptomatic patient, atropine may improve AV node conduction. A temporary pacemaker may be required for long-term relief of symptoms until the rhythm resolves.

When caring for a patient with this block, assess their tolerance for the rhythm and the need for treatment to improve cardiac output. Evaluate the patient for possible causes of the block, including the use of certain medications or the presence of ischemia.

Check the ECG frequently to see if a more severe type of AV block develops. Make sure the patient has a patent intravenous (IV) line. Teach them about temporary pacemaker, if indicated.

Second–degree AV block type II

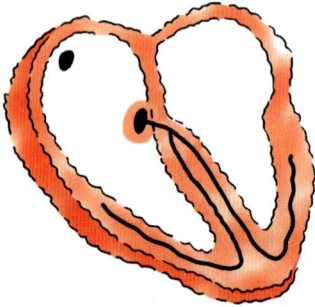

Second-degree AV block Type II, also known as *Mobitz type II block*, is less common than type I but more serious. It occurs when occasional impulses from the SA node fail to conduct to the ventricles.

On an ECG, you won't see the PR interval lengthen before the impulse fails to conduct, as you do with second-degree AV block Type I. You'll see, instead, consistent AV node conduction and an occasional dropped beat. This block is like a line of people passing through a doorway at the same speed, except that, periodically, one of them just can't get through.

How it happens

Second-degree AV block Mobitz type II is usually caused by an anterior wall MI, degenerative changes in the conduction system, or severe coronary artery disease. The arrhythmia indicates a problem at the level of the bundle of His or bundle branches.

Type II block is more serious than type I because the ventricular rate tends to be slower and the cardiac output diminished. It's also more likely to cause symptoms, particularly if the sinus rhythm is slow and the ratio of conducted beats to dropped beats is low, such as 2:1. (See *2:1 AV block*.) Usually chronic, second-degree AV block type II may progress to a more serious form of block. (See *High-grade AV block*, page 173.)

2:1 AV block

In 2:1 second-degree AV block, every other QRS complex is dropped, so there are always two P waves for every QRS complex. The resulting ventricular rhythm is regular.

Keep in mind that type II AV block is more likely to impair cardiac output, lead to symptoms such as syncope, and progress to a more severe form of block. Be sure to monitor the patient carefully.

Don't skip this strip

High-grade AV block

When two or more successive atrial impulses are blocked, the conduction disturbance is called *high-grade AV block*. A high-grade AV block results from either Mobitz 1 or Mobitz II AV block. The rhythm is expressed as a ratio of atrial to ventricular beats (P:QRS), and this block will be at least 3:1, meaning 3 P waves to 1 QRS complex. With the prolonged refractory period of this block, latent pacemakers can discharge. As a result, you'll commonly see idioventricular escape rhythms develop; these ventricular rhythms have a rate of 20 to 40 bpm.

Complications

High-grade AV block causes severe complications. For instance, decreased cardiac output and reduced heart rate can combine to cause Stokes–Adams syncopal attacks. In addition, high-grade AV block usually progresses quickly to third-degree AV block, which is known as complete heart block. Look for these distinguishing characteristics:

Three P waves occur for each QRS complex.

The PR interval remains constant.

- *Rhythm:* Atrial—regular; ventricular—regular or irregular
- *Rate:* Atrial—usually 60 to 100 beats/min; ventricular—usually below 40 beats/min

- *P wave:* Usually normal, but some not followed by a QRS complex
- *PR interval:* Constant, but may be normal or prolonged
- *QRS complex:* Normal or widened periodically absent

- *Other:* None
- *T wave:* Slightly peaked configuration
- *QT interval:* 0.48 seconds

What to look for

When monitoring a rhythm strip, look for an atrial rhythm that's regular and a ventricular rhythm that may be regular or irregular, depending on the block. (See *Identifying second-degree AV block type II.*) If the block is intermittent, the rhythm is irregular. If the block is constant, such as 2:1 or 3:1, the rhythm is regular.

Don't skip this strip

Identifying second-degree AV block type II

This rhythm strip illustrates second-degree AV block type II. Look for these distinguishing characteristics:

The atrial rhythm is regular...

...but the ventricular rhythm is irregular.

The PR interval is constant.

A QRS complex should be here.

- *Rhythm:* Atrial—regular; ventricular—irregular
- *Rate:* Atrial—60 beats/min; ventricular—50 beats/min
- *P wave:* Normal
- *PR interval:* 0.28 seconds
- *QRS complex:* 0.10 seconds
- *T wave:* Normal
- *QT interval:* 0.60 seconds
- *Other:* PR and RR intervals constant before a dropped beat with no warning

Overall, the strip will look as if someone erased some QRS complexes. The PR interval will be constant for all conducted beats but may be prolonged. The QRS complex is usually wide, but normal complexes may occur.

Jumpin' palpitations!

Most patients who experience a few dropped beats remain asymptomatic as long as cardiac output is maintained. As the number of dropped beats increases, patients may experience palpitations, fatigue, dyspnea, chest pain, or lightheadedness. On physical examination, you may note hypotension, and the pulse may be slow and regular or irregular.

How you intervene

If the dropped beats are infrequent and the patient shows no symptoms of decreased cardiac output, the practitioner may choose only to observe the rhythm, particularly if the cause is thought to be reversible. If the patient is hypotensive, treatment aims to improve cardiac output by increasing the heart rate. Atropine, dopamine, or epineph-rine may be given for symptomatic bradycardia. Consider discontinu-ing digoxin or other rate-control negative chronotropic medications (beta-adrenergic blockers, calcium channel blockers), which may be the primary cause of the arrhythmia or exacerbate it. Because the con-duction block occurs in the His–Purkinje system, transcutaneous pac-ing should be initiated quickly.

In the outpatient setting, it's important to order diagnostic tests—including a portable cardiac monitor (Holter or event monitor) that spans from 2 to 30 days, respectively. The monitor helps to assess for underlying arrhythmias, including AV blocks. With arrhythmia, an echocardiogram is also useful to assess for underlying structural issues and overall heart function.

Pacemaker place

Second-degree AV block type II commonly requires the placement of a pacemaker. A temporary pacemaker may be used until a permanent pacemaker can be placed. Assessing patients' tolerance for the rhythm and the need for treatment to improve cardiac output is important. Evaluate for possible correctable causes, such as ischemia.

Keep the patient on bed rest, if indicated, to reduce myocardial oxygen demands. Administer oxygen therapy as ordered. Observe the patient for progression to a more severe form of AV block. If the patient receives a pacemaker, teach the patient and family members about postoperative care, including the signs and symptoms of infec-tion, site care, mobility and lifting restrictions, pacemaker use, and remote monitoring in the outpatient setting.

Third-degree AV block

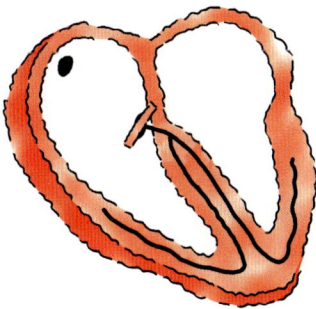

Also called *complete heart block*, third-degree AV block occurs when impulses from the atria are com-pletely blocked at the AV node, inhibiting conduction to the ven-tricles. Maintaining our doorway analogy, this form of block is like a line of people waiting to go through a doorway, but they are barred from progressing forward.

Beats of different drummers

Acting independently, the atria, generally under the control of the SA node, tend to maintain a regular rate of 60 to 100 beats/min.

The ventricular rhythm can originate from the AV node and maintain a rate of 40 to 60 beats/min. Most typically, it originates from the Purkinje system in the ventricles and maintains a rate of 20 to 40 beats/min. The QRS complexes often resemble an escape rhythm.

The rhythm strip will look like a strip of P waves laid independently over a strip of QRS complexes. Note that the P wave doesn't conduct the QRS complex that follows it.

How it happens

Third-degree AV block that originates at the level of the AV node is most commonly a congenital condition. This block may also be caused by coronary artery disease, an anterior or inferior wall MI, degenerative changes in the heart, digoxin toxicity, calcium channel blockers, beta-adrenergic blockers, or surgical injury. It may be temporary or permanent. (See *Heart block after congenital heart repair*)

Because the ventricular rate is so slow, third-degree AV block presents a potentially life-threatening situation because cardiac output can drop dramatically. In addition, the patient loses their atrial kick—up to an extra 30% of blood flow pushed into the ventricles by atrial contraction. That happens as a result of the loss of synchrony between the atrial and ventricular contractions. The loss of atrial kick further decreases cardiac output. Any exertion on the part of the patient can worsen symptoms.

What to look for

When analyzing an ECG for this rhythm, you'll note that the atrial and ventricular rhythms are regular. The P and R waves can be "walked out" across the strip, meaning that they appear to march across the strip in rhythm. (See *Identifying third-degree AV block*, page 177.)

Ages and stages

Heart block after congenital heart repair

After repair of a ventricular septal defect, a child may require a permanent pacemaker if complete heart block develops. This arrhythmia may develop from interference with the bundle of His during surgery.

In third-degree AV block, the patient loses the atrial kick, which presents a potentially life-threatening situation.

Don't skip this strip

Identifying third-degree AV block

This rhythm strip illustrates third-degree AV block. Look for these distinguishing characteristics:

> The atrial rhythm is regular.

> The P wave occurs without a QRS complex.

> The ventricular rhythm is regular.

- *Rhythm:* Regular
- *Rate:* Atrial—90 beats/min; ventricular—30 beats/min
- *P wave:* Normal
- *PR interval:* Varies
- *QRS complex:* 0.16 seconds
- *T wave:* Normal
- *QT interval:* 0.56 seconds
- *Other:* P waves without QRS complex

Some P waves may be buried in QRS complexes or T waves. The PR interval will vary, with no pattern or regularity. If the resulting rhythm, called the *escape rhythm*, originates in the AV node, the QRS complex will be normal and the ventricular rate will be 40 to 60 beats/min. If the escape rhythm originates in the Purkinje system, the QRS complex will be wide, with a ventricular rate below 40 beats/ min.

Escape!

The PR interval varies because the atria and ventricles beat independently of each other. The QRS complex is determined by the site of the escape rhythm. Usually, the duration and configuration are normal; however, with an idioventricular escape rhythm (an escape rhythm originating in the ventricles), the duration is greater than 0.12 seconds, and the complex is distorted.

Although atrial and ventricular rates can vary with third-degree block, they're nearly the same with complete AV dissociation, a similar rhythm. (See *Complete AV dissociation*, page 178.)

Don't skip this strip

Complete AV dissociation

With both third-degree AV block and complete AV dissociation, the atria and ventricles beat independently, each controlled by its own pacemaker. *The key difference:* In third-degree AV block, the atrial rate is faster than the ventricular rate. With complete AV dissociation, the two rates are usually about the same, with the ventricular rate slightly faster.

Rhythm disturbances

Never the primary problem, complete AV dissociation results from one of three underlying rhythm disturbances:
• slowed or impaired sinus impulse formation or SA conduction, as in sinus bradycardia or sinus arrest
• accelerated impulse formation in the AV junction or the ventricle, as in accelerated junctional or ventricular tachycardia
• AV conduction disturbance, as in complete AV block

When to treat

The clinical significance of complete AV dissociation—as well as treatment for the arrhythmia—depends on the underlying cause and its effect on the patient. If the underlying rhythm decreases cardiac output, the patient will need treatment to correct the arrhythmia.

Depending on the underlying cause, the patient may be treated with an antiarrhythmic, such as atropine and isoproterenol, to restore synchrony. Alternatively, the patient may be given a pacemaker to support a slow ventricular rate. If drug toxicity caused the original disturbance, the drug should be discontinued.

Serious signs and symptoms

Most patients with third-degree AV block experience significant symptoms, including severe fatigue, lightheadedness, changes in mental status, dyspnea, chest pain, pulmonary edema, and loss of consciousness. You may note hypotension, pallor, diaphoresis, bradycardia, and a variation in the intensity of the pulse.

A few patients will be relatively free from symptoms, complaining only that they are unable tolerate exercise and are tired for no apparent reason. The severity of symptoms depends, to a great extent, on the resulting ventricular rate.

How you intervene

If cardiac output is inadequate or the patient's condition deteriorates, therapy aims to improve the ventricular rate. Atropine may be given, or a temporary pacemaker may be used to restore adequate cardiac output. Dopamine and epinephrine may also be indicated.

Temporary pacing may be required until the cause of the block resolves or until a permanent pacemaker can be inserted. A permanent block requires the placement of a permanent pacemaker.

With all heart blocks, it is important to reconcile all patient medications and check if these directly induce or exacerbate bradycardia or if there are drug-to-drug interactions that produce this effect. Of note, widely known medications that we've discussed include digoxin, beta-adrenergic blockers (also consider eye drops, which can have systemic effects), calcium channel blockers, and antiarrhythmics. However, realize that psychoactives (selective serotonin reuptake inhibitors, tricyclic antidepressants, donepezil, lithium, opioids), anesthetic agents, cannabis, and muscle relaxants also produce an undesirable effect in the context of heart blocks.

Bundles of troubles

The patient with an anterior wall MI is more likely to have permanent third-degree AV block if the MI involved the bundle of His or the bundle branches than if it involved other areas of the myocardium. Those patients commonly require prompt placement of a permanent pacemaker.

An AV block in a patient with an inferior wall MI is more likely to be temporary, as a result of injury to the AV node. Placement of a permanent pacemaker is usually delayed in such cases to evaluate recovery of the conduction system.

Check it out...

When caring for a patient with third-degree heart block, immediately assess the patient's tolerance of the rhythm and the need for treatment to support cardiac output and relieve symptoms. Make sure the patient has a patent IV catheter. Administer oxygen therapy as ordered. Evaluate for possible correctable causes of the arrhythmia, such as medications or ischemia. Minimize the patient's activity and maintain bed rest.

That's a wrap!

AV blocks review

AV blocks
- Result from an interruption in impulse conduction between the atria and the ventricles
- Possibly occurring at the level of the AV node, the bundle of His, or the bundle branches
- Atrial rate commonly normal (60 to 100 beats/min) with slowed ventricular rate
- Classified according to severity, not location

First-degree AV block
- Occurs when impulses from the atria are consistently delayed during conduction through the AV node
- Can progress to a more severe block

Characteristics
- ECG shows normal sinus rhythm, except for prolonged PR interval
- *Rhythms:* Regular
- *P wave:* Normal
- *PR interval:* Consistent for each beat; greater than 0.20 seconds
- *QRS complex:* Normal; occasionally widened because of bundle branch block
- *QT interval:* Normal

Treatment
- Correction of the underlying cause

Second-degree AV block type I
- Also called *Mobitz type I block*

Characteristics
- *Rhythms:* Atrial—regular; ventricular—irregular
- *Rates:* Atrial rate exceeds ventricular rate

- *P wave:* Normal
- *PR interval:* Gradually gets longer with each beat until P wave fails to conduct to the ventricles
- *QRS complex:* Usually normal
- *T wave:* Normal

Treatment
- No treatment if asymptomatic
- Atropine to improve AV conduction
- Temporary pacemaker insertion

Second-degree AV block type II
- Also known as *Mobitz II block*
- Occasional impulses from the SA node fail to conduct to the ventricles

Characteristics
- *Rhythms:* Atrial—regular; ventricular—irregular if block is intermittent, regular if block is constant (such as 2:1 or 3:1)
- *PR interval:* Constant for all conducted beats, may be prolonged in some cases
- *QRS complex:* Usually wide
- *T wave:* Normal
- *Other:* PR and RR intervals constant before a dropped beat with no warning

Treatment
- Temporary or permanent pacemaker insertion
- Atropine, dopamine, or epinephrine for symptomatic bradycardia
- Discontinuation of digoxin if appropriate

Third-degree AV block
- Also known as *complete heart block*
- Impulses from the atria completely blocked at the AV node and not conducted to the ventricles

AV blocks review (*continued*)

Characteristics
- *Rhythms:* Atrial—regular; ventricular—regular
- *Rates:* Atrial rate exceeding ventricular rate
- *P wave:* Normal
- *PR interval:* Variations with no regularity; no relation between P waves and QRS complexes
- *QRS complex:* Normal (junctional pacemaker) or wide and bizarre (ventricular pacemaker)
- *T wave:* Normal
- *Other:* P waves without QRS complex

Treatment
- Correction of the underlying cause
- Temporary or permanent pacemaker
- Atropine, dopamine, or epinephrine for symptomatic bradycardia

Complete AV dissociation
- Atria and ventricles beat independently and asynchronously, each controlled by its own pacemaker

Characteristics
- *Rates:* Atrial and ventricular rates nearly equal, with ventricular rate slightly faster
- *Rhythms:* Regular
- *P wave:* No relation to QRS
- *QRS complex:* Usually normal; may be wide and bizarre

Treatment
- Correction of the underlying cause
- Atropine or isoproterenol to restore synchrony
- Pacemaker insertion

Quick quiz

1. No treatment is necessary if the patient has the form of AV block known as:
    A. first-degree AV block.
    B. Second-degree AV block type II.
    C. third-degree AV block.
    D. complete AV dissociation.

Answer: A. A patient with first-degree AV block rarely experiences symptoms and usually requires only monitoring for progression of the block.

2. In second-degree AV block Mobitz type I, also known as Wenckebach, the PR interval:
    A. varies according to the ventricular response rate.
    B. progressively lengthens until a QRS complex is dropped.
    C. remains constant despite an irregular ventricular rhythm.
    D. is typically unmeasurable.

Answer: B. Progressive lengthening of the PR interval creates an irregular ventricular rhythm with a repeating pattern of groups of QRS complexes. Those groups are followed by a dropped beat in which the P wave isn't followed by a QRS complex. The PR interval following that dropped beat is the shortest.

3. Myocardial ischemia may cause cells in the AV node to repolarize:
    A. in a normal manner.
    B. more quickly than normal.
    C. more slowly than normal.
    D. in a retrograde manner.

Answer: C. Injured cells conduct impulses slowly or inconsistently. Relief of the ischemia can restore normal function to the AV node.

4. Second-degree AV block type II is generally considered more serious than type I because in most cases of type II, the:
    A. cardiac output is diminished.
    B. ventricular rate rises above 100 beats/min.
    C. peripheral vascular system shuts down almost as soon as the arrhythmia begins.
    D. atrial rate rises above 100 beats/min.

Answer: A. This form of AV block causes a decrease in cardiac output, particularly if the sinus rhythm is slow and the ratio of conducted beats to dropped beats is low, such as 2:1.

5. AV block can be caused by inadvertent damage to the heart's conduction system during cardiac surgery. Damage is most likely to occur in surgery involving which area of the heart?
    A. Pulmonic or tricuspid valve.
    B. Mitral or pulmonic valve.
    C. Aortic or mitral valve.
    D. Mitral or tricuspid valve.

Answer: D. AV block can be caused by surgery involving the mitral or tricuspid valve or in the closure of a ventricular septal defect.

6. A main component of the treatment for third-degree AV block is the use of:
    A. a pacemaker.
    B. calcium channel blockers.
    C. oxygen and antiarrhythmics.
    D. beta-adrenergic blockers.

Answer: A. Temporary pacing may be required for this rhythm disturbance until the cause of the block resolves or until a permanent pacemaker can be implanted. A permanent third-degree AV block requires the placement of a permanent pacemaker.

7.   Treatment of first-degree AV block is aimed at correcting the underlying cause. Which of the following may cause first-degree AV block?
  A.   Stress.
  B.   Digoxin.
  C.   Angiotensin-converting enzyme inhibitors.
  D.   Strenuous physical exertion.

Answer: B. First-degree AV block may be caused by MI or ischemia, myocarditis, degenerative changes in the heart, and negative chrono-trope medications, such as digoxin, calcium channel blockers, and beta-adrenergic blockers.

Test strips

Okay, try these test strips. Using the eight-step method for interpretation, fill in the blanks below with the particular characteristics of the strip. Then check your answers with ours.

Strip 1

Atrial rhythm: _____

Ventricular rhythm: _____

Atrial rate: _____

Ventricular rate: _____

P wave: _____

PR interval: _____

QRS complex: _____

T wave: _____

QT interval: _____

Other: _____

Interpretation: _____

Strip 2

Atrial rhythm: _____

Ventricular rhythm: _____

Atrial rate: _____

Ventricular rate: _____

P wave: _____

PR interval: _____

QRS complex: _____

T wave: _____

QT interval: _____

Other: _____

Interpretation: _____

Strip 3

Atrial rhythm: _____

Ventricular rhythm: _____

Atrial rate: _____

Ventricular rate: _____

P wave: _____

PR interval: _____

QRS complex: _____

T wave: _____

QT interval: _____

Other: _____

Interpretation: _____

Answers to test strips

1. Rhythm: Regular atrial and ventricular rhythms
    Rate: 75 beats/min
    P wave: Normal size and configuration
    PR interval: 0.34 seconds
    QRS complex: 0.08 seconds
    T wave: Normal configuration
    QT interval: 0.42 seconds
    Other: None
    Interpretation: Normal sinus rhythm with first-degree AV block

2. Rhythm: Regular atrial and ventricular rhythms
    Rate: Atrial rates 100 beats/min; ventricular rates 50 beats/min
    P wave: Normal size and configuration
    PR interval: 0.14 seconds
    QRS complex: 0.06 seconds
    T wave: Normal configuration
    QT interval: 0.44 seconds
    Other: Two P waves for each QRS
    Interpretation: Second-degree AV block type II

3. Rhythm: Regular atrial and ventricular rhythms
    Rate: Atrial rates 75 beats/min; ventricular rates 36 beats/min
    P wave: Normal size; no constant relationship to QRS complex
    PR interval: None
    QRS complex: 0.16 seconds; wide and bizarre
    T wave: Normal, except for the second beat distorted by a P wave
    QT interval: 0.42 seconds
    Interpretation: Third-degree AV block

Scoring

☆☆☆ If you correctly answered all seven questions and filled in all the blanks, way to go! We're willing to bet 2:1 that you're aces when it comes to AV block.

☆☆ If you answered six questions correctly and correctly filled in most of the blanks, good job!

☆ If you answered fewer than six questions correctly and missed most of the blanks, give it another go. We certainly won't block your impulse to reread the chapter.

Selected references

Chandler, S. F., Fynn-Thompson, F., Mah, D. Y. (2017). Role of cardiac pacing in congenital complete heart block. *Expert Review Cardiovascular Therapy, 15*(11), 853–861. https://doi.org/10.1080/14779072.2017.1376655

Chen, L. Y., Ribeiro, A. L. P., Platonov, P. G., Cygankiewicz, I., Soliman, E. Z., Gorenek, B., Ikeda, T., Vassilikos, V. P., Steinberg, J. S., Varma, N., Bayés-de-Luna, A., & Baranchuk, A. (2022). P wave parameters and indices: A critical appraisal of clinical utility, challenges, and future research-A consensus document endorsed by the International Society of Electrocardiology and the International Society for Holter and Noninvasive Electrocardiology. *Circulation. Arrhythmia and electrophysiology, 15*(4), e010435. https://doi.org/10.1161/CIRCEP.121.010435

Kusumoto, F. M., Schoenfeld, M. H., Barrett, C., Edgerton, J. R., Ellenbogen, K. A., Gold, M. R., Goldschlager, N. F., Hamilton, R. M., Joglar, J. A., Kim, R. J., Lee, R., Marine, J. E., McLeod, C. J., Oken, K. R., Patton, K. K., Pellegrini, C. N., Selzman, K. A., Thompson, A., & Varosy, P. D. (2019). 2018 ACC/AHA/HRS Guideline on the evaluation and management of patients with bradycardia and cardiac conduction delay: Executive summary: A report of the American College of Cardiology/American Heart Association Task Force on clinical practice guidelines, and the Heart Rhythm Society. *Journal of the American College of Cardiology, 74*(7), 932–987. https://doi.org/10.1016/j.jacc.2018.10.043

McLaughlin, M. A. (2018). *Cardiovascular care made incredibly visual* (3rd ed.). Wolters Kluwer.

Panchal, A. R., Berg, K. M., Kudenchuk, P. J., DelRios, M., Hirsch, K. G., Link, M. S., Kurz, M. C., Chan, P. S., Cabañas, J. G., Morley, P. T., Hazinski, M. F., & Donnino, M. W. (2018). 2018 American Heart Association focused update on advanced cardiovascular life support use of antiarrythmic drugs during and immediately after cardiac arrest: An update to the American Heart Association Guidelines for cardiopulmonary resuscitation and emergency cardiovascular care. *Circulation, 138*(23), e740–e249. https://doi.org/10.1161/CIR.0000000000000613

Samesima, N., God, E. G., Kruse, J. C. L., Leal, M. G., Pinho, C., França, F. F. A. C., Pimenta, J., Cardoso, A. F., Paixão, A., Fonseca, A., Pérez-Riera, A. R., Ribeiro, A. L. P., Madaloso, B. A., Luna Filho, B., Oliveira, C. A. R., Grupi, C. J., Moreira, D. A. R., Kaiser, E., Paixão, G. M. M., ... Pastore, C. A. (2022). Brazilian Society of Cardiology Guidelines on the analysis and issuance of electrocardiographic reports—2022. Diretriz da Sociedade Brasileira de Cardiologia sobre a Análise e Emissão de Laudos Eletrocardiográficos—2022. *Arquivos brasileiros de cardiologia, 119*(4), 638–680. https://doi.org/10.36660/abc.20220623

Sole, M. L., Klein, D. G., & Moseley, M. J. (2020). *Introduction to critical care nursing* (8th ed.). Saunders.

Part III

Treating arrhythmias

Nonpharmacologic treatments

Just the facts

In this chapter, you'll learn:

◆ nonpharmacologic treatments of arrhythmias and how they work

◆ ways to identify and treat complications of nonpharmacologic treatments

◆ nursing care for patients receiving nonpharmacologic treatments

◆ patient teaching points for nonpharmacologic treatments.

A look at pacemakers

Keep up to pace with pacemaker information!

A pacemaker is an artificial device that electrically stimulates the myocardium to depolarize, which begins a contraction.

Pacemakers are usually used for (1) bradycardia caused by sinus node dysfunction (SND), medications, or atrioventricular (AV) block (AVB) and (2) cardiac dyssynchrony because of advanced heart failure. The device may be temporary or permanent, depending on the patient's condition. Pacemakers are commonly necessary for the aging heart and following myocardial infarction or cardiac surgery.

And the beat goes on...

Pacemakers work by generating an impulse from a power source and transmitting that impulse to the heart muscle. The impulse flows throughout the heart and causes the heart muscle to depolarize. Pacemakers usually consist of three components: the pulse generator, the pacing leads, and the electrodes at the tips of the pacing leads.

Making the pacer work

The pulse generator contains the pacemaker's power source and circuitry. The lithium battery in a permanent or implanted pacemaker is its power source and lasts about 10 years. The circuitry of the pacemaker is a microchip that guides heart pacing.

189

A temporary pacemaker, which is an external device, is about the size of a large cell phone or a telemetry box and is powered by alkaline batteries. These units also contain a microchip and are programmed by a touchpad or dials.

A stimulus on the move

An electrical stimulus from the pulse generator moves through wires (referred to as *pacing leads* or *leads*) to the electrode tips. The leads for a pacemaker designed to stimulate a single heart chamber are placed in either the atrium or the ventricle. For dual-chamber, or AV, pacing, the leads are placed in both chambers, usually on the right side of the heart.

One pole or two

The electrodes—one on a unipolar lead or two on a bipolar lead—send information about electrical impulses in the myocardium back to the pulse generator. The pulse generator senses the heart's electrical activity and responds according to how it has been programmed.

A look at pacing leads

Pacing leads have either one (unipolar) or two (bipolar) electrodes. These illustrations show the difference between the two leads.

Unipolar lead

In a unipolar system, electric current moves from the pulse generator through the pacing lead to the negative pole at the tip of the pacing lead. From there, it stimulates the heart and returns to the pulse generator's metal surface (the positive pole) to complete the circuit.

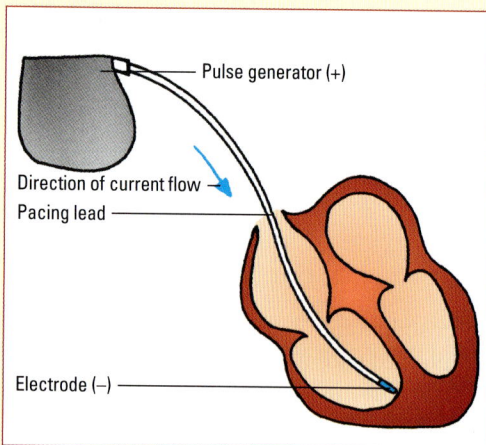

Bipolar lead

In a bipolar system, current flows from the pulse generator through the pacing lead to the negative pole at the tip. At that point, it stimulates the heart and then travels to the positive pole within the pacing lead to complete the circuit.

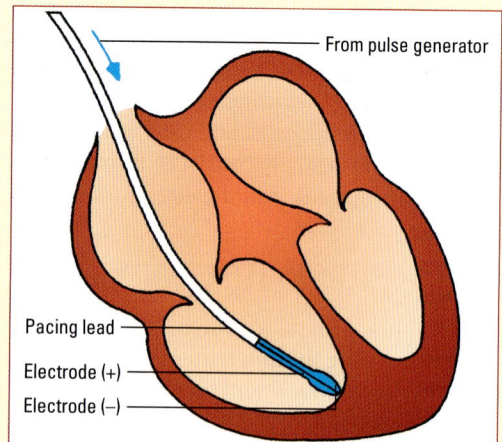

Pulse generator (+)

Direction of current flow

Pacing lead

Electrode (−)

From pulse generator

Pacing lead

Electrode (+)

Electrode (−)

A unipolar lead system is more sensitive to the heart's intrinsic electrical activity than a bipolar system. A bipolar system isn't as easily affected by electrical activity outside the heart and the generator (e.g., from skeletal muscle contraction or magnetic fields). (See *A look at pacing leads*, page 190.)

Working with pacemakers

On an ECG, you'll notice the spike from a unipolar system right away. (See *Pacemaker spikes.*) It occurs when the pacemaker sends an electrical impulse to the heart muscle. That impulse appears as a vertical line or spike. The spike with a bipolar system can sometimes be difficult to see.

Depending on the position of the electrode, the spike appears in different locations on the waveform.

- When the atria are stimulated by the pacemaker, the spike is followed by a P wave and then the paced or patient's intrinsic QRS complex, then the T wave. This series of waveforms represents the successful capture of the atrial myocardium. The P wave may look different from the patient's intrinsic P wave.
- When the ventricles are stimulated by a pacemaker, the spike is followed by a QRS complex and a T wave. The paced QRS complex usually appears wider than the patient's intrinsic QRS complex because of the longer time it takes the ventricles to depolarize when paced.
- When the pacemaker stimulates both the atria and the ventricles, the first spike is followed by a P wave, then another spike, and then a QRS complex. Be aware that the type of pacemaker used and the patient's condition may affect whether every beat is paced.

Permanent and temporary pacemakers

Depending on the patient's needs, a permanent or a temporary pacemaker can be used to maintain heart rhythm. Pacing lead placement varies according to the patient's specific needs.

Permanent pacemakers

A permanent pacemaker is used to treat chronic heart conditions, such as SND, AVB, or dyssynchrony. SND causing symptomatic bradycardia can be because of advanced age or drug therapy. AVB is commonly because of cardiomyopathy, cardiac surgery, or septal ablation. Dyssynchrony between all the chambers and within the left ventricle is caused by advanced cardiomyopathy. Permanent pacemakers are surgically implanted, usually under local anesthesia. Conscious sedation or general anesthesia is used in addition to local anesthesia. (See *Placing a permanent pacemaker with pacing leads*, page 192.)

Pacemaker spikes

Pacemaker impulses—the stimuli that travel from the pacemaker to the heart—are visible on the patient's ECG tracing as spikes. Large or small, pacemaker spikes appear above or below the isoelectric line. This example shows an atrial and a ventricular pacemaker spike.

- P wave
- QRS complex
- Ventricular pacemaker spike
- Atrial pacemaker spike

Placing a permanent pacemaker with pacing leads

The practitioner who implants the endocardial pacemaker usually selects a transvenous route and begins pacing lead placement by inserting a catheter percutaneously or by venous cutdown. Then, with a stylet and fluoroscopic guidance, the catheter is threaded through the vein until the tip reaches the endocardium.

Lead placements

For pacing lead placement in the atrium, the tip is usually anchored in the right atrial appendage or to the right atrial septum. For placement in the right ventricle, it is usually anchored within the right ventricular septum or in one of the interior muscular ridges, or *trabeculae* in the apex. Resynchronization therapy with a biventricular pacemaker requires a pacing lead to be placed in the coronary sinus that lies over the left ventricle. This enables the capture of the left ventricular myocardium through the wall of the coronary sinus. Biventricular pacing improves outcomes and reduces mortality in certain patients. With the relatively new use of His bundle pacing, the right ventricular lead is placed in the right atrium next to the His–Purkinje network. This allows for depolarization of both ventricles via a normal conduction pathway. Both biventricular and His bundle pacing are an attempt to result in more physiologic pacing.

Placing a leadless permanent pacemaker

A leadless pacemaker is inserted percutaneously through a large (27 Fr) catheter in the femoral vein and placed in the right ventricle.

Implanting the generator

When the pacing lead is in the proper position, the pulse generator is secured in a subcutaneous pocket of tissue just below the clavicle. Changing the pacemaker's battery or microchip circuitry requires the whole generator to be replaced. However, only a shallow incision over the previously made pocket and a quick generator exchange are done (and generally, the leads remain intact). If the leads require revision, this is a separate procedure performed at the same time as the generator replacement. On occasion, a decision is made ahead to upgrade the device depending upon the patient's clinical status.

Subclavian vein

Generator in subcutaneous pocket

Right atrial lead

Right ventricular lead

Pocket generator

The generator consists of a battery and microchip circuitry enclosed in a titanium case. It is implanted in a pocket made from subcutaneous tissue. The pocket is usually constructed under the clavicle. Permanent pacemakers are initially programmed during implantation. The programming determines how the pacemaker functions and can be adjusted externally using a Programmer, which is a manufacturer-specific device designed to receive and transmit data from implantable devices and allows both temporary and permanent programming of the device.

Permanent pacing leads

Permanent pacing leads are usually placed transvenously. They are positioned in the appropriate chambers and then anchored to the endocardium or in the coronary sinus for left ventricular pacing. Some patients may require permanent epicardial pacing leads that are placed during cardiac surgery. This is common for patients with tricuspid valve surgery and for patients who require left ventricular pacing but for whom a coronary sinus lead was unable to be placed transvenously. (See *Placing a permanent pacemaker with pacing leads*, page 192.)

Leadless pacemakers

This is a self-contained pacemaker the size and shape of a large capsule of medicine. It is placed within the right ventricle via the femoral vein. Therefore, there is no chest incision or lead wire. It paces and senses only the right ventricle. It is indicated for people in whom atrial pacing is not needed. For example, for patients with:

- symptomatic high-grade AVB in the presence of atrial fibrillation
- symptomatic high-grade AVB or SND and when an atrial lead implant is difficult, high risk, or not needed

Currently, there are devices in clinical trials that are dual-chamber leadless pacemakers. These devices use a proprietary technology, which allows two devices across two chambers to communicate with each other.

Temporary pacemakers

A temporary pacemaker is commonly inserted in an emergency. The patient may show signs of decreased cardiac output, such as hypotension or syncope. The temporary pacemaker supports the patient until the condition resolves.

A temporary pacemaker can also serve as a bridge until a permanent pacemaker is inserted, for example, immediately following cardiac surgery or while awaiting resolution of a bloodstream infection. Temporary pacemakers are used for patients with heart block, sinus bradycardia, or low cardiac output. Several types of temporary pacemakers are available, including transvenous, epicardial, and transcutaneous.

Temporary pacemakers should have the batteries, pacing thresholds, and connections between the pacing leads and the generator routinely checked. The insertion sites should be kept sterile and be regularly monitored. Unit-based guidelines need to exist for this routine care.

Going the transvenous way

The transvenous approach is used when inserting a temporary pacemaker in nonsurgical environments. In this method, the pacing leads are commonly inserted through the subclavian or internal jugular vein. The transvenous pacemaker is probably the most common and reliable type of temporary pacemaker. It's usually inserted at the bedside or in a fluoroscopy suite. The pacing lead is typically advanced through a catheter into the right ventricle and then connected to an external pulse generator.

Taking the epicardial route

Epicardial pacemakers are commonly placed while patients are undergoing cardiac surgery. The doctor attaches the tips of the pacing leads (thin wires) to the surface of the heart and then brings the wires through the chest wall, below the incision. They're then attached to an external pulse generator. The pacing wires are usually cut or removed several days after surgery or when the patient no longer requires them.

> A temporary pacemaker can serve as a bridge until a permanent one can be placed. Types include transvenous, epicardial, and transcutaneous.

Following the transcutaneous path

The use of an external or transcutaneous pacemaker has become commonplace. In this noninvasive method, one electrode pad is placed over the heart on the patient's anterior chest wall, and a second is applied behind the heart on the back. An external pulse generator then emits pacing impulses that travel through the skin, muscle, and bone to the heart muscle. Transcutaneous pacing is also built into many external defibrillators for use in an emergency. In this case, the pacing electrode pads are built into the same electrode pads used for defibrillation.

Transcutaneous pacing is a quick and effective method of pacing heart rhythm and is commonly used in an emergency until a transvenous pacemaker can be inserted. However, some alert patients can't tolerate the painful electrical stimuli produced from pacing at the levels needed to capture the myocardium through the chest wall.

Setting the controls

When your patient has a temporary pacemaker, you'll notice several types of settings on the pulse generator. The rate control regulates how many impulses are generated in 1 minute and is measured in pulses per minute (ppm). The rate is usually set at 60 to 80 ppm. (See *A look at a pulse generator.*) The pacemaker is usually programmed in a demand mode. Thus, it fires only if the patient's heart rate (HR) falls below the rate (e.g., 60) set on the pacemaker. The rate may be set higher in an effort to increase cardiac output or if the patient has a tachyarrhythmia that's being treated with overdrive pacing.

A look at a pulse generator

This is an illustration of a temporary pulse generator with brief descriptions of its various parts. The pacemaker sensitivity control adjusts pacemaker sensitivity in relation to the patient's electrical amplitude or height of P or R waves. The rate control sets the desired HR. An intrinsic HR less than this setting causes pacing.

The pace meter registers every pacing stimulus delivered to the heart.

The sensing meter registers every time an intrinsic depolarization is recognized.

The rate control sets desired HR. An intrinsic HR less than this setting causes pacing.

The pacemaker sensitivity control adjusts pacemaker sensitivity in relation to the patient's electrical amplitude or height of P or R waves.

The output controls determine the amount of electricity sent to the heart (in milliamperes).

The on–off buttons activate and deactivate the pulse generator.

Measuring the output

The electrical output of a temporary pacemaker is measured in milliampere (mA). First, the stimulation threshold, or the minimum amount of energy required to capture or stimulate the cardiac muscle to depolarize, is assessed. Then the pacemaker's output is set 10% higher than the stimulating threshold to ensure myocardial capture under various physiologic conditions, such as hypokalemia.

Sensing the norm

You can also program the pacemaker's sensing or the ability to sense electricity (e.g., P waves and QRS complexes). Sensing is measured and set in millivolt (mV). Most pacemakers are programmed in a demand mode; therefore, only pacing when the heart's own electrical activity is not sensed. Pacing is inhibited when the heart's own P waves and QRS complexes are sensed. This may be referred to as *demand pacing*. So many patients will at times have a paced rhythm, an intrinsic rhythm, or a rhythm with both paced and intrinsic beats at any given time.

Pacemaker codes

The capabilities of permanent pacemakers may be described by a generic five-letter coding system, although three letters are more commonly used. (See *Pacemaker coding system*.)

Introducing letter 1

The first letter of the code identifies the heart chambers that can be paced when necessary. These are the options and the letters used to signify those options:
- V = Ventricle
- A = Atrium
- D = Dual (ventricle and atrium)
- O = None

Learning about letter 2

The second letter of the code signifies the heart chamber in which the pacemaker senses the intrinsic activity:
- V = Ventricle
- A = Atrium
- D = Dual (ventricle and atrium)
- O = No sensing. When a pacemaker doesn't sense intrinsic electricity, it paces, even if intrinsic activity exists. This is referred to as *asynchronous pacing*. Although permanent pacemakers may be programmed this way when the patient is undergoing certain procedures, temporary pacemakers should not be. Asynchronous pacing in the ventricle with a temporary pacemaker can lead to ventricular tachycardia (VT), ventricular fibrillation, or torsades de pointes.

Looking at letter 3

The third letter indicates the pacemaker's response to the intrinsic electrical activity it senses in the atrium or ventricle:
- T = Triggers pacing (For instance, if atrial activity is sensed, ventricular pacing may be triggered.)

- I = Inhibits pacing (If the pacemaker senses intrinsic activity in a chamber, it won't fire in that chamber.)
- D = Dual (The pacemaker can be triggered or inhibited in the atrium, ventricle, or both.)
- O = None (The pacemaker doesn't respond to electrical activity.) If a pacemaker can't sense because the second letter is an O, then the third letter is usually also an O. A pacemaker that can't sense can't respond to an event.

Pacemaker coding system

A coding system for pacemaker functions can provide a simple description of pacemaker capabilities. One commonly used coding system employs three letters to describe functions. The first letter refers to the *chamber paced* by the pacemaker. The second refers to the *chamber sensed* by the pacemaker. The third refers to the *pacemaker's response* to the sensed event.

In the example shown here, both chambers can pace if necessary (represented in the code by the first *D*, for dual). Both chambers are sensed (represented in the code by the second *D*, for dual). Because the third letter is *D*, the pacing will be either inhibited or triggered. If intrinsic electrical activity is sensed in either the atrium or the ventricle, the pacemaker will inhibit (or withhold) pacing in whichever chamber that the electricity is sensed. Sensed electricity in one chamber (e.g., the atrium) can also trigger pacing in the other chamber (e.g., the ventricle).

Figuring out letter 4

The fourth letter of the code describes rate modulation, also known as *rate responsiveness* or *rate-adaptive pacing*:

- R = Rate modulation. (A sensor adjusts the programmed paced HR in response to the patient's physiologic need. For example, increased movement or respiratory rate will increase the paced rate.) This is used for chronotropic incompetence or when the patient's sinus node can't increase the sinus rate during increased physiologic demand.
- O = None (Rate modulation is unavailable or disabled.)

Don't be puzzled by pacemaker codes. Use a three- or four-letter system.

Finally, letter 5

The final letter of the code is rarely used but specifies the location or absence of multisite pacing:

- O = None (No multisite pacing is present.)
- A = Atrium or atria (Multisite pacing in the atrium or atria is present.)
- V = Ventricle or ventricles (Multisite pacing in the ventricle or ventricles is present.)
- D = Dual site (Dual-site pacing in both the atrium and the ventricles is present.)

Pacemaker modes

The mode of a pacemaker indicates its functions. Several different modes may be used during pacing. Here are three of the more commonly used modes and their three-letter abbreviations. (A three-letter code, rather than a five-letter code, is typically used to describe pacemaker function.) Pacemaker rates vary by age (see *Pediatric pacemakers*) and other patient characteristics.

AAI mode

The AAI, or atrial demand, pacemaker is a single-chambered pacemaker that paces and senses the right atrium. When the pacemaker senses intrinsic atrial activity, it inhibits pacing and resets itself. If it does not sense intrinsic atrial activity, it paces. Only the atria are sensed and paced.

Not in block

Because an AAI pacemaker requires a healthy and functioning AV node (AVN) and resulting consistent ventricular conduction, it isn't used in AVB. An AAI pacemaker may be used in patients with sinus bradycardia, as after heart transplant, or with sick sinus syndrome as long as the His–Purkinje system isn't diseased.

VVI mode

The VVI, or ventricular demand, pacemaker paces and senses the ventricles. (See *AAI and VVI pacemakers*, page 199.) When it senses intrinsic ventricular activity, it inhibits pacing. This single-chambered pacemaker benefits patients with complete heart block and those needing rare or less frequent pacing. Because it doesn't affect atrial activity, it may be used for patients with a temporary pacemaker (e.g., postcardiac surgery) who don't need an atrial kick. Atrial kick provides up to a 30% of cardiac output that comes from atrial contraction. The VVI mode is also common for patients with a permanent pacemaker who have long-standing persistent atrial fibrillation.

Ages and stages

Pediatric pacemakers

Many young children don't have AVB. Therefore, they may receive a single-chamber atrial pacemaker. The pulses per minute are initially set at an appropriate rate for the child's age. As the child grows, the HR can be adjusted to a lower rate.

AAI and VVI pacemakers

AAI and VVI pacemakers are single-chamber pacemakers. Typically, the pacing electrode for an AAI is placed in the right atrium and in a pacing lead in the right ventricle for a VVI pacemaker. These rhythm strips show how each pacemaker works.

AAI pacemaker

Note how the AAI pacemaker senses and paces the atria only. Each spike is immediately followed by a P-wave complex, depicting consistent capture. The QRS complex that follows occurs as a result of the heart's own AV conduction.

Each atrial spike…

…is followed by a P wave (atrial depolarization).

The QRS complex results from normal conduction.

VVI pacemaker

The VVI pacemaker senses and paces the ventricles. Each spike is immediately followed by a wide QRS complex, depicting consistent capture. When all QRS complexes are preceded by a spike, as shown here, the rhythm is said to reflect 100% pacing.

Each ventricular spike…

…is followed by a QRS complex (ventricular depolarization).

Unsynchronized activity

If the patient has spontaneous atrial activity, the VVI pacemaker won't synchronize the ventricular activity with it. So, there will be no relationship between the P waves and paced QRS complexes, and tricuspid and mitral regurgitation may develop. Sedentary patients who don't require the atrial kick, or patients with atrial fibrillation, may receive this type of pacemaker.

DDD mode

A DDD pacemaker is used with AVB. Annual incidence of AVB development in people with SND is about 1% to 5%. Therefore, some patients with SND get a dual-chamber pacemaker. (See *DDD pacemaker rhythm strip.*) However, because the pacemaker possesses so many capabilities, it may be hard to troubleshoot problems. Its advantages include its:

* versatility
* programmability

DDD pacemaker rhythm strip

This DDD pacemaker rhythm strip reveals how this pacemaker ensures AV synchrony.

In the atrium: The pacemaker paces in the atrium if it does not sense an intrinsic P wave at a certain beats per minute (bpm) rate, as in beats 6, 9, 11, and 13. Therefore, a paced P wave should and does follow the atrial spike. Sensed P waves cause withholding of pacing in the atrium as in beats 1, 2, 3, 4, and 7. When the patient has an intrinsic P wave, the pacemaker serves only to make sure the ventricles respond.

In the ventricle: The pacemaker paces in the ventricle if it does not sense an intrinsic QRS complex in the ventricle, as in beats 1, 4, 6, 7, 9, and 11. Sensed QRS complexes cause withholding of pacing in the ventricle as in beats 2, 3, 5, 8, 10, and 12.

As you can see, there are several different possible ECG scenarios: AV-paced (e.g., beat 6), AV-sensed (e.g., beat 2), A-paced and V-sensed (e.g., beat 13), and A-sensed and V-paced (e.g., beat 4). This ECG strip has all four possibilities in one strip. However, patients typically have one or two scenarios in one strip, for example, a patient in sinus rhythm with only a very rare, paced beat.

Also of note, these ventricularly paced beats have a QRS complex that is narrower than right ventricularly paced beats. This may be because of pacing lead position (e.g., left ventricular or His bundle pacing) or a QRS complex that is a result of fusion between ventricular pacing and an inherent beat.

The pacemaker is pacing the ventricles only.

This is the patient's own ventricular depolarization.

The pacemaker is pacing both the atria and the ventricles.

- ability to provide a more physiologic cardiac cycle than VVI pacing by pacing the ventricles following atrial activity (P waves) but not above the set maximal rate limit
- ability to change modes automatically. DDD pacemakers can be programmed in an AAI mode that automatically switches to DDD when a P wave is not conducted to the ventricles. This is advantageous for patients with intermittent loss of AV conduction because intrinsic AV conduction, as used in AAI mode, is more physiologic than dual-chamber pacing. However, a patient with AVN disease would not receive a pacemaker that only paces in the atrium. Pacemakers can also automatically change to a nontracking mode if the atrial rate goes too high, as in atrial fibrillation.

Home, home on the rate range

Unlike other pacemakers, the DDD pacemaker is set with a rate range, rather than a single critical rate. It senses atrial activity and ensures that the ventricles track or respond to each atrial stimulation up to an upper ventricular rate limit, thereby maintaining normal AV synchrony. A typical rate range is from 60 to 120 bpm. This causes pacing in the atrium once the atrial rate falls below 60. The ventricles will track (be paced after each P wave) if there is no sensed QRS complex, up to 120 bpm. A pacemaker can't stop a heart's intrinsic conduction. Therefore, even though a pacemaker's upper rate may be 120, the patient's HR may well exceed 120 bpm when there is intact intrinsic AV conduction.

Taking the low road

The DDD pacemaker paces (sometimes referred to as "fires") in the atria when the atrial rate falls below the lower set rate. If the ventricles don't respond to an atrial event, the pacemaker will pace the ventricles. (See *Evaluating a DDD pacemaker rhythm strip.*) You or the telemetry monitor may calculate the HR by averaging 6 or 10 seconds. However, the pacemaker calculates the HR between two consecutive beats. Therefore, although you or a monitor may average the HR as being 60 or higher, the pacemaker will pace if the patient's intrinsic rate is 59 between two consecutive beats.

Taking the high road

The upper set rate acts as a safety mechanism by preventing the pacemaker from following (or tracking) an atrial tachyarrhythmia, such as atrial fibrillation, atrial tachycardia, or atrial flutter. That upper rate limit is usually set at 120 or 130 bpm. One's AVN would normally block the approximate 500 atrial bpm during atrial fibrillation from passing to the ventricle. The AVN is bypassed with a pacemaker, making the upper rate limit necessary with a DDD pacemaker.

Evaluating a DDD pacemaker rhythm strip

Look for these possible events when examining a rhythm strip showing the activities of a DDD pacemaker:
- Intrinsic rhythm—No pacemaker activity occurs because none is needed.
- Intrinsic P wave followed by a ventricular pacemaker spike—The pacemaker is tracking the atrial rate and ensuring a ventricular response.
- Pacemaker spike before a P wave, then an intrinsic ventricular QRS complex—The atrial rate is falling below the lower rate limit, causing the atrial channel to fire. Normal conduction to the ventricles then ensues.
- Pacemaker spike before a P wave and a pacemaker spike before the QRS complex—No intrinsic activity above the lower rate limit occurs in either the atria or the ventricles.

Evaluating pacemakers

Now you're ready to find out if your patient's pacemaker is working correctly. To do this, follow the following procedures.

Read the records

First, determine the pacemaker's mode and settings, particularly the rate setting. If your patient had a permanent pacemaker implanted before admission, ask them whether they have a wallet card from the manufacturer that notes which generator and pacing leads were implanted. It is important to note full details of the device and all leads, which are also important to assess for magnetic resonance imaging (MRI) compatibility at a later date, if needed (the device may be compatible and the leads may not or vice versa).

If the pacemaker was recently implanted, check the patient's records for information. It's imperative to check the ECG tracing and interrogate the device—you might misinterpret the ECG if you don't know the mode or which pacing leads the patient has.

Look at the 12-lead ECG

Next, review the patient's 12-lead ECG. If it isn't available, examine lead V_1 or MCL_1 on telemetry. If there is only one ventricular lead, it is usually in the right ventricle. Therefore, expect a negatively deflected paced QRS complex in V_1 or MCL_1, just as with a left bundle branch block. An upright QRS complex in V_1 or MCL_1 may mean that the pacing lead is out of position, perhaps even perforating the septum and lodging in the left ventricle, or that there is a properly positioned pacing lead in the coronary sinus vein. When the His bundle is paced, the QRS complex should be narrow.

Scrutinize the spikes

Then select a monitoring lead that clearly shows the pacemaker spikes. Some monitors have a filter or bandwidth menu that allows adjustment for seeing larger pacemaker spikes. **Make sure to use the "paced mode" on the telemetry monitor.** If the monitor doesn't "know" it's looking at a rhythm that may have pacemaker spikes, it can interpret a pacemaker spike as a QRS complex. Therefore, a pacemaker spike that is not followed by a QRS complex without the "paced mode" on will NOT cause an important alarm.

Mull over the mode

When looking at the ECG tracing of a patient with a pacemaker, consider the pacemaker mode. Then interpret the paced rhythm. Does it match what you know about the pacemaker?

Unravel the rhythm

Look for information that tells you which chamber is paced. Is there a capture? Is there a P wave or QRS complex after each atrial or ventricular spike?, Or do the P waves and QRS complexes stem from intrinsic activity?

Look for information about the pacemaker's sensing ability. Do you see spikes where you wouldn't expect them—like within or too close after a P wave or QRS complex? Remember if the pacemaker is sensing the electricity causing the P waves and QRS complexes, it should withhold a spike. Look at the rate. What's the pacing rate per minute? Is it appropriate given the pacemaker's upper and lower rate settings? Although you can determine the rate quickly by counting the number of complexes in a 6-second ECG strip, a more accurate method is to count the number of small boxes between two complexes and divide this into 1,500.

Troubleshooting problems

Pacemaker malfunction can lead to arrhythmias and/or loss of AV synchrony. (See *When a temporary pacemaker malfunctions*, page 204.) If you see questionable pacemaker activity for a patient with a permanent pacemaker, call the cardiology or cardiac electrophysiology team. There are actions you should take for patients with temporary pacemakers who have questionable pacemaker activity. Pacemaker problems that can lead to low cardiac output, hypotension, syncope, and death include:

- failure to capture
- failure to pace
- undersensing
- oversensing.

Failure to capture

Failure to capture is indicated on an ECG by a pacemaker spike without the appropriate atrial or ventricular response—a spike without a complex. Think of failure to capture as the pacemaker's inability to stimulate the chamber to contract.

Mixed signals

When a temporary pacemaker malfunctions

Occasionally, pacemakers fail to function properly. When that happens, you need to take immediate action to correct the problem. The following strips are examples of problems that can occur with a temporary pacemaker and corrective actions to take in response.

Failure to capture

- If the patient's condition has changed, notify the practitioner and ask for new settings. Be prepared to initiate cardiopulmonary resuscitation (CPR) if needed.
- If pacemaker settings have been altered by the patient or someone else, return them to their correct positions. If the pacemaker has dials, make sure the face of the pacemaker is covered with its plastic shield and remind the patient not to touch the dials.
- If the heart still doesn't respond, carefully check all connections. You can also increase the milliampere setting slowly (according to your facility's policy or the practitioner's orders), turn the patient from side to side, or change the battery. Keep in mind that the practitioner may order a chest X-ray to determine the position of the pacing lead.

Failure to pace

- If the pacing light is flashing, check the connections to the cable and the patient. The position of the pacing lead in the patient may need to be repositioned (usually under fluoroscopy).
- If the pulse generator is turned on but the indicators aren't flashing, change the battery. If that doesn't help, use a different pulse generator.
- Decrease the sensitivity by increasing the millivolts. The pacemaker may be inhibiting pacing because of oversensing electrical activity from another heart chamber, muscle, or external source.
- Make sure a transcutaneous pacemaker, isoproterenol, and atropine are available in case the patient's HR drops. Be prepared to initiate CPR if needed.

Failure to sense intrinsic beats

- If the pacemaker is undersensing (it fires but at the wrong times or for the wrong reasons), put the sensitivity control to a smaller number.
- Change the battery or pulse generator.
- Remove items in the room that might cause electromechanical interference. Check if the bed is grounded. Unplug each piece of equipment and then check to see if the interference stops.
- If the pacemaker still fires on the T wave, turn off the pacemaker (per facility policy or practitioner's order). Make sure isoproterenol, atropine, and transcutaneous pacemaker are available in case the patient's HR drops, and be prepared to initiate CPR if needed.

There is a pacemaker spike but no response from the heart.

A pacemaker spike should appear here but doesn't.

Undersensing causing inappropriate early pacing, R-on-T, and VT.

V pacing

Intrinsic QRSs

Causes include hypoxia, acidosis, an electrolyte imbalance, fibrosis, an incorrect lead position, a low pacing output setting (milliampere with temporary pacemakers and volts with permanent pacemakers), depletion of the battery, a broken or cracked pacing lead, or perforation of the pacing lead through the myocardium. It can lead to lightheadedness, hypotension, or asystole.

Failure to pace

Failure to pace is indicated by no pacemaker activity or spike at the set rate on an ECG. The problem is caused by battery or circuit failure, cracked or broken pacing leads, loose connections, oversensing, or the pacing output set too low. It can also lead to lightheadedness, hypotension, or asystole.

Undersensing

Undersensing is demonstrated by a pacemaker spike when intrinsic cardiac activity is already present. Undersensing causes the pacemaker to fire even if intrinsic electricity is present. Think of it as help being given when none is needed. With undersensing, spikes occur on the ECG where they shouldn't. Although they may appear in any part of the cardiac cycle, the spikes are especially dangerous with a temporary pacemaker if they fall on the T wave. This can cause "R-on-T," resulting in VT, ventricular fibrillation, or torsades de pointes. The output of a temporary pacemaker is much higher than that of a permanent pacemaker. Therefore, undersensing with a temporary pacemaker as opposed to a permanent pacemaker can lead to a fatal arrhythmia. With a permanent pacemaker, the unneeded pacing would most likely result in early battery depletion.

The problem can be caused by millivoltage set too high, electrolyte imbalances, disconnection or dislodgment of a lead, improper pacing lead placement, edema or fibrosis at the electrode tip, drug interactions, or a depleted or dead pacemaker battery.

Oversensing

If the pacemaker is too sensitive, it can misinterpret other electricity as the heart's electricity and, therefore, withhold pacing. This extraneous electricity can be from myopotentials from nearby muscle movement, electrical events in a different chamber, electricity from nongrounded items, or certain equipment that have a strong magnetic or electrical field. You should wear rubber gloves when handling exposed temporary pacing wires. This will prevent you from transmitting electrical current from static or ungrounded equipment to the patient. Likewise, temporary pacing wires should be covered with something nonconductive, like the finger of a rubber glove. Oversensing causes inhibition of pacing when the patient actually needs it. The HR, AV synchrony, and cardiac output won't be maintained. This can cause asystole, hypotension, lightheadedness, and/or syncope.

Memory jogger

Malfunction of a pacemaker can lead to fatal arrhythmias, hypotension, and syncope. To help you remember common pacemaker problems, think "failure times two, under, over":

Failure to capture—spike without a P wave or QRS complex following it

Failure to pace—no spike on ECG at the rate set

Undersensing—spike when intrinsic activity is already present

Oversensing—no spike when the patient needs it

How you intervene

Make sure you're familiar with different types and modes of pacemakers and how they function. This will save you time and worry during an emergency. When caring for a patient with a pacemaker, follow these guidelines.

Checks and balances

Temporary pacemakers

- Assist with pacemaker insertion as appropriate.
- Regularly check the patient's pacemaker settings, connections, and functions.
- Reposition the patient carefully. Turning may dislodge the pacing wire.
- Avoid potential microshocks to the patient by ensuring that electrical equipment is grounded properly, including the patient's bed.

All pacemakers

- Remember that pacemaker spikes on the monitor don't mean there is capture or that your patient is stable. Be sure to check the vital signs and assess for signs and symptoms of decreased cardiac output, such as hypotension, chest pain, dyspnea, lightheadedness, and syncope.
- Turn the telemetry monitor's "paced mode" on.
- Monitor the patient to see how well they tolerate the pacemaker.

On the alert

- Be alert for signs of local and/or systemic infection.
- Look for pectoral or diaphragmatic muscle twitching or hiccups that occur in synchrony with the pacemaker. Both are signs of stimulation of a structure other than the heart, which may be serious. Notify the practitioner if you note either condition.
- Watch for a perforated ventricle and cardiac tamponade. Signs and symptoms include persistent hiccups, distant heart sounds, pulsus paradoxus (a drop in the strength of a pulse or a drop in systolic blood pressure greater than 10 mm Hg during inspiration), hypotension with narrowed pulse pressure, cyanosis, distended jugular veins, decreased urine output, restlessness, and complaints of fullness in the chest. Notify the practitioner immediately if you note any of these signs and symptoms.
- Watch for pneumothorax signs and symptoms, including shortness of breath, restlessness, and hypoxia. Mental status changes and arrhythmias may also occur. Palpate for subcutaneous air, which feels crunchy under your fingers, around the pacemaker

insertion site. Auscultate for diminished breath sounds over the pneumothorax, usually at the apex of the lung on the side where the pacemaker was placed. Notify the practitioner if you suspect pneumothorax.

- Assess the area around the incision and report swelling, tenderness, drainage, redness, unusual warmth, or hematoma. Patients on anticoagulation or antiplatelet therapy are at higher risk of bleeding at the insertion site, which increases the chances of infection.

What to teach the patient and significant other(s)

Temporary pacemakers:
- Explain why a pacemaker is needed, how it works, and what they can expect.
- Warn the patient with a temporary pacemaker not to get out of bed without assistance.
- Explain that a transcutaneous pacemaker causes twitching of the pectoral muscles. Reassure that you will be asking the patient if medication is desired for the discomfort.
- Instruct the patient not to manipulate the temporary pacemaker wires or pulse generator; and not to "fiddle" with the implanted generator, as this can lead to dislodgement of or damage to the leads.

Permanent pacemakers: In addition to explaining need, function, and expectations, give patients with permanent pacemakers the following:
- Teach how to care for the incision. Advise the patient to avoid tight clothing or other direct pressure over the pulse generator. The patient should observe the incision daily and notify the health care practitioner of redness or other signs of infection, including purulence or fever.
- Give the patient the manufacturer's identification card and tell them to carry it at all times. They should show it to airport or law enforcement personnel as to avoid walking through strong metal detectors or handheld wands used by these staff.
- Inform the patient that they may want to wear a medical identification bracelet indicating that they have an implanted device in case they need medical attention and are unable to speak.
- Emphasize the importance of identifying pacemaker problems via routine remote and in-office checks. Of note, reprogramming the device can only be accomplished with an in-person visit.
- Explain the signs and symptoms of pacemaker malfunction, how to take a pulse, and what to do if any signs or symptoms exist, including notification of the health care practitioner.

- Advise the patient to avoid moving the arm on the side of the pacemaker in an extreme, exaggerated, or repetitive manner for 6 to 8 weeks or per the health care provider who cares for the permanent pacemaker.
- Advise the patient to speak to the practitioner who manages the pacemaker before having MRI, radiation therapy, surgery, or diagnostic studies. The practitioner should also be consulted before the use of power-generating equipment, equipment with antennas, or strong magnets.
- Tell the patient to follow normal routines and to increase exercise as tolerated and as allowed by the practitioner.
- Stress the importance of follow-up care and regular checkups.
- Explain that a remote monitor is frequently used in the patient's home to alert practitioners of rhythms and device function and to reduce the need for some office visits. Stress the importance of keeping the remote monitor plugged in at all times. With certain devices, the monitor is in the form of an app on a smartphone. The app needs to stay open and running in the background at all times. In addition to this, the smartphone's Bluetooth functionality must be turned on.

A look at biventricular pacemakers

Biventricular pacing is used in the treatment of some patients with class III and IV heart failure, with both systolic heart failure and intraventricular conduction delay. Also called *cardiac resynchronization therapy*, biventricular pacing reduces symptoms and improves the quality of life of patients with advanced heart failure. It also records heart failure parameters such as those indicating the amount of fluid in the chest.

Two ventricles, three leads

Unlike other pacemakers, a biventricular pacemaker usually has three leads rather than one or two: one to pace the right atrium, one to pace the right ventricle, and one to pace the left ventricle. Both ventricles are commonly either paced at the same time, or the left ventricle is paced milliseconds before the right ventricle. This causes them to contract about the same time, increasing cardiac output.

Different ventricles, different timing

Under normal conditions, the right and left ventricles contract simultaneously to pump blood to the lungs and body, respectively. However, in heart failure, the damaged ventricles can't pump as forcefully and the amount of blood ejected with each contraction is reduced. If the ventricular conduction pathways are also damaged, electrical impulses reach the ventricles at different times, producing asynchronous contractions. This condition, called *intraventricular conduction defect*, further reduces the amount of blood that the heart pumps, worsening the patient's symptoms.

An important tip

Unlike traditional lead placement, the pacing lead for the left ventricle is placed into a branch of a cardiac vein via the coronary sinus. This vein lies on the exterior of the left ventricle. The left ventricle is paced through the wall of the vein. Because this pacing lead isn't anchored in place, lead displacement may be more likely to occur. (See *Biventricular lead placement*.)

Biventricular lead placement

The biventricular pacemaker uses three leads: one usually to pace the right atrium, one to pace the right ventricle, and one to pace the left ventricle. The left ventricular lead is placed in the coronary sinus. Both ventricles are paced at about the same time, causing them to contract almost simultaneously, improving cardiac output.

Improves symptoms and quality of life

Biventricular pacing produces an improvement in the patient's symptoms and activity tolerance. Moreover, biventricular pacing improves left ventricular remodeling and diastolic function and reduces sympathetic stimulation. As a result, in many patients, the progression of heart failure is slowed and quality of life is improved.

Sympathetic response

To compensate for reduced cardiac output, the sympathetic nervous system releases neurohormones, such as aldosterone, norepinephrine, and vasopressin, to boost the amount of blood ejected with each contraction. The resultant tachycardia and vasoconstriction increase the heart's demand for oxygen, reduce diastolic filling time, promote sodium and water retention, and increase the pressure that the heart must pump against. The effect on the patient is a worsening of symptoms. Resynchronization therapy can reduce symptoms of heart failure, decrease hospitalizations and morbidity, and improve quality of life.

Who's a candidate?

Not all patients with heart failure benefit from biventricular pacing. Candidates should have both systolic heart failure and intraventricular conduction delay along with the following characteristics:
- Symptomatic heart failure despite maximal medical therapy
- Moderate-to-severe heart failure (New York Heart Association class III or IV)
- QRS complex greater than 0.13 seconds
- Left ventricular ejection fraction (EF) of 35% or less.

Many patients who meet criteria for biventricular pacing also meet criteria for a defibrillator. Therefore, patients having defibrillators with biventricular pacing (biventricular implantable cardioverter-defibrillator [ICD]) is very common.

Caring for the patient

Provide the same basic care for the patient with a biventricular pacemaker that you would for a patient with a standard permanent pacemaker. Specific care includes the following guidelines:
- Before the procedure, ask the patient if they have an allergy to iodine or shellfish because contrast medium is used to visualize

the coronary sinus and veins. Notify the practitioner if an allergy exists.

- Because of the position of the left ventricular lead, watch for stimulation of the diaphragm and left chest wall. Ask patients if they feel any thumping in or on their chest. Notify the practitioner if this occurs because the left ventricular pacing lead output or configuration may need to be reprogrammed or the left ventricular lead may need repositioning.
- Observe the ECG for pacemaker spikes. Although both ventricles are paced, usually only one ventricular pacemaker spike is seen.
- Note the presence of positive R waves in lead V_1 and negative R waves in leads I and aVL. Notify the practitioner if this isn't the case or if the R-wave direction changes at any time.

What to teach the patient

Provide the same basic teaching that you would for the patient receiving a permanent pacemaker. In addition, when a patient gets a biventricular pacemaker, be sure to cover the following points:

- Explain to the patient and their family why a biventricular pacemaker is needed, how it works, and what they can expect. Include that it can take 6 months for a patient to notice heart failure symptom improvement and that heart failure medications are still necessary.
- Tell the patient and their family that it's sometimes difficult to place the left ventricular lead and that the procedure can take 4 hours or more.
- Stress the importance of calling the practitioner immediately if the patient develops chest pain, shortness of breath, swelling of the hands or feet, or a weight gain of 3 lb (1.4 kg) in 24 hours or 5 lb (2.3 kg) in 72 hours.

A look at implantable cardioverter-defibrillators

An ICD is an electronic device implanted in the body to provide continuous monitoring of the heart for bradycardia, VT, and ventricular fibrillation. The device then administers override (antitachycardia) pacing beats or shocks to treat the dangerous arrhythmia. Implanted defibrillators are indicated for patients who have had a myocardial infarction and have an EF of 30% or less, or who have had nonsustained VT and an EF of 40% or less.

The placement and procedure for an ICD are usually similar to that of a permanent pacemaker and is usually inserted in an electrophysiology laboratory.

What it is

An ICD consists of a programmable pulse generator, a shocking lead, and one or more pacing leads. The pulse generator is a small battery-powered computer that monitors the heart's electrical signals and delivers electrical therapy when it identifies an abnormal rhythm. The leads are insulated wires that carry the heart's signal to the pulse generator and deliver the electrical energy from the pulse generator to the heart.

Subcutaneous implantable cardioverter-defibrillators

Subcutaneous ICDs (S-ICDs) have a lead wire that is subcutaneous as opposed to transvenous. The lead is parallel and just to the left of the sternum. The generator is placed in the mid- to anterior axillary line, near the sixth rib. It is larger than the traditional transvenous ICD. However, this does not make the ICD more uncomfortable to patients once the sites heal. The main advantage is less chance of complications associated with transvenous leads (e.g., bloodstream infection). S-ICDs are indicated when pacing for bradycardia, resynchronization, or antitachycardia pacing is not needed; and when transvenous lead placement would be difficult or risky, the patient is young and will need lifetime therapy, and after removal of an infected transvenous ICD system. Patients are screened for ECG morphology of sinus rhythm and VT to determine candidacy.

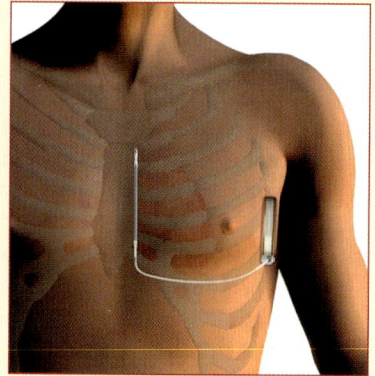

Storing and retrieving information

An ICD also stores information about the heart's activity before, during, and after an arrhythmia, along with tracking which treatment was delivered and the outcome of that treatment. Devices also store electrograms (electrical tracings similar to ECGs). With an interrogation programmer, a specially trained practitioner can retrieve information to evaluate ICD function and battery status and to adjust ICD system settings. Biventricular ICDs, like biventricular pacemakers, store information that aids in heart failure assessment.

Automatic response

Today's advanced devices can detect a wide range of arrhythmias and automatically respond with the appropriate therapy, such as brady-cardia pacing (both single and dual chamber), biventricular pacing, antitachycardia pacing, cardioversion, and defibrillation. ICDs that provide therapy for atrial arrhythmias, such as atrial fibrillation, are also available. (See *Types of ICD therapies*, page 213.) Most ICDs will temporarily pace postshock, if necessary. The S-ICD does not deliver any pacing. Those with transvenous lead wires can also function as a typical pacemaker for chronic bradycardia needs and deliver antitachycardia pacing.

Types of ICD therapies

ICDs can deliver a range of therapies depending on the arrhythmia detected and how the device is programmed. Therapies include antitachycardia pacing, cardioversion, defibrillation, biventricular pacing, and bradycardia pacing.

Therapy	Description
Antitachycardia pacing	This is usually the first line of therapy, when an ICD with lead wires detects a ventricular arrhythmia. A short series of rapid, electrical pacing pulses are used to interrupt monomorphic VT and return the heart to its normal rhythm. This pain-free therapy usually effectively terminates VT.

Therapy	Description
Cardioversion	A low- or high-energy shock (up to 41 J) is timed to the R wave to terminate VT and return the heart to its normal rhythm.
Defibrillation	A high-energy shock (up to 41 J) to the heart is used to terminate ventricular fibrillation and return the heart to its normal rhythm.
Bradycardia pacing	Electrical pacing pulses are used when the heart's natural electrical signals are too slow. ICD systems can pace in any way that a pacemaker can pace, including biventricular pacing.

How it's programmed

When caring for a patient with an ICD, it's important to know how the device is programmed. This information is available through a status report that can be obtained and printed when the specially trained practitioner interrogates the device. This involves placing a small piece of equipment on the skin, over the implanted pulse generator, to retrieve information. The stored information helps to evaluate any arrhythmias that the device was programmed to store, any therapy delivered, and the device function.

Program information includes:
- type and model of the ICD
- status of the arrhythmia detection device and therapy (on or off)
- HRs and ECG morphology that result in a detected arrhythmia
- therapies that will be delivered: bradycardia pacing, antitachycardia pacing, cardioversion, and defibrillation.

Arresting developments

Follow the following guidelines if your patient experiences an arrhythmia:

- If the patient experiences cardiac arrest, initiate CPR and advanced cardiac life support.
- If the ICD delivers a shock while you're performing chest compressions, you may also feel a slight shock. Wear gloves to prevent you from feeling the shock.
- Externally defibrillating the patient is safe as long as the paddles aren't placed directly over the pulse generator. The anteroposterior pad position is preferred.

Be alert

Provide the same basic care for the patient with an ICD that you would for a patient with a permanent pacemaker. Frequently, patients who are biventricularly paced also have an ICD. Specific care for patients with ICDs includes the following:

- Monitor the patient's rhythm for antitachycardia pacing or shocks.
- Patients post-ICD implant may be more sedated than postpacemaker because of the anesthesia administered so the patient does not feel or remember any testing shocks.
- Put the telemetry monitor in "paced mode." All ICDs are programmed to pace once the patient's own HR gets below the programmed set HR, for example, 40 bpm.

What to teach the patient

- Explain to the patient and their family why an ICD is needed, how it works, potential complications, and what they can expect. Make sure they also understand ICD terminology.
- Discuss signs and symptoms to report to the practitioner immediately.
- Explain actions the patient should take if they receive a shock with and without symptoms or get multiple shocks. For example, call their cardiologist when they receive a shock and call 911 if they feel ill after a shock or get sequential shocks.
- Educate family members in emergency techniques (such as dialing 911 and performing CPR) in case the device fails to restore circulation.
- Advise patients to speak with their physician before operating a transport vehicle (e.g., car, bus, plane).

A look at radiofrequency ablation

Radiofrequency ablation is an invasive procedure that may be used to treat arrhythmias in patients who haven't responded to antiarrhythmic drugs or cardioversion or can't tolerate antiarrhythmic drugs. In this procedure, bursts of radiofrequency energy are delivered through a catheter to the heart tissue to destroy the focus of the arrhythmia or block its conduction pathway.

> With radiofrequency ablation, a burst of energy is sent right to the part of me that's causing or supporting the arrhythmia.

Who's a candidate?

Radiofrequency ablation is commonly used in treating patients with atrial tachycardia, atrial fibrillation, atrial flutter, AV nodal reentry tachycardia (AVNRT), inappropriate sinus tachycardia, bypass tracts like Wolff–Parkinson–White (WPW) syndrome, VT, and frequent premature ventricular contractions.

Understanding the procedure

The patient first undergoes an electrophysiology study to identify and map the specific areas of the heart that cause or support the arrhythmia. The ablation catheters are inserted into a vein, usually the femoral vein, and advanced into the heart where short bursts of radiofrequency waves destroy small, targeted areas of heart tissue. The destroyed tissue can no longer conduct electrical impulses. Other types of energy may also be used, such as microwave, sonar, or cryo (freezing).

Hitting the target

Arrhythmias can be categorized by being either focal or reentrant. Examples of focal arrhythmias include atrial tachycardia, inappropriate sinus tachycardia, premature atrial contractions, and right or left ventricular outflow tract VT. The arrhythmia originates from one spot or foci. Reentrant arrhythmias include VT (other than outflow tract), atrial fibrillation, AVNRT, and accessory pathways like WPW syndrome.

WPW is typically a congenital rhythm disorder occurring mainly in young children and adults aged 20 to 35 years. In WPW, an extra conduction pathway develops outside the AV junction and connects the atria with the ventricles. The accessory pathway of impulse conducts through a bypass known as the *bundle of Kent*. Since impulses aren't delayed in the AVN, conduction occurs abnormally fast. Retrograde conduction, circus reentry, and reentrant tachycardia can result in conduction pathways that interfere with each other and may cause lightheadedness, syncope, palpitations, shortness of breath, and cardiac arrest.

Reentrant arrhythmias are supported by abnormal conduction that is typically in a continuous circular path or circuit. Radiofrequency ablation is used to either destroy the source of a focal tachycardia or block the abnormal pathway of the reentrant conduction circuit. (See *Destroying the source or the circuit.*)

Destroying the source or the circuit

In radiofrequency ablation, special catheters are inserted into a vein and advanced to the heart. After the type and source of the arrhythmia are identified, radiofrequency energy is used to either (1) ablate focal tissue or (2) interrupt or isolate a reentry path or circuit. The following illustrations demonstrate two types of catheter ablation.

Sinus node modification

A focal arrhythmia, inappropriate sinus tachycardia, is characterized by a sinus rate out of proportion to physiologic need. It is treated with a sinus node modification in which tissue in the sinus node is destroyed until the desired HR is achieved.

SA node

Radiofrequency catheter

Right atrium

AV node

Radiofrequency energy is used to destroy selected tissue in the SA node.

Atrial fibrillation ablation

In most patients with atrial fibrillation, the tissue inside the pulmonary veins is the source of the arrhythmia. Ablation within the pulmonary veins would cause pulmonary vein stenosis. Therefore, radiofrequency energy is used to destroy the tissue encircling the pulmonary veins to block the path of the abnormal impulses from exiting the pulmonary veins and traveling into the atria and ventricles. Hence, this procedure is commonly referred to as *pulmonary vein isolation*. Other sites within the right and left atria can also targeted. Although some believe that atrial fibrillation may be because of many reentrant circuits, the mechanism is still not understood.

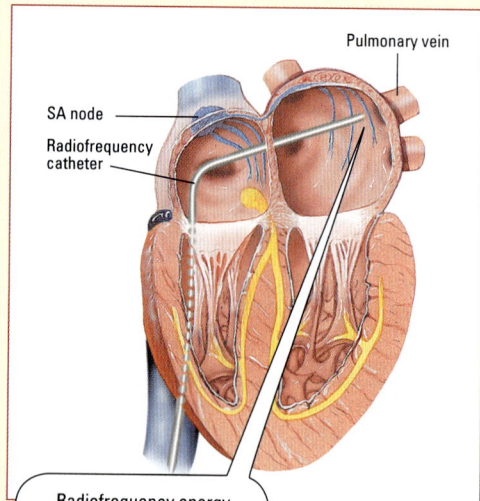

Pulmonary vein

SA node

Radiofrequency catheter

Radiofrequency energy is used to destroy the tissue where the atrium connects to the pulmonary vein.

If a rapid arrhythmia originates above the AVN, the bundle of His in the AVN may be purposefully damaged with ablation to block impulses from reaching the ventricles. This may be done to control the ventricular rate for patients whose intolerable atrial rhythm can't be converted to sinus with chemical or electrical cardioversion or ablation. A permanent pacemaker would be necessary in tandem with this ablation. In addition, anticoagulation therapy may be needed to reduce the risk of stroke.

If the patient has an accessory pathway as in WPW syndrome, electrophysiology studies are used to locate the accessory pathway and ablation can destroy the circuit.

After an ablation, one's HR and/or rhythm should return to normal. Thus, ablation can prevent tachycardia-mediated cardiomyopathy and may restore ventricular pumping function that has been damaged by the effects of prolonged tachycardia. Some ablations can be lifesaving, such as VT ablations.

How you intervene

When caring for a patient after radiofrequency ablation, follow the following guidelines:

- Provide continuous cardiac monitoring, assessing for arrhythmias and ischemic changes.
- Place the patient on bed rest as ordered and keep the affected extremity straight. For example, when a figure-of-eight suture is used, the patients usually remain flat for 4 hours after the suture is placed. Maintain the head of the bed between 15 and 30 degrees.
- Assess the patient's vital signs every 15 minutes for the first hour, then every 30 minutes for 4 hours, unless the patient's condition warrants more frequent checking.
- Assess peripheral pulses distal to the catheter insertion site as well as the color, sensation, temperature, and capillary refill of the affected extremity.
- Check the catheter insertion site for pain, bleeding, bruit, and hematoma formation.
- Medicate for pericardial discomfort.
- Monitor the patient for complications, such as hemorrhage, retroperitoneal bleed, access site hematoma or pseudoaneurysm, stroke, perforation of the heart, cardiac tamponade, phrenic or vagus nerve damage, pericarditis, atrial–esophageal fistula, pulmonic vein stenosis, heart failure, thrombosis, arrhythmias, and sudden death.

Caring for the patient after radiofrequency ablation requires specific guidelines as discussed here.

What to teach the patient

When a patient undergoes radiofrequency ablation, be sure to cover the following points:

- Discuss with the patient and their family why radiofrequency ablation is needed, how it works, and what they can expect.
- Warn the patient and their family that the procedure can be lengthy: an average of 6 hours.
- Explain that the patient may be hospitalized for 24 hours to monitor their heart rhythm and monitor and/or remove intravascular and potential pericardial fluid.
- Advise the patient to continue prescribed medication exactly as directed, especially anticoagulation for stroke prevention. Postdischarge calls to patients can confirm this.
- Have the patient (1) return and demonstrate taking their pulse, (2) describe what an irregular, fast, or slow pulse feels like, and (3) state actions to take with an abnormal pulse.
- Advise the patient to call the team who performed the ablation with any signs or symptoms of complications, such as shortness of breath or edema caused by fluid overload. An extremely rare but often fatal complication of atrial fibrillation ablation is an atrial–esophageal fistula that can cause hemoptysis, fever, malaise, or dysphagia.
- Explain the rationale for temporary limitations per the cardiology team, such as in driving, upper endoscopy, or vigorous activity.
- Provide implanted device teaching if the patient had a pacemaker or ICD inserted. (For more information about pacemaker teaching, see *What to teach the patient and significant other(s)*, page 207.)

Subcutaneous ICD

- Subcutaneous system that defibrillates VT and ventricular fibrillation
- Main advantage is avoidance of vascular access and associated complications.
- Patients must meet selection criteria prior to implant: ECG morphology and no need for bradycardia pacing, antitachycardia pacing, or resynchronization therapy.

That's a wrap!

Nonpharmacologic treatments review

Pacemaker
- A device that electrically stimulates the myocardium to depolarize

Atrial and ventricular stimulation
- *Atrial only:* Spike followed by a P wave and the patient's intrinsic QRS complex and T wave
- *Ventricular only:* Patient's intrinsic atrial rhythm, then a spike followed by a QRS complex and T wave
- *Atrial and ventricular:* First spike followed by a P wave, then a second spike, followed by QRS complex

Pacemaker codes
- The first letter identifies the heart chambers being paced.
- The second letter signifies the heart chamber sensed by the pacemaker.
- The third letter refers to the pacemaker's response to the intrinsic electrical activity of the heart.
- The fourth letter refers to the pacemaker's rate modulation.
- The fifth letter refers to the pacemaker's location or absence of multisite pacing.

Pacemaker modes
- AAI = Single-chamber pacemaker; paces and senses the atria
- VVI = Single-chamber pacemaker; paces and senses the ventricle(s)
- DDD = Dual-chamber pacemaker; paces when the atria or ventricles don't respond on its own; paces the atria when the atrial rate falls below the lower set rate; senses and paces both the atria and the ventricles

Evaluating pacemakers
- Determine the pacemaker's mode and settings.
- Review the patient's 12-lead ECG.
- Select a monitoring lead that clearly shows the pacemaker spikes. Adjust the ECG monitor filter or bandwidth if necessary and if possible.
- Select paced mode to prevent missed alarms for noncapture.
- Interpret the paced rhythm.
- Look for information that tells which chamber is paced and about the pacemaker's sensing ability.

Troubleshooting pacemakers
- Failure to capture: Indicated by a spike without a complex
- Failure to pace: No spike
- Undersensing: Spikes where they don't belong
- Oversensing: No spike when the patient actually needs it

Leadless pacemaker
- Paces the right ventricle only
- Indicated for some patients with high-grade AVB or SND with atrial fibrillation; and when implant of an atrial lead would be difficult or unnecessary

Biventricular pacemaker
- Pacemaker usually has three leads: one to pace the right atrium, one to pace the right ventricle, and one to pace the left ventricle.
- Both ventricles contract in synchrony, increasing cardiac output.

Nonpharmacologic treatments review *(continued)*

Candidates

For treatment of patients with:
- class III and IV heart failure, with both systolic failure and ventricular dyssynchrony
- symptomatic heart failure despite maximal medical therapy
- QRS complex greater than 0.13 seconds
- left ventricular EF of 35% or less

Benefits of biventricular pacing
- Improves symptoms, activity tolerance, and quality of life
- Reverses left ventricular remodeling and diastolic function and reduces sympathetic stimulation

His bundle pacing
- The right ventricular lead is placed in the right atrium next to the His–Purkinje network. This allows for depolarization of both ventricles via a normal conduction pathway, resulting in more physiologic conduction.
- Paced QRS complexes on ECG should be narrow.

Radiofrequency ablation
- Invasive procedure that uses radiofrequency energy to destroy heart tissue or conduction pathway responsible for arrhythmia
- Useful for atrial tachycardia, atrial fibrillation, and flutter; VT; premature ventricular contractions; AVNRT; inappropriate sinus tachycardia; and WPW syndrome

Types of ablation
- Reentrant: Atrial fibrillation ablation (also known as pulmonary vein isolation), VT ablation, and accessory pathway ablation
- Focal: His bundle ablation (with pacemaker insertion), atrial tachycardia ablation, and sinus node modification

Implantable cardioverter-defibrillator
- Implanted device that monitors for bradycardia, VT, and ventricular fibrillation
- Provides pacing for bradycardia, and pacing and shocks to break arrhythmias

Types of therapy
- *Antitachycardia pacing:* Bursts of pacing to interrupt VT
- *Cardioversion:* Shock synchronized to the R wave to terminate VT
- *Defibrillation:* Asynchronized shock to terminate ventricular fibrillation
- *Bradycardia pacing:* Pacing when the HR is below the rate set

Programming information
- Type and model
- Status of tachyarrhythmia therapy (on or off)
- Recorded arrhythmias
- Therapies to be delivered

Quick quiz

1. When using a transcutaneous temporary pacemaker, the energy level should be set at:
    A.   the highest milliampere setting the patient can tolerate.
    B.   10% above the milliampere needed for consistent capture of the myocardium.
    C.   a milliampere setting midway between the setting that causes capture of the myocardium and the setting at which symptoms first appear.
    D.   the milliampere setting that provides an HR of 80 bpm.

Answer: B. Determine the minimum amount of milliamperes required to capture the myocardium (threshold). Then set the milliampere output at 10% above the threshold. This should ensure capture under stressed physiologic conditions while keeping the possibly painful pacing stimuli at a minimum.

2. Failure to capture is represented on the ECG as:
    A.   no pacemaker activity.
    B.   spikes where they shouldn't be.
    C.   a spike on a T wave.
    D.   a spike without a complex.

Answer: D. A spike without a complex indicates the pacemaker's inability to capture or stimulate the chamber.

3. The first letter in the five-letter coding system for pacemakers identifies the:
    A.   chamber in which the pacemaker senses intrinsic activity.
    B.   heart chamber being paced.
    C.   pacemaker's response to the intrinsic electrical activity.
    D.   pacemaker's response to a tachyarrhythmia.

Answer: B. The first letter identifies the heart chamber being paced, the second letter signifies the heart chamber that senses intrinsic activity, the third letter shows the pacemaker's response to that activity, the fourth letter describes the rate modulation, and the fifth letter shows the location or absence of multisite pacing.

4. A patient with a biventricular pacemaker usually has which pacing leads? A lead for:
    A.   both ventricles only.
    B.   each atrium and each ventricle.
    C.   the right atrium and each ventricle.
    D.   both the atria and the left ventricle.

Answer: C. A biventricular pacemaker usually has three leads: one to pace the right atrium, one to pace the right ventricle, and one to pace the left ventricle.

5. After ablation of tissue in the bundle of His, the patient will need a pacemaker because:
   A. impulses can no longer be conducted from the atria to the ventricles.
   B. the sinoatrial node no longer initiates an electrical impulse.
   C. accessory pathways now conduct impulses from the atria to the ventricles.
   D. the AVN begins to fire at its intrinsic rate.

Answer: A. After His bundle ablation, a pacemaker is needed because the electrical impulses from the atria are no longer conducted through the bundle of His in the AVN to the ventricles.

6. When the device delivers a series of rapid electrical pacing pulses, the patient with an ICD receives:
   A. bradycardia pacing.
   B. defibrillation.
   C. cardioversion.
   D. antitachycardia pacing.

Answer: D. Antitachycardia pacing consists of a series of rapid electrical pacing pulses used to interrupt VT and restore normal sinus rhythm.

Test strip

Time to try out a test strip. Ready? Go!

1. In the following ECG strip, the pacemaker is pacing and sensing the ventricles with 100% capture. The mode of response can't be evaluated because of the lack of intrinsic activity. You would determine that the patient probably has a(n):
   A. VVI pacemaker.
   B. DDD pacemaker.
   C. AAI pacemaker.
   D. AOO pacemaker.

Answer: B. The patient has a DDD pacemaker. It senses atrial activity and, therefore, inhibits atrial pacing. The P wave then triggers the pacemaker to try to sense a QRS complex. Because there is no intrinsic QRS complex after the P wave, the pacemaker paces the ventricle.

Scoring

☆☆☆ If you answered all seven questions correctly, all right! You've taken the lead when it comes to nonpharmacologic treatment methods.

☆☆ If you answered six questions correctly, terrific! Keep up the good pace.

☆ If you answered fewer than six questions correctly, no sweat. Go with your impulse to reread the chapter and you're sure to do better next time.

Recommended references

Cohen, B. J., & Hull, L.A. (2019). *Memmler's structure and function of the human body* (12th ed.). Wolters Kluwer.

Ferrick, A. M., Raj, S. R., Deneke, T., Kojodjojo, P., Lopez-Cabanillas, N., Abe, H., Boveda, S., Chew, D. S., Choi, J. I., Dagres, N., Dalal, A. S., Dechert, B. E., Frazier-Mills, C. G., Gilbert, O., Han, J. K., Hewit, S., Kneeland, C., Mirza, S. D., Mittal, S., … Varosy, P. D. (2023). 2023 HRS/EHRA/APHRS/LAHRS expert consensus statement on practical management of the remote device clinic. *Journal of Arrhythmia, 39*(3), 250–302. https://doi.org/10.1002/joa3.12851

Kantharia, B. (2019). *Atrial tachycardia: Practice essentials.* http://emedicine.medscape.com/article/151456-overview

Kiehl, E. L., & Cantillon, D. J. (2016). Leadless cardiac pacing: What primary care providers and non-EP cardiologists should know. *Cleveland Clinic Journal of Medicine, 83*(11 Suppl. 2), S24–S34. https://doi.org/10.3949/ccjm.83.s2.04

Kusumoto, F. M., Bailey, K. R., Chaouki, A. S., Deshmukh, A. J., Gautam, S., Kim, R. J., Kramer, D. B., Lambrakos, L. K., Nasser, N. H., & Sorajja, D. (2018). Systematic review for the 2017 AHA/ACC/HRS guideline for management of patients with ventricular arrhythmias and the prevention of sudden cardiac death: A report of the American College of Cardiology/American Heart Association Task Force on Clinical Practice Guidelines and the Heart Rhythm Society. *Heart Rhythm, 15*(10), e253–e274. https://doi.org/10.1016/j.hrthm.2017.10.037

Kusumoto, F. M., Schoenfeld, M. H., Barrett, C., Edgerton, J. R., Ellenbogen, K. A., Gold, M. R., Goldschlager, N. F., Hamilton, R. M., Joglar, J. A., Kim, R. J., Lee, R., Marine, J. E., McLeod, C. J., Oken, K. R., Patton, K. K., Pellegrini, C. N., Selzman, K. A., Thompson, A., & Varosy, P. D. (2019). 2018 ACC/AHA/HRS guideline on the evaluation and management of patients with bradycardia and cardiac conduction delay: A report of the American College of Cardiology/American Heart Association Task Force on Clinical Practice Guidelines and the Heart Rhythm Society. *Heart Rhythm, 16*(9), e227–e279. https://doi.org/10.1016/j.hrthm.2018.10.036

Malaczynska-Rajpold, K., Elliot, M., Wijesuriya, N., Mehta, V., Wong, T., Rinaldi, C. A., & Behar, J. M. (2023). Leadless cardiac pacing: New Horizons. *Cardiology and Therapy, 12*(1), 21–33. https://doi.org/10.1007/s40119-022-00288-0

McLaughlin, M. A. (Clinical Ed.). (2018). *Cardiovascular care made incredibly visual* (3rd ed.). Wolters Kluwer.

Steffel, J. (2020). The subcutaneous ICD for prevention of sudden cardiac death: Current evidence and future directions. *Pacing and Clinical Electrophysiology: PACE, 43*(12), 1421–1427. https://doi.org/10.1111/pace.14066

Wagner, G. S., & Strauss, D. G. (2021). *Marriott's practical electrocardiology* (13th ed.). Wolters Kluwer.

Writing Group Members, January, C. T., Wann, L. S., Calkins, H., Chen, L. Y., Cigarroa, J. E., Cleveland, J. C., Jr, Ellinor, P. T., Ezekowitz, M. D., Field, M. E., Furie, K. L., Heidenreich, P. A., Murray, K. T., Shea, J. B., Tracy, C. M., & Yancy, C. W. (2019). 2019 AHA/ACC/HRS focused update of the 2014 AHA/ACC/HRS guideline for the management of patients with atrial fibrillation: A report of the American College of Cardiology/American Heart Association Task Force on Clinical Practice Guidelines and the Heart Rhythm Society. *Heart Rhythm, 16*(8), e66–e93. https://doi.org/10.1016/j.hrthm.2019.01.024

Pharmacologic treatments

Just the facts

In this chapter, you'll learn:

◆ basic details about the antiarrhythmic drug classification system (also known as the Vaughan–Williams classification system)

◆ the effects antiarrhythmics have on the cardiovascular system and other body systems

◆ administration techniques and adverse effects of antiarrhythmic drugs

◆ nursing interventions for patients on antiarrhythmic drugs

◆ patient education related to antiarrhythmic administration.

A look at antiarrhythmics

Almost half a million Americans die each year from cardiac arrhythmias; countless others suffer symptoms or lifestyle limitations. Along with other treatments, antiarrhythmic drugs can help alleviate symptoms and improve quality of life. It is important to keep in mind that all of these drugs have potential adverse effects, possibly life-threatening in nature, and must be prescribed with caution and the patients carefully monitored.

Antiarrhythmic drugs affect the movement of ions across the cell membrane and alter the electrophysiology of the cardiac cell. They're classified according to their effect on the cell's electrical activity (action potential) and their mechanism of action. (See *Antiarrhythmics and the action potential*, page 226.)

Drugs in the same class are similar in action and adverse effects. When you identify an antiarrhythmic according to its assigned classification, you'll be better able to remember its specific actions and adverse effects.

Antiarrhythmic drugs can help prolong life.

Classifying antiarrhythmics

The classification system divides antiarrhythmic drugs into four major classes. Let's take a look at each one.

Antiarrhythmics and the action potential

Each class of antiarrhythmic drugs acts, primarily, on a particular phase of the heart's action potential. Here's a run-down of the four classes of antiarrhythmics and how they affect the action potential.

Class IV drugs inhibit calcium's slow influx during phase 2, which lengthens the phase. They also depress phase 4 and lengthen phases 1 and 2.

Phase 1

Phase 2

Classes Ia, Ib, and Ic drugs reduce movement of sodium ions into the cell during phase 0.

Phase 0

Class III drugs prolong phase 3, which increases repolarization and refractoriness.

Phase 3

Phase 4

Phase 4

Class II drugs inhibit adrenergic stimulation of cardiac tissue by depressing phase 4 spontaneous depolarization and slowing sinoatrial node impulses.

Class I blocks sodium

Class I drugs cause moderate blockage of sodium ion influx into the cell during phase 0 (rapid depolarization) of the action potential, which minimizes the chance of sodium reaching its threshold potential and causing cells to depolarize. Because phase 0 is also referred to as the *sodium channel* or *fast channel*, these drugs may also be called *sodium channel blockers* or *fast channel blockers*. Drugs in this class are potentially proarrhythmic, meaning they can cause or worsen arrhythmias.

Antiarrhythmic drugs in this class are further categorized as:

- Class Ia, which prolongs conduction and repolarization (prolongs QTc interval)

- Class Ib, which slows phase 0 depolarization, doesn't affect conduction, and shortens phase 3 repolarization (shortens QTc interval)
- Class Ic, which markedly slows phase 0 depolarization and prolongs conduction, with little effect on repolarization (does not affect QT interval)

Class II blocks beta-receptors

Class II drugs block sympathetic nervous system beta-adrenergic receptors and, thereby, decrease heart rate (HR). Beta-blockers are widely used for HR control with many arrhythmias and are often the first-line of antiarrhythmic use due to their efficacy and safety profile, as well as improvement in patients' symptoms. Phase 4 depolarization is diminished, resulting in depressed sinoatrial (SA) node automaticity and increased atrial and atrioventricular (AV) nodal refractoriness, or resistance to stimulation.

Class III blocks potassium

Class III drugs are called *potassium channel blockers* because they block the movement of potassium during phase 3 of the action potential and prolong repolarization and the refractory period (prolongs QTc interval).

Class IV blocks calcium

Class IV drugs block the movement of calcium during phase 2 of the action potential. Because phase 2 is also called the *calcium channel* or the *slow channel*, drugs that affect phase 2 are also known as *calcium channel blockers* or *slow channel blockers*. These include non-dihydropyridine calcium channel blockers, such as diltiazem and verapamil. They prolong conductivity and increase the refractory period at the AV node.

Some drugs don't fit

Not all drugs fit neatly into these classifications. For example, sotalol possesses characteristics of both Class II and Class III drugs. Some drugs used to treat arrhythmias don't fit into the classification system at all, including adenosine (Adenocard), atropine, digoxin (Lanoxin), epinephrine, and magnesium sulfate. Despite these limitations, the classification system helps health care providers understand how antiarrhythmic drugs prevent and treat arrhythmias.

Drug distribution and clearance

Many patients receive antiarrhythmic drugs by intravenous (IV) bolus or infusion to improve bioavailability over the oral route of administration. The cardiovascular system then distributes the drugs throughout the body, specifically to the site of action.

Memory jogger

To help you remember the four classifications of antiarrhythmic drugs, think of the phrase "Sure Beats Picking Corn." Class I drugs block **sodium**, Class II drugs block **beta-adrenergic receptors**, Class III drugs block **potassium**, and Class IV drugs block **calcium**.

Most drugs are changed, or *biotransformed*, into active or inactive metabolites in the liver. The kidneys are the primary sites for the excretion of those metabolites. When administering these drugs, remember that patients with impaired heart, liver, or kidney function may suffer from inadequate drug effects or toxicity. (See *Drug metabolism and elimination across the lifespan.*)

Antiarrhythmics by class

Broken down by classes, the following section describes commonly used antiarrhythmic drugs. It highlights their dosages, adverse effects, and recommendations for patient care.

Class Ia antiarrhythmics

Class Ia antiarrhythmic drugs are called *sodium channel blockers.* They include quinidine (the prototype drug), procainamide, and disopyramide. These drugs reduce the excitability of the cardiac cell, have an anticholinergic effect, and decrease cardiac contractility. Because these drugs prolong the QT interval, the patient is prone to polymorphic ventricular tachycardia (VT). (See *Effects of Class Ia antiarrhythmics,* page 229.)

Quinidine

Quinidine is effective against supraventricular and ventricular arrhythmias. It is no longer commonly prescribed but was used to treat atrial fibrillation, atrial flutter, paroxysmal supraventricular tachycardia (PSVT), AV node reentrant tachycardia (AVNRT), and Wolff–Parkinson–White (WPW) syndrome.

Quinidine has more recently been studied in patients with life-threatening ventricular arrhythmias, such as idiopathic ventricular fibrillation (VF) and Brugada syndrome, and has been found to be effective.

The drug comes in several forms, including quinidine sulfate and quinidine gluconate.

How to give it

Here's how to administer quinidine:

- To convert atrial flutter or fibrillation—Give 200 mg of quinidine sulfate orally every 2 to 3 hours for five to eight doses, with subsequent daily increases until sinus rhythm is restored or toxic effects develop. NOTE: It is critical to control AV node conduction before administering quinidine, as the drug can slow the atrial rate and increase conduction over the AV node, causing rapid 1:1

Ages and stages

Drug metabolism and elimination across the lifespan

Neonates have a reduced ability to metabolize drugs because of the limited activity of liver enzymes at the time of birth. As the infant grows, drug metabolism improves. The glomerular filtration rate is also reduced at birth, causing neonates to eliminate drugs more slowly than adults.

In older patients, advancing age usually reduces the blood supply to the liver and certain liver enzymes become less active. Consequently, the liver loses some of its ability to metabolize drugs. With reduced liver function, higher drug levels remain in circulation, causing more intense drug effects and increasing the risk of drug toxicity. Because kidney function also diminishes with age, drug elimination may be impaired, resulting in increased drug levels.

Effects of Class Ia antiarrhythmics

Class Ia antiarrhythmic drugs—including drugs such as quinidine, procainamide, and disopyramide—affect the cardiac cycle in specific ways and lead to specific ECG changes, as shown on the rhythm strip. Class Ia antiarrhythmics
- block sodium influx during phase 0, which depresses the rate of depolarization
- prolong repolarization and the duration of the action potential
- lengthen the refractory period (in accessory pathways as well)
- decrease contractility.

The QRS complex is slightly widened.

The QT interval is prolonged.

conduction of atrial arrhythmias. Class II or Class IV medications are used for this purpose.
- Initial dosage for PSVT—Give 400 to 600 mg of quinidine sulfate orally every 6 hours.
- Initial dosage for premature atrial and ventricular contractions, paroxysmal AV junctional rhythm, paroxysmal atrial tachycardia (PAT), paroxysmal VT, or maintenance after cardioversion of atrial fibrillation or flutter—Give 200 mg of quinidine sulfate orally, then 200 to 300 mg orally every 4 to 6 hours, or 300 to 600 mg of extended-release quinidine every 8 to 12 hours. IV quinidine is no longer commercially available.
- Daily dosage for patients with life-threatening VT/VF, such as idiopathic VF or Brugada syndrome, is approximately 900 mg QD (once a day), in divided doses.

What can happen

Adverse cardiovascular effects of quinidine include hypotension, cardiotoxicity, VT, ECG changes (widening of the QRS complex, widened QT and PR intervals), torsades de pointes, AV block, and exacerbation of heart failure. (See *Noncardiac adverse effects of quinidine*, page 230.)

Noncardiac adverse effects of quinidine

In addition to adverse cardiovascular effects of quinidine, other adverse effects include:
• *Central nervous system (CNS)*—anticholinergic effects—vertigo, confusion, lightheadedness, depression, delirium, headache, tinnitus, hearing loss, vision disturbances
• *Respiratory*—acute asthmatic attack, respiratory arrest
• *Gastrointestinal (GI)*—nausea, vomiting, diarrhea, abdominal pain, anorexia, hepatotoxicity
• *Hematologic*—hemolytic anemia, thrombocytopenia, anaphylaxis, or allergic reactions including rash
• *Other*—photosensitivity, angioedema

How you intervene

Keep the following points in mind when caring for a patient taking quinidine:
• Monitor the patient's ECG, HR, and blood pressure closely. Don't give more than 4 g/day. Adjust dosages in patients with heart failure and liver disease.
• Obtain a baseline QT interval measurement before the patient begins therapy. Watch for and notify the practitioner if the patient develops prolongation of the QT interval, a sign that the patient is predisposed to developing polymorphic VT. Also, notify the practitioner if the QRS complex widens by 25% or more.
• Remember that quinidine should be avoided in patients with second- or third-degree AV block who don't have pacemakers. It should also be avoided in patients with profound hypotension, myasthenia gravis, intraventricular conduction defects, or hypersensitivity to the drug. Use it cautiously in older patients and in those with renal disease, hepatic disease, or asthma.
• Avoid rapidly conducted atrial fibrillation or atrial flutter by administering AV nodal blocking agents, such as beta-blockers or calcium channel blockers, before giving quinidine.
• Closely monitor patients receiving quinidine and digoxin for signs and symptoms of digoxin toxicity, such as nausea, vision changes, or arrhythmias. Digoxin levels will be increased.
• Monitor serum drug levels. The therapeutic level for arrhythmia control is 2 to 5 mcg/mL.
• Ask the patient about herb use. Concomitant use with jimsonweed may adversely affect cardiovascular function. Licorice combined with quinidine use may prolong the patient's QT interval.

Herbs can affect the way quinidine works. Ask your patient about herb use.

Procainamide

Procainamide is indicated for supraventricular and ventricular arrhythmias. It is used IV to acutely convert atrial fibrillation, atrial flutter, or VT. It is the drug of choice for atrial fibrillation with conduction over an accessory pathway. It is also used for AVNRT.

How to give it

Here's how to administer procainamide:

- Orally—Initial dosage is 50 mg/kg/day of conventional formulation in divided doses every 3 hours until a therapeutic level is reached. For maintenance, an extended-release form is substituted to deliver the total daily dose divided every 6 hours. An extended-release form may be used to deliver the dose divided every 12 hours.
- IM—Initial daily dosage is 50 mg/kg divided into equal doses every 3 to 6 hours.
- IV—Slow injection of 100 mg is given with the patient in a supine position, no faster than 25 to 50 mg/min until the arrhythmia is suppressed, adverse effects develop, or 500 mg has been given. The usual loading dose is 500 to 600 mg.
- IV infusion—Infuse at 1 to 6 mg/min for a maintenance dosage.

What can happen

Adverse cardiovascular effects of procainamide include bradycardia, hypotension, worsening heart failure, AV block, VF, and asystole. (See *Noncardiac adverse effects of procainamide.*)

Noncardiac adverse effects of procainamide

In addition to adverse cardiovascular effects of procainamide, other dose-related adverse effects include:

- *CNS*—mental depression, hallucinations, seizures, confusion, dizziness
- *GI*—anorexia, nausea, vomiting, diarrhea, bitter taste
- *Hematologic*—agranulocytosis, hemolytic anemia, neutropenia
- *Skin*—rash, urticaria
- *Other*—fever, lupus-like syndrome in long-term therapy, Raynaud's phenomenon

How you intervene

Keep the following points in mind when caring for a patient taking procainamide:

- Monitor the patient's HR, blood pressure, and ECG. Notify the practitioner if the patient has hypotension or if you notice widening of the QRS complex by 50% or more. Also, report a prolonged

QT interval if it's more than one-half of the R-R interval—a sign that the patient is predisposed to developing polymorphic VT.

- Warn the patient taking procainamide orally not to chew it, which causes rapid absorption and intensified drug effect.
- Monitor serum drug levels. (See *Monitoring procainamide*.)

Monitoring procainamide

For patients taking procainamide, you'll need to monitor serum drug levels and the active metabolite *N*-acetylprocainamide (NAPA) to prevent toxic reactions. To suppress ventricular arrhythmias, the therapeutic serum concentration of procainamide should range between 4 and 12 mcg/mL. Therapeutic levels of NAPA should average between 9 and 20 mcg/mL.

- Remember that procainamide should be avoided in patients with second- or third-degree AV block who don't have pacemakers and in patients with blood dyscrasias, myasthenia gravis, profound hypotension, or known hypersensitivity to the drug. Procainamide may also aggravate digoxin toxicity.

Disopyramide

Disopyramide (Norpace) is effective in digitalis-induced arrhythmias, atrial arrhythmias, AVNRT, supraventricular tachycardia (SVT) because of accessory pathways, and ventricular tachyarrhythmias. The negative inotropic action of disopyramide can be useful in neurocardiogenic (vasodepressor) syncope and hypertrophic cardiomyopathy.

How to give it

Here's how to give disopyramide:
- Orally, 100 to 150 mg every 6 hours or 200 to 300 mg every 12 hours (controlled release formula)

What can happen

Adverse cardiovascular effects include sinus bradycardia in patients with sick sinus syndrome (SSS), QRS and QT prolongation by 10% to 15%, variable AV conduction changes, and proarrhythmia including VF and torsades de pointes.

How you intervene

Keep the following points in mind when caring for a patient taking disopyramide:
- Monitor ECG and HR closely.
- Obtain 12-lead ECG for baseline and periodically for accurate interval measurements.

- Give atrioventricular node (AVN) blocking agents before disopyramide, when treating atrial fibrillation or atrial flutter.
- Reduce dose in renal and hepatic dysfunction.
- Do not use in patients with systolic congestive heart failure (CHF).
- Check K+ and magnesium levels before initiating Norpace and replete if necessary.
- Avoid use of erythromycin with Norpace as it can increase levels and lead to torsades de pointes.

Class Ib antiarrhythmics

Class Ib antiarrhythmics in use include such drugs as lidocaine and mexiletine. Because of their actions on ventricular muscle and Purkinje fibers, these drugs are effective in suppressing ventricular ectopy but do not affect atrial muscle. (See *Effects of Class Ib antiarrhythmics.*) These drugs slow phase 0 depolarization and shorten phase 3 repolarization and the action potential. Sinus node automaticity and AV node automaticity and conductivity are not affected by lidocaine.

Effects of Class Ib antiarrhythmics

Class Ib antiarrhythmic drugs—such as lidocaine, tocainide, and mexiletine—may affect the QRS complexes, as shown on the rhythm strip. These drugs
- block sodium influx during phase 0, which depresses the rate of depolarization
- shorten repolarization and the duration of the action potential
- suppress ventricular automaticity in ischemic tissue.

The QRS complex is slightly widened.

Lidocaine

Lidocaine was once the drug of choice for suppressing ventricular arrhythmias; however, amiodarone is now favored. When lidocaine is used, a patient is generally first given a loading dose and then an infusion.

How to give it

Here's how to administer lidocaine:

- IV bolus injection—Administer 1 to 1.5 mg/kg (usually 50 to 100 mg) at 25 to 50 mg/min and repeat every 3 to 5 minutes to a maximum of 300-mg total bolus during a 1-hour period.
- IV infusion immediately following the bolus dose—Infuse at 1 to 4 mg/min.

What can happen

Cardiovascular adverse effects of lidocaine include hypotension, bradycardia, and cardiac arrest. (See *Noncardiac adverse effects of lidocaine.*)

How you intervene

Keep the following points in mind when caring for a patient receiving lidocaine:

- Monitor the patient's HR, blood pressure, and ECG.
- Watch for signs and symptoms of drug toxicity. Seizures may be the first sign of toxicity. The potential for toxicity is increased if the patient has liver disease, is older adult, is taking cimetidine (Tagamet) or propranolol (Inderal), or receives an infusion of the drug for longer than 24 hours.
- Avoid use of the drug in patients known to be hypersensitive to it or in severe sinus node disease, AV block or intraventricular block in the absence of an artificial pacemaker.
- Administer cautiously with other antiarrhythmics.

Mexiletine

Mexiletine is an oral congener of lidocaine, used in the treatment of ventricular arrhythmias. It has no activity against atrial arrhythmias.

How to give it

150 to 200 mg every 8 hours to a maximum dose of 400 mg every 8 hours. Decrease dose in hepatic disease. No adjustment required in renal disease or with CHF.

> As ordered, administer an antiarrhythmic such as lidocaine to help suppress ventricular ectopy.

Noncardiac adverse effects of lidocaine

In addition to adverse cardiovascular effects of lidocaine, other adverse effects (mostly dose-related) include:
- *CNS*—seizures, confusion, drowsiness, dizziness, tremors, restlessness, lightheadedness, paresthesia, tinnitus, double vision
- *Respiratory*—respiratory arrest, status asthmaticus
- *GI*—nausea, vomiting
- *Other*—anaphylaxis.

What can happen

- Proarrhythmia is very rare, about 1.3%.
- Very little effect on HR, blood pressure, or cardiac output
- Exacerbation of CHF is rare, about 2%.
- Monitor for GI side effects including nausea and CNS effects of tremor, blurred vision, dysarthria, ataxia, and confusion.

How you intervene

- Monitor ECG for efficacy in controlling ventricular arrhythmias.
- Give medication with food to avoid GI effects.

Class Ic antiarrhythmics

Class Ic antiarrhythmic drugs include flecainide (Tambocor) and propafenone (Rythmol). These drugs decrease intracardiac conduction in all parts of the heart. (See *Effects of Class Ic antiarrhythmics.*) These drugs are primarily used for supraventricular arrhythmias. Because of their proarrhythmic potential, they are avoided in patients with structural heart disease such as coronary artery disease, cardiomyopathy, and CHF.

Effects of Class Ic antiarrhythmics

Class Ic antiarrhythmic drugs—including flecainide and propafenone—cause the effects shown later on an ECG by exerting particular actions on the cardiac cycle. Class Ic antiarrhythmics block sodium influx during phase 0, which depresses the rate of depolarization. Repolarization is not affected.

The PR interval is prolonged.

The QT interval is prolonged.

The QRS complex is widened.

Flecainide

Flecainide is used to treat paroxysmal atrial fibrillation or flutter in patients without structural heart disease. It is also used to prevent PSVT.

How to give it

The dosage for flecainide is 50 to 200 mg orally every 12 hours, to a maximum of 400 mg/day.

What can happen

Adverse cardiovascular effects of flecainide include bradycardia (in the presence of sinus node disease), chest pain, palpitations, heart failure, new or worsened arrhythmias, and cardiac arrest.

Flecainide can decrease the atrial rate in atrial fibrillation or atrial flutter, facilitating AV node conduction and faster ventricular rate. Class II or IV antiarrhythmic medication is given to slow AV conduction and prevent rapid ventricular response when using flecainide for atrial arrhythmias. (See *Noncardiac adverse effects of flecainide*.)

> Flecainide helps me take it easy. It slows conduction without affecting the duration of the action potential.

Noncardiac adverse effects of flecainide

In addition to adverse cardiovascular effects of flecainide, other adverse effects include:
- *CNS*—headache, drowsiness, dizziness, syncope, fatigue, blurred vision, tremor, ataxia, vertigo, lightheadedness, paresthesia, flushing
- *Respiratory*—dyspnea
- *GI*—nausea, vomiting, constipation, abdominal pain, diarrhea, anorexia
- *Hematologic*—neutropenia.

How you intervene

Keep the following points in mind when caring for a patient taking flecainide:
- Monitor the patient's HR, blood pressure, and ECG. Report widening of the QRS complex by 25% or more and watch closely for signs of heart failure.
- Use flecainide cautiously in SSS or in patients with heart, kidney, or liver failure. Avoid its use entirely in second- or third-degree AV block and use caution in bifascicular block.
- Administer flecainide cautiously in patients receiving cimetidine, digoxin, or propranolol.
- Correct electrolyte imbalances before starting flecainide therapy.
- Administer AV node blocking agents (Class II or IV medications) with flecainide, to avoid rapid ventricular conduction of atrial flutter or atrial fibrillation.

Propafenone

Propafenone slows conduction in all cardiac tissues. The drug is used for the treatment of SVT, including atrial fibrillation, atrial flutter, AVNRT, and arrhythmias because of accessory pathways.

How to give it

The usual dosage of propafenone is 150 to 300 mg orally every 8 hours, to a maximum dosage of 900 mg/day.

What can happen

Propafenone's adverse effects on the cardiovascular system include exacerbation of heart failure, AV block, and proarrhythmia (VT, VF, and premature ventricular contraction [PVCs]). However, proarrhythmia is rare in patients treated for SVT, with a structurally normal heart. (See *Noncardiac adverse effects of propafenone*.)

Noncardiac adverse effects of propafenone

In addition to adverse cardiovascular effects of propafenone, other adverse effects include:
- *CNS*—dizziness, blurred vision, fatigue, headache, paresthesia, anxiety, ataxia, drowsiness, insomnia, syncope, tremors
- *Respiratory*—dyspnea, exacerbation of asthma
- *GI*—unusual taste, nausea, vomiting, dyspepsia, constipation, diarrhea, abdominal pain, dry mouth, flatulence.

How you intervene

Keep the following points in mind when caring for a patient taking propafenone:
- Monitor the patient's HR, blood pressure, and ECG. Report widening of the QRS complex greater than 25%. If widening occurs, the dosage may need to be reduced. Monitor the patient closely for exacerbation of heart failure.
- Correct electrolyte imbalances before starting propafenone therapy.
- Remember that propafenone should be avoided in patients with a structurally abnormal heart (low ejection fraction, previous myocardial infarction [MI], cardiomyopathy or significant left ventricular hypertrophy), bronchospastic disorders, hypotension, or sinus node disease, AV, block, or bifascicular blocks.
- Propafenone is contraindicated in the presence of CHF and cardiogenic shock, as well as in SA, AV, and intraventricular conduction disorders in the absence of an artificial pacemaker.
- Administer propafenone cautiously in patients also receiving cimetidine, propranolol, or metoprolol.
- Be aware that patients receiving digoxin along with propafenone may have increased plasma concentration of digoxin, leading to digoxin toxicity.
- Use cautiously in patients also taking warfarin (Coumadin); propafenone can increase the plasma concentration of the anticoagulant.

Class II antiarrhythmics

Class II antiarrhythmic drugs are used to treat supraventricular and ventricular arrhythmias, especially those caused by excess catecholamines. The drugs are called *beta-adrenergic blockers* because they block beta-adrenergic receptors in the sympathetic nervous system. (See *Effects of Class II antiarrhythmics*.)

Effects of Class II antiarrhythmics

Class II antiarrhythmic drugs—including such beta-adrenergic blockers as propranolol, esmolol, acebutolol, and sotalol—cause certain effects on an ECG (as shown here) by exerting particular actions on the cardiac cycle. Class II antiarrhythmics

- depress SA node automaticity
- shorten the duration of the action potential
- increase the refractory period of atrial and AV junctional tissues, which slows conduction
- inhibit sympathetic activity.

The PR interval is slightly prolonged.

The QT interval is slightly shortened.

Two types of beta-adrenergic receptors exist: beta$_1$ and beta$_2$. Beta$_1$-adrenergic receptors increase HR, contractility, and conductivity. Blocking those receptors decreases the actions listed earlier.

Beta$_2$-adrenergic receptors relax smooth muscle in the bronchi and blood vessels. Keep in mind that blocking these receptors may result in vasoconstriction and bronchospasm.

Beta-adrenergic blockers that block only beta$_1$-adrenergic receptors are referred to as *cardioselective*. Those that block both beta$_1$-adrenergic and beta$_2$-adrenergic receptors are referred to as *noncardioselective*. Cardioselective formulations are preferred in patients with asthma.

Beta-blockers depress the slope of phase 4 depolarization, suppress automaticity, and prolong AV node conduction. These drugs are used to control ventricular rate in atrial fibrillation and atrial flutter,

Smooth muscle in the bronchi and blood vessels are relaxed by beta$_2$-adrenergic receptors.

reduce the risk of sudden cardiac death (SCD) in patients with non-sustained VT and structural heart disease, reduce SCD in patients post-MI, prevent SCD in long QT interval syndrome, prevent recurrence of SVT, and to slow HR in PAT.

Beta–adrenergic blockers

The following beta-adrenergic blockers are approved by the US Food and Drug Administration for use as antiarrhythmics:

- Acebutolol (Sectral), which is classified as cardioselective and decreases contractility, HR, and blood pressure
- Propranolol (Inderal), which is classified as noncardioselective; decreases HR, contractility, and blood pressure; and reduces the incidence of SCD after MI
- Esmolol (Brevibloc), which is a short-acting, cardioselective drug administered by IV titration that decreases HR, contractility, and blood pressure
- Sotalol (Betapace), which is a noncardioselective drug that also has Class III characteristics, decreases HR, slows AV conduction, decreases cardiac output, and has proarrhythmic effects and increases the QT interval. It has little effect on blood pressure. It is used primarily to maintain sinus rhythm (SR) with atrial fibrillation or atrial flutter.

Other beta-blockers often used to treat arrhythmias include metoprolol, atenolol, nadolol, bisoprolol, and nebivolol. These agents are briefly described:

- Metoprolol (cardioselective) is available in short-acting (metoprolol tartrate) or extended-release (metoprolol succinate) oral formulations, as well as in IV form. This is the most commonly used medication to slow AV node conduction and to treat atrial and ventricular ectopy.
- Atenolol (cardioselective) is desirable for its once-daily dosing. It has become less preferred to other drugs in this class but is still used.
- Nadolol (noncardioselective) is the preferred beta-blocker in treating potentially life-threatening ventricular arrhythmias in patients with some forms of long QT syndrome (LQTS).
- Bisoprolol (cardioselective) is sometimes used when other beta-blocking medications cause significant adverse reactions, as this formulation is often associated with improved tolerance.
- Nebivolol (cardioselective, at low doses), like bisoprolol, is often better tolerated than other agents in this class.

How to give it

These four beta-adrenergic blockers should be administered as follows:

- Acebutolol—The normal dosage is 200 mg orally twice daily, increased as needed to a usual dosage of 600 to 1,200 mg daily.
- Propranolol—It may be given orally or IV. The oral dosage is 10 to 30 mg three or four times daily. The IV dose is 0.5 to 3.0 mg, at a rate not to exceed 1 mg/min. If necessary, a second IV dose may be administered after 2 minutes; subsequent doses may be given no sooner than every 4 hours.
- Esmolol—The loading dose is 500 mcg/kg over 1 minute, then 50 mcg/kg/min for 4 minutes. If an adequate response doesn't occur within 5 minutes, repeat the loading dose and infuse 100 mcg/kg/min for 4 minutes. If needed, increase infusion to a maximum of 200 mcg/kg/min.
- Sotalol—The initial dosage is 80 mg orally twice daily. Most patients respond to a daily dose of 160 to 320 mg.

What can happen

The adverse effects of beta-adrenergic blockers on the cardiovascular system may vary, but they include bradycardia, hypotension, and AV block. (See *Noncardiac adverse effects of Class II beta-adrenergic blockers.*)

Noncardiac adverse effects of Class II beta-adrenergic blockers

In addition to adverse cardiovascular effects of Class II beta-adrenergic blockers, other adverse effects include:
- *CNS*—insomnia, syncope, mental depression, emotional lability, fatigue, headache, dizziness, lethargy, vivid dreams, hallucinations, lightheadedness
- *Respiratory*—dyspnea, bronchospasm, especially in patients with asthma or other bronchospastic disease.

How you intervene

Keep the following points in mind when caring for a patient taking a beta-adrenergic blocker:
- Monitor the patient's HR, blood pressure, and ECG.
- Remember that beta-adrenergic blockers should be avoided in patients with symptomatic bradycardia, second- or third-degree AV block without a pacemaker, and shock. Use them cautiously in patients with diabetes mellitus (they mask the signs of hypoglycemia), heart failure, kidney disease, liver disease, myasthenia gravis, peripheral vascular disease, and hypotension.
- Keep in mind that noncardioselective beta-adrenergic blockers are contraindicated in patients with asthma or other bronchospastic disease.

- Correct electrolyte imbalances before starting therapy with a beta-adrenergic blocker.
- Remember that beta-adrenergic blockers diminish the patient's ability to withstand exercise because the HR can't increase. These drugs also block sympathetic response to shock.

Class III antiarrhythmics

Class III antiarrhythmics are called *potassium channel blockers.* (See *Effects of Class III antiarrhythmics* below.) They include amiodarone hydrochloride (Cordarone), ibutilide (Corvert), dofetilide (Tikosyn), and dronedarone (Multaq). Sotalol has qualities of both Class II and Class III antiarrhythmics. All Class III antiarrhythmics have proarrhythmic potential.

Effects of Class III antiarrhythmics

Class III antiarrhythmic drugs—including amiodarone, sotalol, and ibutilide—cause the effects shown later below by exerting particular actions on the cardiac cycle. Class III antiarrhythmics
- block potassium movement during phase 3
- increase duration of the action potential
- prolong the effective refractory period.

The PR interval is prolonged.

The QRS complex is widened.

The QT interval is prolonged.

Amiodarone

Amiodarone is used to treat supraventricular arrhythmias, including atrial fibrillation and atrial flutter, as well as ventricular arrhythmias.

How to give it

Here's how to administer amiodarone:
- Orally—Give 800 to 1,600 mg daily in divided doses for 1 to 3 weeks, followed by 400 to 800 mg/day for 4 weeks, followed by 200 to 400 mg/day as a maintenance dosage.

- IV infusion—Infuse 150 mg over 10 minutes (15 mg/min); then infuse 360 mg over the next 6 hours (1 mg/min), followed by 540 mg infused over 18 hours (0.5 mg/min). After the first 24 hours, a maintenance IV infusion of 720 mg per 24 hours (0.5 mg/min) should be continued.

What can happen

Adverse cardiovascular effects of amiodarone given by IV infusion include bradycardia, hypotension, AV block, heart failure, asystole, and pulseless electrical activity.

Long-term oral therapy can be associated with bradycardia, pulmonary fibrosis, thyroid dysfunction, elevated liver function tests, and corneal deposits, not usually leading to visual disturbances. (See *Noncardiac adverse effects of amiodarone*.)

Noncardiac adverse effects of amiodarone

In addition to adverse cardiovascular effects of amiodarone, other adverse effects include:
- *CNS*—malaise, fatigue, dizziness, peripheral neuropathy, ataxia, paresthesia, tremors, headache, vision disturbances
- *Respiratory*—pulmonary toxicity (progressive dyspnea, cough, fever, pleuritic chest pain)
- *GI*—nausea, vomiting, constipation, anorexia, elevated liver function tests
- *Other*—photosensitivity, abnormal taste and smell, hypothyroidism or hyperthyroidism, bleeding disorders, muscle weakness.

How you intervene

Keep the following points in mind when caring for a patient taking amiodarone:
- Monitor the patient's vital signs, ECG, and respiratory status.
- Monitor laboratory test results, such as electrolyte levels, liver function studies, thyroid function studies, pulmonary function studies, and chest X-rays.
- Check for signs of digoxin toxicity or increased prothrombin time. Amiodarone can increase the serum levels of digoxin and warfarin.
- Remember that amiodarone should be avoided in patients with hypersensitivity to the drug, cardiogenic shock, marked sinus bradycardia, and second- or third-degree AV block without a pacemaker. Use the drug cautiously in patients with cardiomegaly, preexisting bradycardia or sinus node disease, conduction disturbances, or depressed ventricular function.

- Be aware that the drug has a long half-life (56 days, with a range from 13 to 103 days) and therefore takes weeks to reach therapeutic levels and possibly up to 3 months to be cleared by the body.
- Know that amiodarone may increase theophylline levels in patients taking theophylline. Monitor the patient for signs of theophylline toxicity.
- Be aware that amiodarone may increase phenytoin (Dilantin) levels. Monitor phenytoin levels closely.
- Instruct the patient to wear sunscreen and protective clothing to avoid photosensitivity reactions. A blue-gray discoloration of exposed skin may occur.
- Recommend that the patient have yearly ophthalmic examinations. Within 1 to 4 months after beginning amiodarone therapy, most patients show corneal microdeposits upon slit-lamp ophthalmic examination. Instillation of methylcellulose ophthalmic solution minimizes corneal microdeposits.
- Administer the IV drug through a central venous access device to avoid phlebitis.
- The lowest possible effective maintenance dose should be used to avoid toxicity.

Ibutilide

Ibutilide is used for the rapid conversion of recent-onset atrial fibrillation or flutter to sinus rhythm. The drug increases atrial and ventricular refractoriness.

How to give it

If your adult patient weighs greater than 132 lb (60 kg) or more, they will receive 1 mg of ibutilide IV over 10 minutes. If they weigh less than 132 lb, the dose is 0.01 mg/kg.

If the arrhythmia is still present 10 minutes after the infusion is complete, the dose may be repeated.

What can happen

Adverse cardiovascular effects of ibutilide include PVCs, nonsustained VT, sustained polymorphic VT, hypotension, bundle branch block, AV block, hypertension, bradycardia, tachycardia, palpitations, heart failure, and lengthening of the QT interval. Noncardiac adverse effects include headache, nausea, and renal failure.

How you intervene

Keep these points in mind when giving ibutilide:
- Correct electrolyte abnormalities before administering ibutilide.
- Monitor the patient's vital signs and ECG continuously during the infusion and for at least 4 hours afterward. The infusion will be

Adverse effects of ibutilide include PVCs, VT, hypotension (gulp), AV block (gulp) ... Is it getting hot in here?

stopped if the arrhythmia terminates or if the patient develops VT or marked prolongation of the QT interval, which signals the risk of polymorphic VT.

- Have emergency equipment and medication nearby for the treatment of sustained VT.
- Don't give ibutilide to patients with a history of polymorphic VT.
- Give the drug cautiously in patients receiving digoxin (Lanoxin) because it can mask signs and symptoms of cardiotoxicity associated with excessive digoxin levels.
- Don't administer ibutilide at the same time or within 4 hours of Class Ia or other Class III antiarrhythmics.
- Don't give ibutilide with other drugs that prolong the QT interval, such as phenothiazines and tricyclic or tetracyclic antidepressants.
- Be aware that patients with atrial fibrillation that has lasted longer than 24 to 48 hours must receive anticoagulants for at least 3 weeks before the initiation of ibutilide therapy, unless atrial thrombosis is confirmed negative by transesophageal echocardiogram.

Dofetilide (Tikosyn)

Dofetilide is used to maintain normal sinus rhythm in patients with symptomatic atrial fibrillation or atrial flutter. It is also used to convert atrial fibrillation and atrial flutter to normal sinus rhythm.

How to give it

Dosage is based on creatinine clearance and QTc interval, which must be determined before the first dose (QT interval should be used if the HR is less than 60 beats/min). The usual recommended dosage is 500 mcg orally twice per day for patients with a creatinine clearance greater than 60 mL/min. The dose is 250 mcg twice daily if the creatinine clearance is 40 to 60 mL/min and 125 mcg twice daily if the creatinine clearance is 20 to 40 mL/min. QTc should be less than 440 milliseconds before administration of the first dose of dofetilide.

Dofetilide is initiated in the hospital setting, with continuous cardiac monitoring, for 72 hours. The possibility of life-threatening ventricular arrhythmias is greatest during this time. Twelve-lead ECG tracings are obtained frequently to assess medication effect on the QTc interval, and dose adjustments made as indicated.

What can happen

Adverse cardiovascular effects of dofetilide include VF, VT, torsades de pointes, AV block, bundle branch block, heart block, bradycardia, chest pain, edema, cardiac arrest, and MI. (See *Noncardiac adverse effects of dofetilide*, page 245.)

Noncardiac adverse effects of dofetilide

In addition to adverse cardiovascular effects of dofetilide, other adverse effects include:

- *CNS*—headache, dizziness, insomnia, migraine, paresthesia
- *GI*—nausea, diarrhea, abdominal pain
- *Respiratory*—respiratory tract infection, dyspnea
- *Skin*—rash
- *Other*—angioedema.

How you intervene

Remember these facts when giving dofetilide:

- Use cautiously in patients with severe hepatic impairment.
- Provide continuous ECG monitoring for at least 3 days.
- Avoid discharging the patient within 12 hours of conversion to normal sinus rhythm.
- Monitor the patient for prolonged diarrhea, sweating, and vomiting. Report these signs to the practitioner because electrolyte imbalance may increase the potential for arrhythmia development.
- Assess for hypokalemia and hypomagnesemia if the patient is receiving potassium-depleting diuretics, which increase the risk of torsades de pointes. Potassium level should be within normal range before giving dofetilide and kept in normal range. Use of hydrochlorothiazide should be avoided in patients treated with dofetilide.
- Stop antiarrhythmic therapy under careful monitoring for a minimum of three plasma half-lives before starting dofetilide.
- Don't give dofetilide after amiodarone therapy until the amiodarone level is below 0.3 mcg/mL or until amiodarone has been stopped for at least 3 months.
- Provide a washout period of at least 2 days before starting other drug therapy if dofetilide is stopped to allow treatment with other drugs (such as those that interact with dofetilide).
- Don't give dofetilide with grapefruit juice; it may decrease hepatic metabolism and increase the drug level.
- Don't give with drugs that prolong the QT interval, such as phenothiazines, tricyclic or tetracyclic antidepressants, and erythromycin.
- Avoid using with cimetidine (Tagamet), ketoconazole (Nizoral), co-trimoxazole (Bactrim), verapamil (Calan), and inhibitors of CYP3A4, such as amiodarone (Cordarone), diltiazem (Cardizem), norfloxacin (Noroxin), and selective serotonin reuptake inhibitors.

When giving dofetilide, skip the grapefruit juice and go for water instead. Grapefruit juice can affect metabolism of this drug.

- Avoid using with inhibitors of renal cationic secretion, such as megestrol (Megace), amiloride (Midamor), metformin (Glucophage), and triamterene (Dyrenium).

Dronedarone (Multaq)

Dronedarone is used to maintain normal sinus rhythm in patients with paroxysmal atrial fibrillation. It should not be used in persistent atrial fibrillation due to lack of efficacy and increased risk of side effects.

How to give it

Dronedarone has only one dosage and route. It is given 400 mg twice daily orally with meals. There is no dose adjustment for renal impairment. It is contraindicated for hepatic impairment. It can be started on an outpatient basis, and there is no need for hospitalization upon initiation of the drug.

What can happen

Multaq can increase QT intervals causing ventricular arrhythmias. It can also increase the risk of heart failure, especially in patients with preexisting heart failure.

Noncardiac adverse effects of dronedarone

In additional to heart failure and ventricular arrhythmias, dronedarone has other adverse effects:
- *GI*—nausea, vomiting, diarrhea, abdominal pain
- *Skin*—rash, itching, hives
- *Respiratory*—cough, fluid retention, and shortness of breath
- *Liver*—dronedarone has been associated with liver injury
- *Vision*—blurred vision and visual disturbances.

How you intervene

- Do not use in patients with preexisting hepatic impairment. Check hepatic panel before initiation of dronedarone and routinely if the patient continues therapy long term.
- Check QT interval on a 12-lead ECG, monitor for ventricular arrhythmias.
- Advise patients to take with meals to prevent GI side effects.
- Consider heart failure workup in patients who experience shortness of breath, cough, fluid retention.
- Caution when given to patients who are on warfarin or digoxin as dronedarone increases international normalized ratio (INR) and increases digoxin levels. Follow levels closely.

Class IV antiarrhythmics

Class IV antiarrhythmic drugs are called *calcium channel blockers*. They include verapamil and diltiazem. These drugs prolong conduction time and the refractory period in the AV node. (See *Effects of Class IV antiarrhythmics*.)

Effects of Class IV antiarrhythmics

Class IV antiarrhythmic drugs—including such calcium channel blockers as verapamil and diltiazem—affect the cardiac cycle in specific ways and may lead to the ECG change shown here. Class IV antiarrhythmics
- block calcium movement during phase 2
- prolong the conduction time and increase the refractory period in the AV node
- decrease contractility.

The PR interval is prolonged.

Other calcium channel blockers, including nifedipine (Procardia) and amlodipine (Norvasc) are used primarily to treat hypertension rather than antiarrhythmic or electrophysiologic management.

Verapamil

Verapamil is used for PSVT because of its effect on the AV node. It also slows the ventricular response in atrial fibrillation and flutter.

How to give it

Here's how to administer verapamil:
- Orally for chronic atrial fibrillation—Give 80 to 120 mg three or four times per day to a maximum of 480 mg/day.
- IV injection for supraventricular arrhythmias—Give 0.075 to 0.15 mg/kg (usually 5 to 10 mg) over 2 minutes; you can repeat in 30 minutes if no response occurs.

What can happen

Cardiovascular adverse effects of verapamil include bradycardia, AV block, hypotension, heart failure, edema, and VF. (See *Noncardiac adverse effects of verapamil.*)

Noncardiac adverse effects of verapamil

In addition to adverse cardiovascular effects of verapamil, other adverse effects include:
- *CNS*—headache, dizziness
- *Respiratory*—dyspnea, pulmonary edema
- *GI*—nausea, constipation, elevated liver enzymes
- *Skin*—rash.

How you intervene

Keep the following points in mind when caring for a patient taking verapamil:
- Monitor the patient's HR, blood pressure, and ECG. Also, monitor liver function studies.
- Note that calcium may be given before verapamil to prevent hypotension.
- Advise the patient to change position slowly to avoid orthostatic hypotension.
- Remember that verapamil should be avoided in SSS or second- or third-degree AV block without a pacemaker and in atrial fibrillation or flutter in a patient with WPW syndrome. It also should be avoided in patients with hypersensitivity to the drug, advanced heart failure, cardiogenic shock, profound hypotension, acute MI, or pulmonary edema.
- Give the drug cautiously to patients receiving digoxin or oral beta-adrenergic blockers, older patients, and patients with heart failure, hypotension, liver disease, or kidney disease. Don't give verapamil to patients receiving IV beta-adrenergic blockers.

Diltiazem

Diltiazem is administered IV to treat PSVT and for ventricular rate control with atrial fibrillation or flutter.

How to give it

Here's how to give diltiazem:
- IV injection—Give 0.25 mg/kg (usually 20 mg) over 2 minutes; you can repeat in 15 minutes at 0.35 mg/kg (usually 25 mg) over 2 minutes.

- IV infusion—Infuse at a rate of 5 to 15 mg/hour; increase dose by 5 mg/hour increments. Continuous infusion should generally be used for 24 hours or less, because of drug accumulation.
- Oral dosing—Start immediate-release oral formulation 1 hour before stopping the IV infusion. Immediate-release doses are given four times daily. Usual effective total daily dose is 360 mg, in divided doses. Once stable daily dose is reached, extended-release dosing can be given once or twice daily, depending on formulation.

What can happen
Adverse cardiovascular effects of diltiazem include edema, flushing, bradycardia, hypotension, heart failure, arrhythmias, conduction abnormalities, sinus node dysfunction, and AV block. (See *Noncardiac adverse effects of diltiazem.*)

Noncardiac adverse effects of diltiazem
In addition to adverse cardiovascular effects of diltiazem, other adverse effects include:
- *CNS*—headache, dizziness
- *GI*—nausea, transient elevation of liver enzymes, constipation, abdominal discomfort, acute hepatic injury
- *Skin*—rash.

How you intervene
Keep the following points in mind when caring for a patient receiving diltiazem:
- Monitor the patient's HR, blood pressure, and ECG.
- Diltiazem should be avoided in patients with SSS or second- or third-degree AV block without a pacemaker, atrial fibrillation or flutter with WPW syndrome, advanced heart failure, cardiogenic shock, profound hypotension, acute MI, pulmonary edema, or sensitivity to the drug.
- Use cautiously in older patients; in patients with heart failure, hypotension, or liver or kidney disease; and in those receiving digoxin or beta-adrenergic blockers. (See *Prolonged effects in older patients*, page 250.)
- Give cautiously to patients receiving IV beta-adrenergic blockers. IV diltiazem and IV beta-adrenergic blockers should be given separately and several hours apart from one another.
- Advise the patient to change position slowly to avoid orthostatic hypotension.

Patients taking diltiazem should change position slowly.

Unclassified antiarrhythmics

Some antiarrhythmic drugs defy categorization. Let's look at some of those drugs, which are called unclassified or miscellaneous antiarrhythmic drugs.

Adenosine

Adenosine is a naturally occurring nucleoside used to treat PSVT. It acts on the AV node to slow conduction and inhibit reentry pathways. It's also useful in treating PSVT associated with WPW syndrome.

Although adenosine isn't effective for atrial fibrillation or atrial flutter, it does slow conduction through the AV node enough to determine the atrial rhythm and to allow for appropriate treatment of the arrhythmia.

How to give it

Administer 6 mg of adenosine IV over 1 to 2 seconds, immediately followed by a rapid flush with 20-mL normal saline solution. Because the drug's half-life is less than 10 seconds, it needs to reach the circulation quickly. The IV line should be placed at the antecubital space, rather than more distal to the heart. Repeat with an IV injection of 12 mg of adenosine if the rhythm doesn't convert within 1 to 2 minutes.

What can happen

Adverse cardiovascular effects of adenosine include transient arrhythmias such as a short asystolic pause at the time of conversion. Other adverse effects include hypotension (if large doses are used), facial flushing, diaphoresis, chest pressure, and recurrence of the arrhythmia. (See *Noncardiac adverse effects of adenosine*.)

Prolonged effects in older patients

Administer diltiazem cautiously to an older adult because the half-life of the drug may be prolonged. Be especially careful if the older adult also has heart failure or impaired hepatic or renal function.

Noncardiac adverse effects of adenosine

In addition to adverse cardiovascular effects of adenosine, other adverse effects include:
* *CNS*—anxiety, lightheadedness, burning sensation, headache, numbness and tingling in arms
* *Respiratory*—dyspnea
* *GI*—nausea.

How you intervene

Keep the following points in mind when caring for a patient receiving adenosine:
* Monitor the patient's HR, blood pressure, ECG, ventilatory rate and depth, and breath sounds for wheezes.
* Remember that adenosine should be avoided in patients with hypersensitivity to the drug, second- or third-degree AV block, or

SSS without a pacemaker. Use cautiously in older adults and in patients with asthma or those receiving dipyridamole (Persantine) or carbamazepine (Tegretol).

- Store adenosine at room temperature.
- Be aware that the patient may require a higher dose or may not respond to therapy at all if they are also taking aminophylline or another xanthine derivative.

Atropine

Atropine is an anticholinergic drug that blocks vagal effects on the SA and AV nodes. This enhances conduction through the AV node and speeds the HR. Atropine is used to treat symptomatic bradycardia and asystole. However, atropine is ineffective in patients following dissection of the vagus nerve during heart transplant surgery. Isoproterenol (Isuprel) can be used to treat symptomatic bradycardia in these patients.

How to give it

Administer atropine by a 0.5- to 1-mg IV injection repeated as needed at 3- to 5-minute intervals, to a maximum dose of 2 mg. The initial dose for asystole is 1 mg. The maximum dose is 3 mg.

What can happen

Adverse cardiovascular effects of atropine include tachycardia (with high doses), palpitations, bradycardia if given slowly or in a dose of less than 0.5 mg, hypotension, and chest pain and increased myocardial oxygen consumption in patients with coronary artery disease. (See *Noncardiac adverse effects of atropine.*)

Noncardiac adverse effects of atropine

In addition to cardiovascular effects of atropine, other adverse effects include:
- *CNS*—ataxia, disorientation, delirium, agitation, confusion, headache, restlessness, insomnia, dizziness, blurred vision, dilated pupils, photophobia
- *GI*—dry mouth, constipation, paralytic ileus, nausea, vomiting
- *Genitourinary*—urine retention
- *Other*—increased intraocular pressure, anaphylaxis, urticaria.

How you intervene

Keep the following points in mind when caring for a patient receiving atropine:

- Monitor the patient's HR, blood pressure, ECG, urine output, and bowel sounds.

- Remember that atropine should be avoided in patients with hyper-sensitivity to belladonna, acute angle closure glaucoma, GI obstruction, obstructive uropathy, myasthenia gravis, and tachyarrhythmias.
- Use atropine cautiously in patients with renal disease, heart failure, hyperthyroidism, hepatic disease, hypertension, and acute MI. Don't give atropine for bradycardia unless the patient is symptomatic.

Digoxin

Digoxin (Lanoxin) was historically used to treat PSVT, atrial fibrillation, and atrial flutter for the purpose of decreasing HR. It provides antiarrhythmic effects by enhancing vagal tone and slowing conduction through the SA and AV nodes. Class II and IV drugs are now the preferred medications for controlling HR. Digoxin has visible effects on the patient's ECG. (See *Effects of digoxin*.)

Effects of digoxin

Digoxin affects the cardiac cycle in various ways and may lead to the ECG changes shown here.

Gradual sloping occurs, causing the ST-segment depression in the direction opposite that of the QR deflection.

The P wave may be notched.

Don't forget to check for signs of digoxin toxicity.

How to give it

To administer digoxin rapidly and orally or IV, give a digitalizing dose of 0.5 to 1 mg divided into two or more doses every 6 to 8 hours. The usual maintenance dosage is 0.125 to 0.5 mg daily. The dose is reduced, or the medication avoided, in the patient with renal insufficiency or renal failure.

What can happen

Too much digoxin in the body causes toxicity. Toxic cardiac effects include SA and AV blocks and junctional and ventricular arrhythmias.

Digoxin toxicity is treated by discontinuing digoxin; correcting oxygenation and electrolyte imbalances; treating arrhythmias with phenytoin, lidocaine, atropine, or a pacemaker; giving digoxin immune fab (Digibind) to reverse life-threatening arrhythmias or blocks (reversal occurs within 30 to 60 minutes of administration); and correcting the potassium level before giving digoxin immune fab. (See *Noncardiac adverse effects of digoxin.*)

Noncardiac adverse effects of digoxin

In addition to adverse cardiovascular effects of digoxin, other adverse effects resulting from toxicity include:
• *CNS*—headache, vision disturbances, hallucinations, fatigue, muscle weakness, agitation, malaise, dizziness, stupor, paresthesia
• *GI*—anorexia, nausea, vomiting, diarrhea
• *Other*—yellow-green halos around visual images, blurred vision, light flashes, photophobia, diplopia.

How you intervene
Keep the following points in mind when caring for a patient receiving digoxin:
• Check for signs of digoxin toxicity, especially in patients with hypokalemia, hypocalcemia, hypercalcemia, or hypomagnesemia. Monitor serum electrolyte levels as ordered.
• Monitor the patient's apical HR and ECG. A HR below 60 beats/min or a change in rhythm can signal digoxin toxicity. If this occurs, notify the practitioner.
• Remember that digoxin should be avoided in patients with known hypersensitivity to the drug; SSS, SA, or AV block (without an implanted cardiac pacemaker); VT; hypertrophic cardiomyopathy; or WPW syndrome. Use cautiously in older adults and in patients with acute MI, liver or kidney disease, or hypothyroidism.
• Withhold digoxin for 1 to 2 days before performing electrical cardioversion.
• Be sure to question the patient about herbal preparation use because digoxin reacts with many preparations. Fumitory, lily of the valley, goldenseal, motherwort, shepherd's purse, and rue may enhance the cardiac effects of digoxin. Licorice, oleander, Siberian ginseng, foxglove, and squill may increase the risk of digoxin toxicity.

Epinephrine
Epinephrine is a naturally occurring catecholamine. It acts directly on alpha- and beta-adrenergic receptor sites of the sympathetic nervous system, and it's used to help restore cardiac rhythm in cardiac arrest

and to treat symptomatic bradycardia. Its actions include increasing the systolic blood pressure, slightly decreasing diastolic blood pressure, and increasing HR and cardiac output.

How to give it

To restore sinus rhythm in cardiac arrest in adults, administer epinephrine by IV injection as a 1 mg dose (10 mL of 1:10,000 solution). Each dose given by peripheral IV injection should be followed by a 20-mL flush of IV fluid to ensure quick delivery of the drug. Doses may be repeated every 3 to 5 minutes as needed. (Some practitioners advocate doses of up to 5 mg, especially for patients who don't respond to the usual IV dose.) After initial IV administration, an infusion may be given at 1 to 4 mcg/min.

What can happen

Adverse cardiovascular effects include palpitations, hypertension, tachycardia, VF, anginal pain, shock, and ECG changes, including a decreased T-wave amplitude. (See *Noncardiac adverse effects of epinephrine.*)

Noncardiac adverse effects of epinephrine

In addition to adverse cardiovascular effects of epinephrine, other adverse effects include:

• *CNS*—nervousness, tremor, dizziness, vertigo, headache, disorientation, agitation, fear, pallor, weakness, cerebral hemorrhage, increased rigidity and tremor (in patients with Parkinson disease)
• *Respiratory*—dyspnea
• *GI*—nausea, vomiting
• *Other*—tissue necrosis.

How you intervene

Keep these points in mind when administering epinephrine:
- Be sure to document the concentration of the epinephrine solution used. (Remember that 1 mg equals 1 mL of 1:1,000 or 10 mL of 1:10,000 concentration.)
- When administering IV epinephrine, monitor the patient's HR, ECG rhythm, and blood pressure throughout therapy.
- Don't mix the drug with alkaline solutions. Use D_5W, lactated Ringer solution, or normal saline solution or a combination of dextrose and saline solution.
- Remember that some epinephrine products contain sulfites. Use of those products usually should be avoided in patients with sulfite allergies. The only exception is when epinephrine is being used in an emergency.

- Know that the use of epinephrine with digoxin (Lanoxin) or such general anesthetics as cyclopropane or a halogenated hydrocarbon like halothane (Fluothane) may increase the risk of ventricular arrhythmias.
- Avoid giving epinephrine with other drugs that exert a similar effect. Doing so can cause severe adverse cardiovascular effects.

Magnesium sulfate

Magnesium sulfate is used to treat ventricular arrhythmias, especially polymorphic VT and PAT. Magnesium sulfate acts similarly to Class III antiarrhythmic drugs because it decreases myocardial cell excitability and conduction. It slows conduction through the AV node and prolongs the refractory period in the atria and ventricles.

How to give it

For life-threatening arrhythmias, administer 1- to 2-g magnesium sulfate over 5 to 60 minutes. Follow with an infusion of 0.5 to 1 g/hour. The dosage and duration of therapy depend on the patient's response and serum magnesium levels. The optimum dosage is still under study.

What can happen

Adverse cardiovascular effects of magnesium sulfate include diaphoresis, flushing, depressed cardiac function, bradycardia, hypotension, and circulatory collapse. (See *Noncardiac adverse effects of magnesium sulfate*.)

> Avoid administering magnesium sulfate to patients with renal disease.

Noncardiac adverse effects of magnesium sulfate

In addition to adverse cardiovascular effects of magnesium sulfate, other adverse effects include:
- *CNS*—drowsiness, depressed reflexes, flaccid paralysis, hypothermia
- *Respiratory*—respiratory paralysis
- *Other*—hypocalcemia.

How you intervene

Keep the following points in mind when caring for a patient receiving magnesium sulfate:
- Monitor the patient's HR, blood pressure, ventilatory rate, ECG, urine output, deep tendon reflexes, and mental status.
- Remember that magnesium sulfate should be avoided in patients with renal disease. Use it cautiously in patients with renal insufficiency and in those taking digoxin.
- Monitor closely for signs and symptoms of hypermagnesemia, such as hypotension, AV block, CNS depression, depressed or

absent deep tendon reflexes, muscle weakness or paralysis, and respiratory arrest.
- Have IV calcium available to counteract the effects of hypermagnesemia.
- Have intubation equipment and a mechanical ventilator available.
- Magnesium sulfate is contraindicated in heart block.

Teaching about antiarrhythmics

Here are some important points to emphasize when teaching your patient about antiarrhythmic drugs:
- Take the drug exactly as prescribed. Don't stop taking the drug without consulting your practitioner.
- Call the practitioner if you experience chest pain, shortness of breath, cough, palpitations, dizziness, fatigue, a weight gain of more than 2 lb (0.9 kg) per day, a very fast or slow HR, or a change in the regularity of the heartbeat or if you notice persistent changes you feel might be related to drug therapy.
- See your practitioner for regular checkups, as scheduled. Periodic physical examinations, ECGs, chest X-rays, and laboratory studies will help evaluate the effectiveness of therapy.
- Use herbal preparations with care. Some preparations can cause life-threatening interactions. Notify your provider of any herbal or over-the-counter medications you are taking.

That's a wrap!

Pharmacologic treatments review

Antiarrhythmic drugs
- Classified according to effect on the cell's electrical activity (action potential) and mechanism of action

Class Ia antiarrhythmics
- Are called sodium channel blockers
- Reduce excitability of cardiac cells and decrease contractility
- Have anticholinergic and proarrhythmic effects
- Show widened QRS complex and prolonged QT intervals on ECG

Quinidine
- Used for supraventricular and ventricular arrhythmias

Procainamide hydrochloride
- Used for supraventricular and ventricular arrhythmias

Class Ib antiarrhythmics
- Suppress ventricular ectopy
- Slow phase 0 depolarization
- Shorten phase 3 repolarization and action potential

Pharmacologic treatments review (*continued*)

Lidocaine hydrochloride
• Former drug of choice for suppressing ventricular arrhythmias

Mexiletine
• Oral congener of lidocaine, used to treat ventricular arrhythmias

Class Ic antiarrhythmics
• Slow conduction in all cardiac tissue

Flecainide acetate
• Used for paroxysmal atrial fibrillation or flutter in patients without structural heart disease; prevents SVT

Propafenone hydrochloride
• Used for paroxysmal atrial fibrillation or flutter in patients without structural heart disease; prevents SVT

Class II antiarrhythmics
• Are called beta-adrenergic blockers
• Block sympathetic nervous system beta-receptors and decrease HR
• Used to treat supraventricular and ventricular arrhythmias
• Include acebutolol, propranolol, esmolol, and sotalol

Class III antiarrhythmics
• Are called potassium channel blockers
• Block potassium movement during phase 3
• Increase the duration of the action potential
• Prolong the effective refractory period
• Show prolonged PR and QT intervals and widened QRS complex on ECG

Amiodarone
• Used for supraventricular arrhythmias, atrial fibrillation, and atrial flutter; PSVT

caused by accessory pathway conduction (as in WPW syndrome); and ventricular arrhythmias

Ibutilide fumarate
• Rapidly converts recent-onset atrial fibrillation or flutter

Dofetilide
• Used for maintenance of normal sinus rhythm in patients with atrial fibrillation or flutter
• Used to convert atrial fibrillation and flutter to normal sinus rhythm

Class IV antiarrhythmics
• Are called calcium channel blockers
• Prolong conduction time and refractory period in the AV node
• Decrease contractility
• Show PR interval prolonged on ECG

Verapamil
• Used for PSVT and to slow ventricular response in atrial fibrillation and flutter

Diltiazem
• Used for PSVT and atrial fibrillation or flutter

Unclassified antiarrhythmics
• Also called miscellaneous antiarrhythmics

Adenosine
• Slows AV node conduction and inhibits reentry pathways
• Used to treat PSVT

Atropine
• Anticholinergic drug that blocks vagal effects on the SA and AV nodes
• Used to treat symptomatic bradycardia and asystole

Pharmacologic treatments review *(continued)*

Digoxin
- Enhances vagal tone and slows conduction through the SA and AV nodes
- Shows ST-segment depression opposite the QRS deflection on ECG; P wave may be notched.
- Historically used to treat PSVT and ventricular rate with atrial fibrillation and flutter

Epinephrine
- Catecholamine that acts on alpha-adrenergic and beta-adrenergic receptor sites of the sympathetic nervous system
- Used for symptomatic bradycardia and to restore cardiac rhythm in cardiac arrest

Magnesium sulfate
- Decreases cardiac cell excitability and conduction; slows conduction through the AV node, and prolongs the refractory period
- Used to treat ventricular arrhythmias.

Quick quiz

1. Antiarrhythmic drugs that depress the rate of depolarization belong to class:
    A. I.
    B. II.
    C. III.
    D. IV.

Answer: A. Class I antiarrhythmic drugs block sodium influx during phase 0, depressing the rate of depolarization.

2. The drug that blocks vagal stimulation and increases the HR is:
    A. magnesium sulfate.
    B. diltiazem.
    C. verapamil.
    D. atropine.

Answer: D. Atropine blocks vagal effects on the SA node, enhances conduction through the node, and speeds the HR. The drug is used to treat symptomatic bradycardia.

3. The Class III antiarrhythmic drug used for the rapid conversion of recent-onset atrial fibrillation or flutter to sinus rhythm is:
    A. digoxin.
    B. ibutilide fumarate.
    C. procainamide.
    D. verapamil.

Answer: B. Ibutilide fumarate increases atrial and ventricular refractoriness and is used for the rapid conversion of recent-onset atrial fibrillation or flutter.

4. A drug known for lowering the resting HR is:
   A. quinidine.
   B. amiodarone.
   C. propranolol.
   D. lidocaine.

Answer: C. Beta-adrenergic blockers, such as propranolol, block sympathetic nervous system and lower HR, contractility, and conduction.

Scoring

⭐⭐⭐ If you answered all four questions correctly, just say "wow"! You're the antiarrhythmic drug czar.

⭐⭐ If you answered three questions correctly, great job! You're the deputy antiarrhythmic drug czar.

⭐ If you answered fewer than three questions correctly, don't fret. Get into the rhythm of antiarrhythmics by reviewing this chapter again.

Selected references

CAAD-VT investigators; Bennett, R. G., Campbell, T., Garikapati, K., Kotake, Y., Turnbull, S., Kanawati, J., Wong, M. S., Qian, P., Thomas, S. P., Chow, C. K., Kovoor, P., Robert Denniss, A., Chik, W., Marschner, S., Kistler, P., Haqqani, H., Rowe, M., Voskoboinik, A., . . . Kumar, S. (2023). A prospective, multicentre randomised controlled trial comparing catheter ablation versus antiarrhythmic drugs in patients with structural heart disease related ventricular tachycardia: The CAAD-VT trial protocol. *Heart, Lung & Circulation, 32*(2), 184–196. https://doi.org/10.1016/j.hlc.2022.09.006

Camm, A. J., & Lüscher, T. F., Maurer, G., and Serruys, P. (2019). *ESC CardioMed—Clinical cardiology: Current practice guidelines* (3rd ed.).

Camm, A. J., Naccarelli, G. V., Mittal, S., Crijns, H. J. G. M., Hohnloser, S. H., Ma, C. S., Natale, A., Turakhia, M. P., & Kirchhof, P. (2022). The increasing role of rhythm control in patients with atrial fibrillation: JACC state-of-the-art review. *Journal of the American College of Cardiology, 79*(19), 1932–1948. https://doi.org/10.1016/j.jacc.2022.03.337

Cohen, B. J., & Taylor, J. R. (2022). *Memmler's structure and function of the human body* (13th ed.). Wolters Kluwer.

Frishman, W. H., Cheng-Lai, A., & Hoffman, B. B. (2021). *Cardiovascular pharmacotherapeutics manual*. Wolters Kluwer.

Heidenreich, P. A., Bozkurt, B., Aguilar, D., Allen, L. A., Byun, J. J., Colvin, M. M., Deswal, A., Drazner, M. H., Dunlay, S. M., Evers, L. R., Fang, J. C., Fedson, S. E., Fonarow, G. C., Hayek, S. S., Hernandez, A. F., Khazanie, P., Kittleson, M. M., Lee, C. S., Link, M. S., Milano, C. A., . . . Yancy, C. W. (2022). 2022 AHA/ACC/HFSA Guideline for the Management of Heart Failure: A Report of the American College of Cardiology/American Heart Association Joint Committee on Clinical Practice Guidelines. *Circulation, 145*(18), e895–e1032. https://doi.org/10.1161/CIR.0000000000001063

Khachatryan, A., Merino, J. L., de Abajo, F. J., Botto, G. L., Kirchhof, P., Breithardt, G., Stambler, B., Abenhaim, L., & Grimaldi-Bensouda, L. (2022). International cohort study on the effectiveness of dronedarone and other antiarrhythmic drugs for atrial fibrillation in real-world practice (EFFECT-AF). *Europace, 24*(6), 899–909. https://doi.org/10.1093/europace/euab262

Ommen, S. R., Ho, C. Y., Asif, I. M., Balaji, S., Burke, M. A., Day, S. M., Dearani, J. A., Epps, K. C., Evanovich, L., Ferrari, V. A., Joglar, J. A., Khan, S. S., Kim, J. J., Kittleson, M. M., Krittanawong, C., Martinez, M. W., Mital, S., Naidu, S. S., Saberi, S., Semsarian, C., ... Waldman, C. B. (2024). 2024 AHA/ACC/AMSSM/HRS/PACES/SCMR Guideline for the Management of Hypertrophic Cardiomyopathy: A Report of the American Heart Association/American College of Cardiology Joint Committee on Clinical Practice Guidelines. *Circulation, 149*(23), e1239–e1311. https://doi.org/10.1161/CIR.0000000000001250

Li, D. L., Cox, Z. L., Richardson, T. D., Kanagasundram, A. N., Saavedra, P. J., Shen, S. T., Montgomery, J. A., Murray, K. T., Roden, D. M., & Stevenson, W. G. (2021). Quinidine in the management of recurrent ventricular arrhythmias: A reappraisal. *JACC Clinical Electrophysiology, 7*(10), 1254–1263. https://doi.org/10.1016/j.jacep.2021.03.024

Lippincott Williams & Wilkins. (2021). *Cardiovascular care made incredibly easy!* (5th ed.). Wolters Kluwer.

Luthra, A., & Justin Purcell, R. (2020). *Management of atrial fibrillation and atrial flutter: A practical guide.* Wiley-Blackwell.

Mann, D. L., Zipes, D. P., Libby, P., & Bonow, R. O. (Eds.). (2019). *Braunwald's heart disease: A textbook of cardiovascular medicine* (11th ed.). Elsevier.

Mark Estes, N. A., & Rod Gimbel, J. (2019). *Atrial tachycardia: Clinical cardiology monographs.* Springer.

Urden, L. D., Stacy, K. M., & Lough, M. E. (2021). *Critical care nursing: Diagnosis and management* (9th ed.). Elsevier.

Wagner, G. S., Strauss, D. G., & Morrison, D. A. (2021). *Marriott's practical electrocardiography* (14th ed.). Wolters Kluwer.

Part IV

The 12–lead ECG

Obtaining a 12-lead ECG

Just the facts

In this chapter, you'll learn:

◆ the role of 12-lead ECG in diagnosing pathologic conditions

◆ the relationship between the heart's electrical axis and the 12-lead ECG

◆ the proper technique for preparing your patient, placing the electrodes, and recording the ECG

◆ the diagnostic purposes of the posterior-lead ECG and the right chest–lead ECG

◆ the function of a signal-averaged ECG.

A look at the 12-lead ECG

The 12-lead ECG is a diagnostic test that records the heart's activity by measuring electrical currents through the heart muscle. A 12-lead ECG recording of the heart's rate and rhythm may identify a medical emergency such as, an acute myocardial infarction (AMI), a dangerous abnormal heart rhythm, or may signal cardiovascular heart disease. The 12-lead ECG gives a more complete view of the heart's electrical activity than a rhythm strip does. The ECG records electrical activity from 12 recording lead directions and provides a snapshot in time of the heart rate, rhythm, size, and position. Patients with other conditions that affect the heart's electrical system may also benefit from a 12-lead ECG. (See *Why a 12-lead ECG?*.)

Why a 12-lead ECG?

A 12-lead ECG is performed on patients having a myocardial infarction (MI). It may also be ordered for patients with other conditions that affect the heart, including:

• angina
• arrhythmias

(continued)

Why a 12-lead ECG? *(continued)*

- heart chamber enlargement
- digoxin or other drug toxicity
- electrolyte imbalances
- pulmonary embolism
- pericarditis
- hypothermia.

Now that's one heck of a charge card!

Interdependent evidence

Just like other diagnostic tests, a 12-lead ECG must be viewed alongside other clinical evidence. Always correlate the patient's ECG results with their history, physical assessment findings, laboratory results, and medication regimen.

In addition to a 12-lead ECG, it is possible to monitor the heart's electrical activity while the patient is going about their everyday activities. Ambulatory ECG recorders are an invaluable tool for identifying arrhythmias that may occur infrequently and unpredictably outside the clinical setting. There are several types of ambulatory ECG monitors, including Holter monitors, external cardiac event recorders, and implantable loop recorders.

A Holter monitor is worn for 24 to 48 hours. It continuously records the heart's rate and rhythm. If symptomatic, the patient may press the Holter recorder button and simultaneously note their activity in a diary. There is no real-time detection of arrhythmias. A complete analysis is performed after the monitor is returned. Holter monitors give the most detailed information of all the external ECG monitors.

Unlike Holter monitors, cardiac event recorders may be worn for longer periods of time (several weeks/months) and do not attempt to record every heartbeat. The earliest cardiac event recorders, still in use today, require the patient to take an action by activating the recorder to initiate an ECG recording. The patient will send the recording over a landline phone to the monitoring company. (See *Transtelephonic cardiac monitoring*, page 265.)

With advancements in technology, newer generation external cardiac event recorders and implantable loop recorders (inserted under the skin) have the added ability to automatically detect cardiac arrhythmias and transmit ECG recordings wirelessly over a mobile network for analysis and correlation with reported symptoms.

It's important for nurses to remind patients that cardiac event recorders (external and/or internal) are **not** designed to trigger an emergency response. If a patient experiences a symptom, the patient should generate a recording; document the date, time, and symptoms; and if needed, contact their health care provider.

Cardiac event recorders are increasingly important as a tool for assessing cardiac arrhythmias in symptomatic and asymptomatic patients outside the clinical settings.

Transtelephonic cardiac monitoring

Using a special recorder–transmitter, patients at home can transmit ECGs by telephone to a central monitoring center for immediate interpretation. This technique, called *transtelephonic cardiac monitoring* (TTM), reduces health care costs and is widely used.

Nurses play an important role in TTM. Besides performing extensive patient and family teaching, they also run the central monitoring center and help interpret ECGs sent by patients.

TTM allows the practitioner to assess transient conditions that cause symptoms such as palpitations, light-headedness, syncope, confusion, paroxysmal dyspnea, and chest pain. Such conditions commonly aren't apparent while the patient is in the presence of a practitioner, which can make diagnosis difficult and costly.

With TTM, the patient can transmit an ECG recording from their home when symptoms appear, avoiding the need to go to the hospital for diagnosis and offering a greater opportunity for early diagnosis. Even if symptoms don't appear often, the patient can keep the equipment for long periods of time, which further aids in the diagnosis of the patient's condition.

Home care

TTM can also be used by patients who have cardiac rehabilitation at home. The patient is called regularly during this period to receive transmissions and assess progress. This monitoring can help reduce the anxiety felt by the patient and family members after discharge, especially if the patient suffered a MI.

TTM is especially valuable for assessing the effects of drugs and for diagnosing and managing paroxysmal arrhythmias. In both cases, TTM can eliminate the need for admitting the patient for evaluation and a potentially lengthy hospital stay.

Understanding TTM equipment

TTM requires three main pieces of equipment: an ECG recorder–transmitter, a standard telephone line, and a receiver. The ECG recorder–transmitter converts electrical activity transferred from the patient's heart into acoustic waves. Some models contain built-in memory that stores a recording of the activity so the patient can transmit it at a later date.

A standard telephone line is used to transmit information. The receiver converts the acoustic waves transmitted over the telephone line into ECG activity, which is then recorded on ECG paper for interpretation and documentation in the patient's medical record. The recorder–transmitter uses an electrode applied to the finger, chest, or a wrist bracelet. These electrodes produce ECG tracings similar to those of a standard 12-lead ECG.

Credit card–size recorder

One type of recorder operates on a battery and is about the size of a credit card. When a patient becomes symptomatic, they hold the back of the card firmly to the center of their chest and push the start button. Four electrodes located on the back of the card sense electrical activity and record it. The card can store 30 seconds of activity and can later transmit the recording across phone lines for evaluation by a practitioner.

Other transtelephonic monitors are approximately the size of a beeper and store lengths of ECGs on a digital chip, which can then be transmitted over the phone line and recorded on paper.

How leads work

The 12-lead ECG records the heart's electrical activity using a series of electrodes placed on the patient's extremities and chest wall. The 12 leads include three bipolar limb leads (I, II, and III), three unipolar augmented limb leads (aV_R, aV_L, and aV_F), and six unipolar precordial, or chest, leads (V_1, V_2, V_3, V_4, V_5, and V_6). These leads provide 12 different views of the heart's electrical activity. (See *A look at the leads*.)

A look at the leads

Each of the 12 leads views the heart from a different angle. The following illustrations show the direction of each lead relative to the wave of depolarization (shown in color) and list the 12 views of the heart.

Views reflected on a 12-lead ECG	Leads	View of the heart
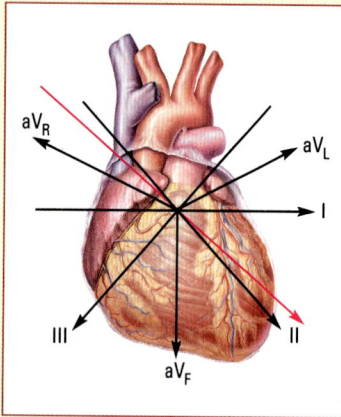	**Standard limb leads (bipolar)**	
	I	Lateral wall
	II	Inferior wall
	III	Inferior wall
	Augmented limb leads (unipolar)	
	aV_R	No specific view
	aV_L	Lateral wall
	aV_F	Inferior wall
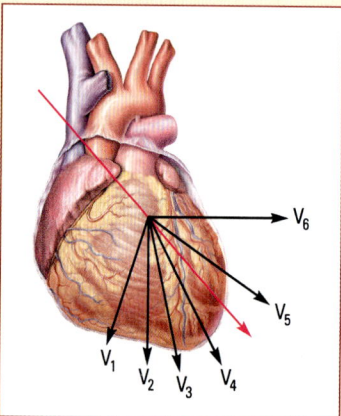	**Precordial, or chest, leads (unipolar)**	
	V_1	Septal wall
	V_2	Septal wall
	V_3	Anterior wall
	V_4	Anterior wall
	V_5	Lateral wall
	V_6	Lateral wall

Up, down, and across

Scanning up, down, and across the heart, each lead transmits information about a different area. The waveforms obtained from each lead vary depending on the location of the lead in relation to the wave of depolarization, or electrical stimulus, passing through the myocardium.

Limb leads

The six limb leads record electrical activity in the heart's frontal plane. This plane is a vertical view through the middle of the heart from top to bottom. Electrical activity is recorded from the anterior to the posterior axis.

Precordial leads

The six precordial leads provide information on electrical activity in the heart's horizontal plane, a transverse view through the middle of the heart, dividing it into upper and lower portions. Electrical activity is recorded from either a superior or an inferior approach.

The electrical axis

Besides assessing 12 different leads, a 12-lead ECG records the heart's electrical axis. The axis is a measurement of electrical impulses flowing through the heart.

As impulses travel through the heart, they generate small electrical forces called *instantaneous vectors*. The mean of these vectors represents the force and direction of the wave of depolarization through the heart. That mean is called the *electrical axis*. It's also called the *mean instantaneous vector* and the *mean QRS vector*.

Havin' a heart wave

In a healthy heart, impulses originate in the sinoatrial node, travel through the atria to the atrioventricular node, and then to the ventricles. Most of the movement of the impulses is downward and to the left, the direction of a normal axis.

Swingin' on an axis

In an unhealthy heart, axis direction varies. That's because the direction of electrical activity swings away from areas of damage or necrosis and toward areas of hypertrophy. Knowing the normal deflection of each lead will help you evaluate whether the electrical axis is normal or abnormal.

Obtaining a 12-lead ECG

To obtain an ECG, you'll need to:
- gather the appropriate supplies
- explain the procedure to the patient
- attach the electrodes properly
- know how to use the ECG machine.

Let's take a closer look at obtaining an ECG

Explain the procedure

Tell the patient that the practitioner has ordered an ECG and explain the procedure. Emphasize that the test takes only a few minutes and that it's a safe, painless, and risk-free way to evaluate cardiac function.

Answer the patient's questions and offer reassurance. Preparing the patient well helps alleviate anxiety and promote cooperation.

Prepare the patient

Ask the patient to lie in a supine or semi-Fowlers position with their arms at their sides. If there are patient mobility issues, modifications to this position can be made. Ensure privacy, and expose the patient's arms, legs, and chest, draping for comfort. Make sure the patient's legs are uncrossed. Remove electrical devices, including cell phones, from the area because of the interference they may cause. (See *Obtaining a pediatric ECG*.)

Skin preparation

Select the areas where you'll attach the electrodes. Choose spots that are flat and fleshy, and avoid areas that are muscular or bony. Dry the skin if it is wet or diaphoretic. Clip the area if it's excessively hairy. Clean excess oil or other substances from the skin to enhance electrode contact. Follow your hospital policy for any additional skin preparation, such as the use of a nonalcohol wipe or abrasive skin prep pad. Remember—the better the electrode contact, the better the recording.

Make the recording

The 12-lead ECG offers 12 different views of the heart, just as 12 photographers snapping the same picture would produce 12 different snapshots. To help ensure an accurate recording—or set of "pictures"—the electrodes must be applied correctly. Inaccurate placement of an electrode by greater than 5/8″ (1.5 cm) from its standardized position may lead to inaccurate waveforms and an incorrect ECG interpretation.

The 12-lead ECG requires a total of 10 electrodes: four electrodes on the limbs, known as *limb* leads, and six precordial leads, which are placed across the front of the chest wall. However, even though there are 10 electrodes, these actually provide 12 views of electrical cardiac activity.

Obtaining a pediatric ECG

You'll need patience when obtaining a pediatric ECG. With the help of the parents, if possible, try distracting the attention of a young child. If artifact from arm and leg movement is a problem, place the electrodes in a more proximal position on the extremity.

Going out on a limb lead

To record the bipolar limb leads I, II, and III and the unipolar limb leads aV_R, aV_L, and aV_F, place electrodes on both of the patient's arms and on their left leg. The right leg also receives an electrode, but that electrode acts as a ground and doesn't contribute to the waveform.

Where the wires go

Finding where to place the electrodes on the patient is easy because each lead wire is labeled or color coded. (See *Monitoring the limb leads*.) For example, a wire—usually white—might be labeled "RA" for right arm. Another wire—usually red—might be labeled "LL" for left leg. Precordial leads are also labeled or color coded according to which wire corresponds to which lead.

Monitoring the limb leads

These diagrams show electrode placement for the six limb leads. RA indicates right arm; LA, left arm; RL, right leg; and LL, left leg. The plus sign (+) indicates the positive pole, the minus sign (−) indicates the negative pole, and G indicates the ground. Each diagram is a sample ECG recording for that lead.

Lead I

This lead connects the right arm (negative pole) with the left arm (positive pole).

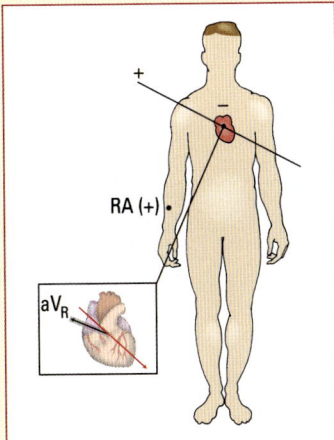

Lead II

This lead connects the right arm (negative pole) with the left leg (positive pole).

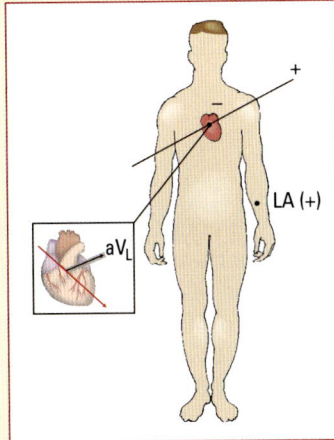

Lead III

This lead connects the left arm (negative pole) with the left leg (positive pole).

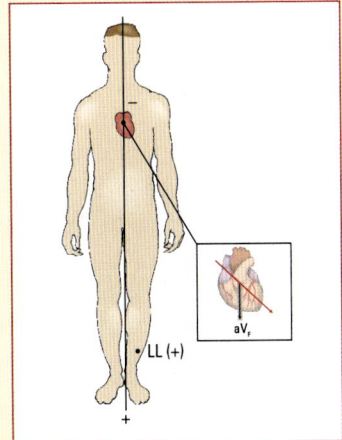

(continued)

Monitoring the limb leads *(continued)*

Lead aV$_R$	Lead aV$_L$	Lead aV$_F$
This lead connects the right arm (positive pole) with the heart (negative pole).	This lead connects the left arm (positive pole) with the heart (negative pole).	This lead connects the left leg (positive pole) with the heart (negative pole).

No low leads allowed

To record the six precordial leads (V$_1$ through V$_6$), position the electrodes on specific areas of the anterior chest wall. It is vital that the practitioner knows the exact placement of each electrode on the patient as incorrect placement can lead to a false diagnosis of infarction or negative changes on the ECG. (See *Positioning precordial electrodes,* page 271.)

- Place lead V$_1$ over the fourth intercostal space at the right sternal border. To find the space, locate the sternal notch at the second rib and feel your way down along the sternal border until you reach the fourth intercostal space (V$_1$ and V$_2$ electrodes that are placed in a more superior location can mimic an anterior wall MI and cause T-wave inversion).

Positioning precordial electrodes

The precordial leads complement the limb leads to provide a complete view of the heart. To record the precordial leads, place the electrodes as shown here.

- Place lead V_2 just opposite V_1, over the fourth intercostal space at the left sternal border.
- Place lead V_3 midway between V_2 and V_4. *Tip:* Placing lead V_4 before lead V_3 makes it easier to see where to place lead V_3.
- Place lead V_4 over the fifth intercostal space at the left midclavicular line.
- Place lead V_5 over the fifth intercostal space at the left anterior axillary line.
- Place lead V_6 over the fifth intercostal space at the left midaxillary line. If you've placed leads V_4 through V_6 correctly, they should line up horizontally.

Give me more electrodes!

In addition to the 12-lead ECG, two other ECGs may be used for diagnostic purposes: the posterior-lead ECG and the right chest–lead ECG. These ECGs use chest leads to assess areas that standard 12-lead ECGs are unable to.

Precordial leads (V_1 through V_6) that are misplaced inferiorly or laterally can alter the amplitude and lead to a misdiagnosis.

Seeing behind your back

Because of lung and muscle barriers, the usual chest leads can't "see" the heart's posterior surface to record myocardial damage there. Some practitioners add three posterior leads to the 12-lead ECG: leads V_7, V_8, and V_9. These leads are placed opposite anterior leads V_4, V_5, and V_6, on the left side of the patient's back, following the same horizontal line.

On rare occasions, a practitioner may request right-sided posterior leads. These leads are labeled V_{7R}, V_{8R}, and V_{9R} and are placed on the right side of the patient's back. Their placement is a mirror image of the electrodes on the left side of the back. This type of ECG provides information on the right posterior area of the heart.

Checking out the right chest

The usual 12-lead ECG evaluates only the left ventricle. If the right ventricle needs to be assessed for damage or dysfunction, the practitioner may order a right chest–lead ECG. For example, a patient with an inferior wall MI might have a right chest–lead ECG to rule out right ventricular involvement.

With this type of ECG, the six leads are placed on the right side of the chest in a mirror image of the standard precordial lead placement. Electrodes start at the left sternal border and swing down under the right breast area.

Know your machine

After you understand how to position the electrodes, familiarize yourself with the ECG machine. Machines come in two types: multichannel recorders and single-channel recorders. Because single-channel recorders are rarely used, we'll only discuss a multichannel recorder.

With a multichannel recorder, attach all electrodes to the patient at once and the machine prints a simultaneous view of all leads. To begin recording the patient's ECG, follow these steps:
- Plug the cord of the ECG machine into a grounded outlet. If the machine operates on a charged battery, it may not need to be plugged in.
- Enter the patient's identification data as prompted by the ECG machine or via an electronic medical record as an order.
- Prepare the patient's skin and then place the electrodes on the patient's chest, arms, and legs.
- Make sure all leads are securely attached.
- Instruct the patient to relax, lie still, and breathe normally. Ask them not to talk during the recording to prevent respiratory waveform distortion of the ECG tracing.

- Verify that the ECG paper speed selector is set to 25 mm/sec. If necessary, calibrate or standardize the machine according to the manufacturer's instructions.
- Press the appropriate button to record the ECG. When performing a right chest–lead ECG, select the appropriate button for recording or note it on the ECG hardcopy.
- Observe the quality of the tracing. When the machine finishes the recording, turn it off.
- Remove the electrodes and, if necessary, clean the patient's skin. If the ECG machine transmits a copy to a central monitoring area or software system, ensure that the copy has been transmitted.

Interpreting the recording

ECG tracings from multichannel machines will all look the same. (See *Multichannel ECG recording*.) The printout will show the patient's name and identification number. At the top of the printout, the patient's heart rate and wave durations will be measured in seconds.

Multichannel ECG recording

The top of a 12-lead ECG recording usually shows patient identification information along with the interpretation done by the machine. A rhythm strip is usually included at the bottom of the recording.

Standardization marks
Look for the standardization marks on the recording, normally 10 small squares high. If the patient has high voltage complexes, the marks will be half as high. Notice that lead markers separate the lead recordings on the paper and that each lead is labeled.

ECG tracing layout
Also familiarize yourself with the order in which the leads are arranged on the ECG tracing. Getting accustomed to the layout of the tracing will help you interpret the ECG more quickly and accurately.

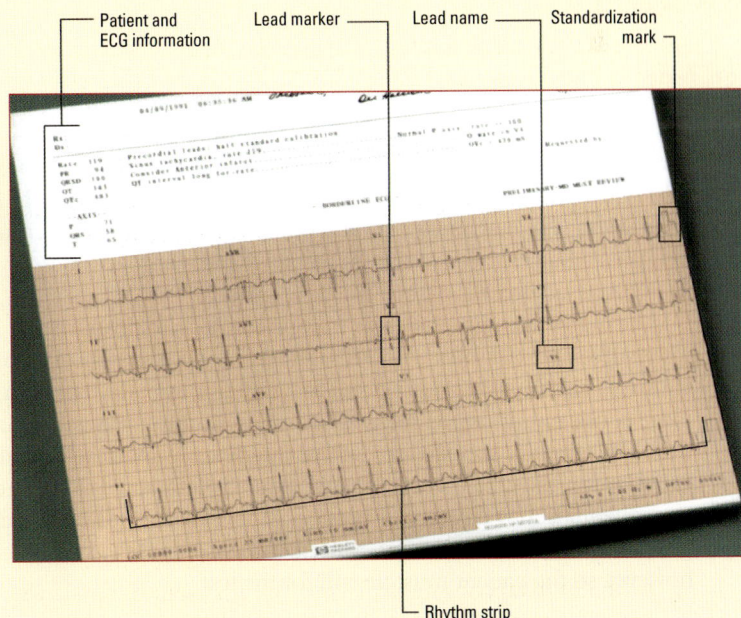

Patient and ECG information — Lead marker — Lead name — Standardization mark

Rhythm strip

Some machines can also record ST-segment elevation and depression. The name of the lead appears next to each 6-second strip.

Remember, ECGs are legal documents. They belong on the patient's medical record and must be saved for future reference and comparison with baseline strips.

Signal–averaged ECG

Although a 12-lead ECG is beneficial as a diagnostic indicator for most patients, an SAECG may also be useful. This simple, noninvasive test helps identify patients at risk for sudden death from sustained ventricular tachycardia.

The test uses a computer to identify late electrical potentials—tiny impulses that follow normal depolarization. Late electrical potentials are not detected by a 12-lead ECG.

Who gets the signal?

Patients prone to ventricular tachycardia—those who have had a recent MI, coronary heart disease, cardiomyopathy, or unexplained syncope, for example—are good candidates for an SAECG. Keep in mind that a 12-lead ECG should be done when the patient is free from arrhythmias.

Noise-free

An SAECG is a noise-free, surface ECG recording taken from three specialized leads for several hundred heartbeats. (See *Electrode placement for a signal-averaged ECG*, page 275.) The test takes approximately 7 to 10 minutes. The machine's computer detects late electrical potentials and then enlarges them so they're recognizable. The electrodes for an SAECG are labeled X^-, X^+, Y^-, Y^+, Z^-, Z^+, and G.

The machine averages signals from these leads to produce one representative QRS complex without artifacts. This process cancels noise, electrical impulses that don't occur as a repetitious pattern or with the same consistent timing as the QRS complex. Multiple electric signals from the heart are averaged to remove interference and reveal small variations in the QRS complex, usually called "late potentials." These late potentials may represent a predisposition toward potentially dangerous ventricular arrhythmias. Muscle noise is unable to be filtered, however, so the patient must lie still for the test.

Memory jogger

To help you remember the electrodes for the signal-averaged ECG (SAECG), think of the phrase "XYZ times 2 and G." The electrodes are X^-, X^+, Y^-, Y^+, Z^-, Z^+, and G (ground).

Electrode placement for an SAECG

Electrodes are placed much differently for an SAECG than they are for a 12-lead ECG. Here's one method:

1. Place the positive X electrode at the left fourth intercostal space, midaxillary line.

2. Place the negative X electrode at the right fourth intercostal space, midaxillary line.

3. Place the positive Y electrode at the left iliac crest.

4. Place the negative Y electrode at the superior aspect of the manubrium of the sternum.

5. Place the positive Z electrode at the fourth intercostal space left of the sternum.

6. Place the ground (G) on the lower right at the eighth rib.

7. Reposition the patient on their side or have them sit forward. Then place the negative Z electrode on the patient's back, directly posterior to the positive Z electrode.

8. Attach all the leads to the electrodes, being careful not to dislodge the posterior lead.

Now, you can obtain the tracing.

Anterior chest

Posterior chest

That's a wrap!

Obtaining a 12-lead ECG

12-lead ECG basics
- Provides 12 different views of the heart's electrical activity

The limb leads
- Three bipolar limb leads: I, II, and III
- Three unipolar limb leads: aV_R, aV_L, and aV_F
- Record electrical activity in the heart's frontal vertical plane, providing a view through the middle of the heart from top to bottom

The precordial leads
- Six unipolar precordial (chest) leads: V_1 through V_6

- Record electrical activity in the heart's horizontal plane, providing a transverse view through the middle of the heart, dividing it into upper and lower portions

Electrical axis
- Measurement of the electrical impulses flowing through the heart
- Normal axis downward and to the left
- Direction of electrical activity swings away from areas of damage or necrosis and toward areas of hypertrophy

Placing the leads
- Bipolar and unipolar limb leads: Electrodes on both arms and the left leg, ground on the right leg

Obtaining a 12-lead ECG *(continued)*

- V_1: Over fourth intercostal space at the right sternal border
- V_2: Over fourth intercostal space at the left sternal border
- V_3: Midway between leads V_2 and V_4
- V_4: Over fifth intercostal space at the left midclavicular line
- V_5: Over fifth intercostal space at the left anterior axillary line
- V_6: Over fifth intercostal space at the left midaxillary line

Views of the heart walls

- Lead I: Lateral wall
- Lead II: Inferior wall
- Lead III: Inferior wall
- Lead aV_R: No specific view
- Lead aV_L: Lateral wall
- Lead aV_F: Inferior wall
- Lead V_1: Septal wall
- Lead V_2: Septal wall
- Lead V_3: Anterior wall

- Lead V_4: Anterior wall
- Lead V_5: Lateral wall
- Lead V_6: Lateral wall

Other lead placements

- Posterior leads: V_7, V_8, and V_9 are placed opposite V_4, V_5, and V_6 on the left side of the back to view the posterior surface of the heart
- Right chest leads: Placed on the right chest in the mirror image of standard precordial leads to view the right ventricle

Types of ECGs

- Multichannel ECG: All electrodes are attached at one time to provide simultaneous views of all leads
- SAECG: Uses a computer to identify late electrical potentials from three specialized leads over hundreds of beats; identifies patients at risk for sudden cardiac death from ventricular tachycardia

Quick quiz

1. The precordial leads are placed on the:
   A. anterior chest starting with the fourth intercostal space at the right sternal border.
   B. lateral chest starting with the fourth intercostal space at the left midaxillary line.
   C. posterior chest wall starting with the fourth intercostal space at the midscapular line.
   D. left leg and both arms.

Answer: A. Lead V_1 is placed anteriorly between the fourth and fifth ribs at the right sternal border. Leads V_2 to V_6 are then placed accordingly.

2. A 12-lead ECG is used to assess the function of the:
   A. right ventricle.
   B. left ventricle.
   C. right and left ventricles simultaneously.
   D. right and left atria simultaneously.

Answer: B. A 12-lead ECG gives a more complete view of the heart's electrical activity than a rhythm strip and is used to assess left ventricular function.

3. A posterior-lead ECG is used to assess:
    A. posterior myocardial damage.
    B. inferior myocardial damage.
    C. damage to the interventricular septum.
    D. damage to the base of the heart.

Answer: A. The posterior-lead ECG assesses damage to the posterior surface of the heart, an area a standard 12-lead ECG can't detect.

4. When recording a 12-lead ECG, the paper speed should be set at:
    A. 10 mm/sec.
    B. 20 mm/sec.
    C. 25 mm/sec.
    D. 50 mm/sec.

Answer: C. The correct paper speed for a 12-lead ECG is 25 mm/sec.

5. A signal-averaged ECG (SAECG) measures:
    A. electrical impulses from the sinoatrial node.
    B. electrical impulses arriving at the atrioventricular node.
    C. action potentials of individual cardiac cells.
    D. late electrical potentials throughout the heart.

Answer: D. Signal-averaged ECGs (SAECGs) measure late electrical potentials, tiny electrical impulses that occur after depolarization and can cause ventricular tachycardia.

6. To record the bipolar limb leads I, II, and III and the unipolar limb leads aV_R, aV_L, and aV_F, place electrodes on:
    A. both of the patient's arms and left leg, with a ground on their right leg.
    B. the patient's right arm and left leg, with a ground on their left arm.
    C. both of the patient's legs and their left arm, with a ground on their right arm.
    D. both of the patient's arms and their right leg, with a ground on their left leg.

Answer: A. To record these bipolar and unipolar limb leads, place electrodes on both of the patient's arms and left leg, with a ground on their right leg.

7. Transtelephonic (TTM) cardiac monitoring:
    A. is a process whereby the patient can transmit their own ECG from home to a central monitoring center for interpretation.
    B. is a costly procedure.
    C. utilizes a special telephone line.
    D. is not as accurate as a standard 12-lead ECG.

Answer: A. It is a process whereby the patient can transmit their own ECG from home to a central monitoring center for interpretation.

Scoring

☆☆☆ If you answered all seven questions correctly, great job! You're the new leader of the 12-lead ECG pack.

☆☆ If you answered six questions correctly, we're impressed! Your leadership qualities are obvious, and you should be next in line for a top job.

☆ If you answered fewer than six questions correctly, that's okay! You'll be sure to take the lead in the next chapter.

Recommended references

Cohen, B. J., & Hull, K. (2019). *Memmler's structure and function of the human body* (12th ed.). Wolters Kluwer.

Fogoros, R. (2022). What you should know about ambulatory ECG monitoring. *Verywell Health.* https://www.verywellhealth.com/ambulatory-ecg-monitoring-4171275

Katritsis, D. G., Gersch, B. J., & Camm, A. J. (2016). *Clinical cardiology: Current practice guidelines.* Oxford University Press.

Libby, P., Bonow, R. O., Mann, D. L., Tomaselli, G. F., Bhatt, D. L., Solomon, S. D., & Braunwald, E. (2022). *Braunwald's heart disease: A textbook of cardiovascular medicine* (12th ed.). Saunders/Elsevier.

McLaughlin, M. A. (Clinical Ed.). (2019). *Cardiovascular care made incredibly easy* (4th ed.). Wolters Kluwer.

Urden, L., Stacy, K. M., & Lough, M. E. (2021). *Critical care nursing* (9th ed.). Mosby/Elsevier.

Interpreting a 12-lead ECG

Just the facts

In this chapter, you'll learn:

♦ to examine each lead's waveforms for abnormalities

♦ to determine techniques that evaluate the heart's electrical axis

♦ ECG changes in patients with angina

♦ ECG characteristics to differentiate types of acute myocardial infarction (MI)

♦ 12-lead ECG changes that occur with a bundle branch block.

A look at 12–lead ECG interpretation

To interpret a 12-lead ECG, use the systematic approach outlined here. Compare the patient's previous ECG, if available, with the current one to help you identify changes.

1. Check the ECG tracing to ensure the baseline is free from electrical interference and drift.
2. Lead aV_R is typically negative. If it is not negative, the leads may be placed incorrectly.
3. Locate the lead markers on the waveform. Lead markers are the points where one lead changes to another.
4. Check the standardization markings to make sure all leads were recorded with the ECG machine's amplitude at the same setting. Standardization markings are usually located at the beginning of the strip.
5. Assess the heart rate and rhythm as you learned in earlier chapters.
6. Determine the heart's electrical axis. Use either the quadrant method or the degree method, described later in this chapter.
7. Examine the limb leads: I, II, and III. The R wave in leads I and II should be dominant with upright P and T waves. The R wave in lead III may be dominant or absent, with upright, flat, or inverted P and T waves. Each lead should have flat ST segments, and pathologic Q waves should be absent.

8. Examine the augmented leads: aV_L, aV_F, and aV_R. The tracings from leads aV_L and aV_F should be similar, but lead aV_F should have taller P and R waves. Lead aV_R has little diagnostic value. Its P wave, QRS complex, and T wave should be deflected downward.
9. Examine the R wave in the precordial leads, V_1 to V_6. Normally, the R wave—the first positive deflection of the QRS complex—gets progressively taller from lead V_1 to lead V_5, then it gets slightly smaller in lead V_6. (See *R-wave progression.*)
10. Examine the S wave—the negative deflection after an R wave—in the precordial leads. It appears extremely deep in lead V_1 and becomes progressively shallower, usually disappearing at lead V_5 or V_6.

That's progress!

R-wave progression

These waveforms show normal R-wave progression through the precordial leads. Note that the R wave is the first positive deflection in the QRS complex. Also note that the S wave gets smaller, or regresses, from lead V_1 to V_6 until it finally disappears.

Ages and stages

Normal findings in pediatric ECGs

In a neonate, dominant R waves in the chest leads and upright T waves are normal findings. By the end of the first week of life, the T wave in lead V_1 becomes inverted and remains inverted through age 7.

All about waves

As you examine each lead, note where changes occur so you can identify the area of the heart that's affected. Remember that P waves should be upright; however, they may be inverted in lead aV_R or biphasic or inverted in leads III, aV_L, and V_1.

PR intervals should always be constant, just like QRS-complex durations. QRS-complex deflections will vary in different leads. Observe for pathologic Q waves. (See *Normal findings in pediatric ECGs.*)

Elevated 1 minute, depressed the next

ST segments should be iso-electric or have minimal deviation. ST-segment elevation greater than 1 mm above the baseline and ST-segment depression greater than 0.5 mm below the baseline are considered abnormal. Leads facing an injured area will have ST-segment elevations, and leads facing away will display ST-segment depressions.

Downsloping ST   Upsloping ST   Horizontal ST

J point

That old, changeable T wave

The T wave should be slightly rounded and upright. It normally deflects upward in leads I, II, and V_3 through V_6. It may also be inverted in leads III, aV_R, aV_F, aV_L, and V_1. T waves should not be tall, peaked, or notched. There are numerous reasons for T-wave changes, which are not always the cause for alarm. Excessively tall, flat, or inverted T waves or ST–T wave changes with accompanying cardiac symptoms, such as chest pain, may indicate myocardial ischemia.

Split-second duration

A normal Q wave generally has a duration of less than 0.04 seconds. An abnormal Q wave has either a duration of 0.04 seconds or more, a depth greater than 4 mm, or a height one fourth of the R wave.

Abnormal Q waves indicate myocardial necrosis. These waves develop when depolarization does not take its normal path because of damaged tissue in the area. Remember that lead aV_R normally has a large Q wave, so disregard this lead when searching for abnormal Q waves.

Finding the electrical axis

The electrical axis is the average direction of the heart's electrical activity during ventricular depolarization. Leads placed on the body sense the sum of the heart's electrical activity and record it as waveforms.

Cross my heart

You can determine your patient's electrical axis by examining the waveforms recorded from the six frontal plane leads: I, II, III, aV_R, aV_L, and aV_F. Imaginary lines drawn from each of the leads intersect the center of the heart and form a diagram known as the hexaxial reference system. (See *Hexaxial reference system*, page 282.)

Hexaxial reference system

The hexaxial reference system consists of six bisecting lines, each representing one of the six limb leads, and a circle representing the heart. The intersection of all lines divides the circle into equal, 30-degree segments.

Shifting degrees

Note that +0 degree appears at the 3 o'clock position (positive pole lead I). Moving counterclockwise, the degrees become increasingly negative, until reaching ±180 degrees, at the 9 o'clock position (negative pole lead I).

The bottom half of the circle contains the corresponding positive degrees. However, a positive-degree designation does not necessarily mean that the pole is positive.

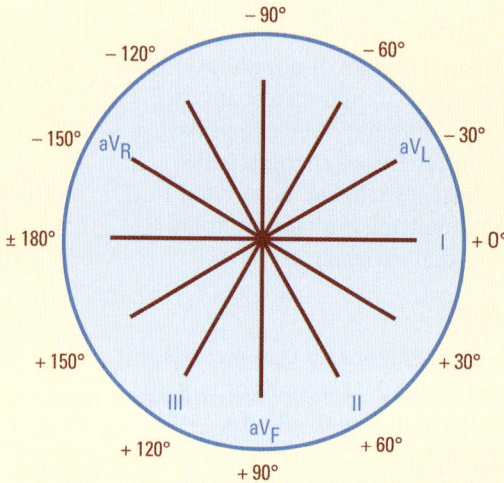

Axis deviation across the lifespan

Right-axis deviation, between +60 and +160 degrees, is normal in a neonate because of the dominance of the right ventricle. By age 1, the axis shifts to fall between +10 and +100 degrees as the left ventricle becomes dominant.

Left-axis deviation commonly occurs in elderly people. This axis shift may result from fibrosis of the anterior fascicle of the left bundle branch or thickness of the left ventricular wall, which increases by 25% between ages 30 and 80.

Where the axis falls

An axis that falls between 0 and +90 degrees (some references concede −30 to +90) is considered normal. An axis between +90 and +180 degrees indicates right-axis deviation, and one between 0 and −90 degrees indicates left-axis deviation. An axis between +180 and −90 degrees indicates extreme-axis deviation and is called an *indeterminate axis*.

To determine your patient's electrical axis, use one of the two methods described here: the quadrant method or the degree method. (See *Axis deviation across the lifespan*.)

This diagram is called the hexaxial reference system. Use it to determine your patient's electrical axis.

Quadrant method

The quadrant method, a fast, easy way to plot the heart's axis, involves observing the main deflection of the QRS complex in leads I and aV$_F$. (See *Quadrant method*.) Lead I indicates whether impulses are moving to the right or the left, and lead aV$_F$ indicates whether they are moving up or down.

Quadrant method

This chart helps you quickly determine the direction of a patient's electrical axis. Just observe the deflections of the QRS complexes in leads I and aV$_F$. Then check the chart to determine whether the patient's axis is normal or has a left-, right-, or extreme-axis deviation.

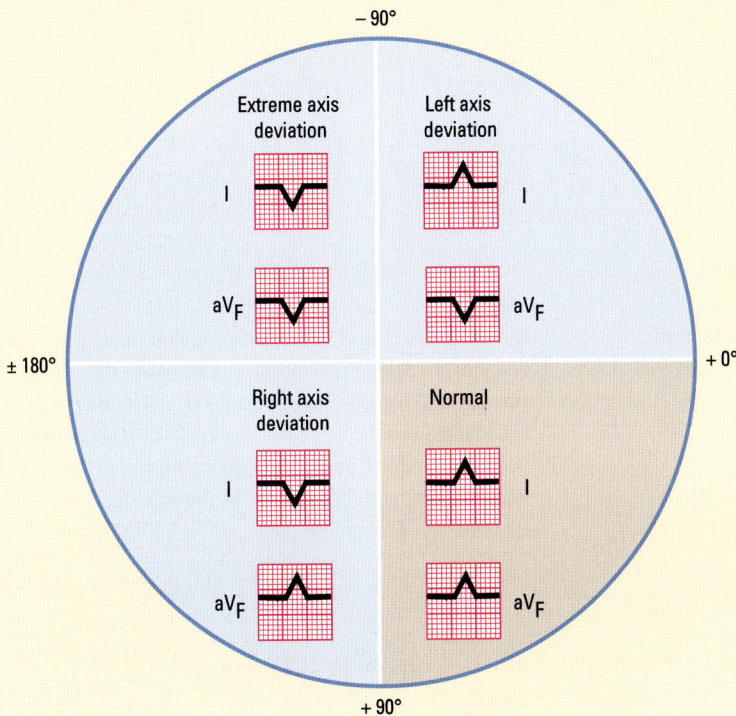

If the QRS-complex deflection is positive or upright in both leads, the electrical axis is normal. If lead I is upright and lead aV$_F$ points down, left-axis deviation exists.

Right on and right in

When lead I points downward and lead aV$_F$ is upright, right-axis deviation exists. Both waves pointing down signal extreme-axis deviation.

Memory jogger

Think of the QRS-complex deflections in leads I and aVF as thumbs pointing up or down. Two thumbs pointing up indicate normal; anything else is abnormal.

Degree method

A more precise axis calculation, the degree method gives an exact degree measurement of the electrical axis. (See *Degree method*.) It also allows you to determine the axis even if the QRS complex isn't clearly positive or negative in leads I and aV_F. To use this method, follow these steps:

Degree method

The degree method of determining axis deviation allows you to identify a patient's electrical axis by degrees on the hexaxial system, not just by quadrant. To use this method, follow the following steps:

Step 1

Identify the lead with the smallest QRS complex or the equiphasic QRS complex. In this example, it is lead III.

Lead I	Lead II	Lead III	Lead aV_R	Lead aV_L	Lead aV_F

Step 2

Locate the axis for lead III on the hexaxial diagram. Then find the axis perpendicular to it, which is the axis for lead aV_R.

Step 3

Now, examine the QRS complex in lead aV_R, noting whether the deflection is positive or negative. As you can see, the QRS complex for this lead is negative. This tells you that the electric current is moving toward the negative pole of aV_R, which, on the hexaxial diagram, is in the right lower quadrant at +30 degrees. So, the electrical axis here is normal at +30 degrees.

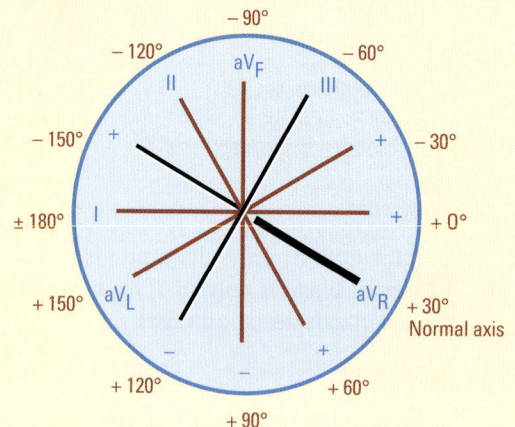

1. Review all six leads and identify the one that contains either the smallest QRS complex or the complex with an equal deflection above and below the baseline.
2. Use the hexaxial diagram to identify the lead perpendicular to this lead. For example, if lead I has the smallest QRS complex, then the lead perpendicular to the line representing lead I would be lead aV$_F$.
3. After you have identified the perpendicular lead, examine its QRS complex. If the electrical activity is moving toward the positive pole of a lead, the QRS complex deflects upward. If it is moving away from the positive pole of a lead, the QRS complex deflects downward.
4. Plot this information on the hexaxial diagram to determine the direction of the electrical axis.

Axis deviation

Finding a patient's electrical axis can help confirm a diagnosis or narrow the range of possible diagnoses. (See *Causes of axis deviation*.) Factors that influence the location of the axis include the heart's position in the chest, the heart's size, the patient's body size or type, the conduction pathways, and the force of the electrical impulses being generated.

> Heart size can influence the location of the electrical axis. Tell me, how does my size look to you…?

Causes of axis deviation

This list covers common causes of right- and left-axis deviation.

Left	Right
• Aging	• Acute pulmonary embolism
• Hyperkalemia	• Dextrocardia
• Inferior wall myocardial infarction (MI)	• Emphysema/chronic obstructive pulmonary disease (COPD)
• Left anterior hemiblock	• Lateral wall MI
• Left bundle branch block (LBBB)	• Left posterior hemiblock
• Left ventricular hypertrophy	• Normal variation
• Mechanical shifts (ascites, pregnancy, tumors)	• Right and left arm lead reversal
• Normal variation	• Right bundle branch block (RBBB)
• Pacemaker-generated rhythm or paced rhythm	• Right ventricular hypertrophy
• Wolff–Parkinson–White syndrome (WPW)	• Ventricular rhythm disturbances (ventricular tachycardia, accelerated idioventricular)

Remember that electrical activity in the heart swings away from areas of damage or necrosis, so the damaged part of the heart will be the last area to be depolarized. For example, in RBBB, the impulse travels quickly down the normal left side and then moves slowly down the right side. This shifts the electrical forces to the right, causing right-axis deviation.

No worries

Axis deviation is not always the cause for alarm, and it may not result from a cardiac origin. For example, infants and children normally have right-axis deviation. Pregnant women normally have left-axis deviation. However, it is important to further investigate the origin with cardiac diagnostic testing, particularly if this is a new finding.

Disorders affecting a 12–lead ECG

A 12-lead ECG is used to diagnose conditions such as angina, bundle branch block, and MI. By reviewing sample ECGs, you will know what classic signs to look for. The following is a synopsis of these three common cardiac conditions with clues for 12-lead ECG signs to look for.

Angina

During an episode of angina, the myocardium demands more oxygen than the coronary arteries can deliver. The arteries are unable to deliver enough oxygenated blood to the heart, commonly as a result of atherosclerosis seen in coronary artery disease (CAD), whereby arteries narrow over time due to plaque deposition and calcification. The pathophysiologic process is inflammatory in nature and is further complicated by platelet aggregation, thrombus formation, and/or vasospasm.

An episode of angina usually lasts a few minutes and may be a precursor to MI.

Angina pain that lasts close to 30 minutes most likely signals an MI.

Stable, unstable, variant?

You may hear the term *stable, unstable,* or *variant angina* applied to certain conditions. In stable angina, an episode of pain is triggered by exertion or stress and is usually relieved by rest or with medicine. Each episode follows the same pattern and may be associated with chest pain that radiates to the arms, back, or other areas.

Unstable angina, which is one of the syndromes related to acute coronary syndrome (ACS), is more easily provoked and usually wakes the patient. It is also unpredictable, worsens over time, is not well ameliorated by rest or medications, and lasts for a longer period of time as compared to stable angina. Chest pain associated with unstable angina may present as epigastric discomfort or substernal burning, pain, or pressure with radiation to common sites, including the shoulder, neck, jaw, left arm, or scapula. These symptoms may be associated with shortness of breath, dyspnea on exertion, diaphoresis, lightheadedness, nausea, or vomiting. The patient with unstable angina is treated as a medical emergency as the onset is a common precursor to MI.

Prinzmetal or variant angina usually arises at rest, frequently from midnight to early morning. Younger patients experience this type of angina caused by coronary artery spasm triggered by cold weather, emotional stress, exertion, smoking, cocaine use, or medicine. People with comorbid conditions of Raynaud phenomenon or migraine headaches may also suffer from Prinzmetal angina. These patients may benefit from nitrates and calcium channel blockers.

Fleeting change of heart

Ischemic changes are evident on the ECG during the episodes of angina and may resolve to some degree when the angina subsides. (See *ECG changes associated with angina*.) Because these changes may be fleeting, always obtain an order for, and perform, a 12-lead ECG as soon as the patient reports chest pain.

ECG changes associated with angina

Here are some classic ECG changes involving the T wave and ST segment that you may see when monitoring a patient with angina.

| Peaked T wave | Flattened T wave | T-wave inversion | ST-segment depression with T-wave inversion | ST-segment depression without T-wave inversion |

The 12-lead ECG will allow you to analyze the electrical activity associated with the myocardium, in order to further determine the culprit coronary artery(ies) involved. By recognizing danger early, you may be able to prevent morbidity or mortality associated with MI.

Pharmacologic agents are a key component of anginal treatment and may include nitrates, beta-adrenergic blockers, calcium channel blockers, aspirin or glycoprotein IIb/IIIa inhibitors to reduce platelet aggregation, nitrates, and ranolazine. With persistent anginal symptoms, revascularization should be considered to improve symptoms.

Bundle branch block

One potential complication of an MI is a bundle branch block. In this disorder, either the left or right bundle branch fails to conduct impulses. A bundle branch block that occurs farther down the left bundle, in the posterior or anterior fasciculus, is called a *hemiblock*.

Some blocks require treatment with a temporary pacemaker. In other cases, blocks are monitored to detect whether they progress to a more complete heart block.

Impulsive behavior

In a bundle branch block, the impulse travels down the unaffected bundle branch and then from one myocardial cell to the next to depolarize the ventricle.

Because this cell-to-cell conduction progresses much more slowly than the conduction along the specialized cells of the conduction system, ventricular depolarization is prolonged.

Wide world of complexes

Prolonged ventricular depolarization means that the QRS complex is widened. The normal width of the complex is 0.06 to 0.12 seconds. If the width increases to greater than 0.12 seconds, a bundle branch block is present.

After you identify a bundle branch block, examine lead V_1, which lies to the right of the heart, and lead V_6, which lies to the left of the heart. You will use these leads to determine whether the block is in the right or left bundle.

Right bundle branch block

RBBB occurs with conditions such as anterior wall MI, CAD, cardiomyopathy, cor pulmonale, and pulmonary embolism. It may also occur without cardiac disease. If this block develops as the heart rate increases, it is called *rate-related RBBB.* (See *How RBBB occurs.*)

In this disorder, the QRS complex is greater than 0.12 seconds and has a different configuration, sometimes resembling rabbit ears or the

How RBBB occurs

In RBBB, the initial impulse activates the interventricular septum from left to right, just as in normal activation. Next, the left bundle branch activates the left ventricle. The impulse then crosses the interventricular septum to activate the right ventricle.

letter "M." (See *Recognizing RBBB,* page 290.) Septal depolarization is not affected in lead V_1, so the initial small R wave remains.

The R wave is followed by an S wave, which represents left ventricular depolarization, and a tall R wave (called *R prime,* or *R'*), which

Recognizing RBBB

This 12-lead ECG shows the characteristic changes of RBBB. In lead V_1, note the rsR' pattern and T-wave inversion. In lead V_6, see the widened S wave and the upright T wave. Also note the prolonged QRS complexes.

Lead I

Lead aV_R

Lead V_1

Lead V_4

Lead II

Lead aV_L

Lead V_2

Lead V_5

Lead III

Lead aV_F

Lead V_3

Lead V_6

represents late right ventricular depolarization. The T wave is negative in this lead. However, that deflection is called a *secondary T-wave change* and is of no clinical significance.

Opposing moves

The opposite occurs in lead V_6. A small Q wave is followed by depolarization of the left ventricle, which produces a tall R wave. Depolarization of the right ventricle then causes a broad S wave. In lead V_6, the T wave should be positive.

Left bundle branch block

Left bundle-branch block (LBBB) develops from underlying pathology often caused by hypertensive heart disease, aortic stenosis, degenerative changes of the conduction system, or CAD. (See *How LBBB occurs.*) When it occurs in conjunction with an anterior wall MI, it usually signals complete heart block requiring insertion of a pacemaker.

How LBBB occurs

In LBBB, the impulse first travels down the right bundle branch. Then the impulse activates the interventricular septum from right to left, the opposite of normal activation. Finally, the impulse activates the left ventricle.

Block

In LBBB, the S wave may be preceded by a Q wave or R wave.

One ventricle after another

In LBBB, the QRS complex will be greater than 0.12 seconds because the ventricles are activated sequentially, not simultaneously. (See *Recognizing LBBB*, page 292.) As the wave of depolarization spreads from the right ventricle to the left, a wide S wave is produced in lead V_1, with a positive T wave. The S wave may be preceded by a Q wave or a small R wave.

Recognizing LBBB

This 12-lead ECG shows characteristic changes of LBBB. All leads have prolonged QRS complexes. In lead V_1, note the QS-wave pattern. In lead V_6, you will see the slurred R- and T-wave inversion. The elevated ST segments and upright T waves in leads V_1 to V_4 are also common in LBBB.

Lead I

Lead aV_R

Lead V_1

Lead V_4

Lead II

Lead aV_L

Lead V_2

Lead V_5

Lead III

Lead aV_F

Lead V_3

Lead V_6
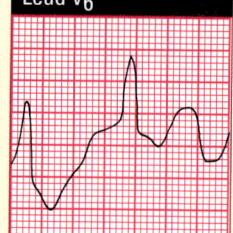

Slurring your R waves

In lead V_6, no initial Q wave occurs. A tall, notched R wave, or a slurred one, is produced as the impulse spreads from right to left. This initial positive deflection is a sign of LBBB. The T wave is negative.

Myocardial infarction

Unlike stable angina, pain associated with an MI lasts from several minutes up to several hours and is unrelieved by rest. Frequently, anginal pain escalates in frequency and duration consistent with ACS prodrome. The location of the MI varies depending upon the culprit coronary artery.

For as long as the myocardium is deprived of an oxygen-rich blood supply, an ECG will reflect the three pathologic changes of an MI: ischemia, injury, and infarction. (See *Reciprocal changes in an MI*.)

Reciprocal changes in an MI

Ischemia, injury, and infarction—the three I's of a MI—produce characteristic ECG changes. Changes shown by the leads that reflect electrical activity in damaged areas are shown on the right of the illustration.

Reciprocal leads, those opposite the damaged area, will show opposite ECG changes, as shown to the left of the illustration.

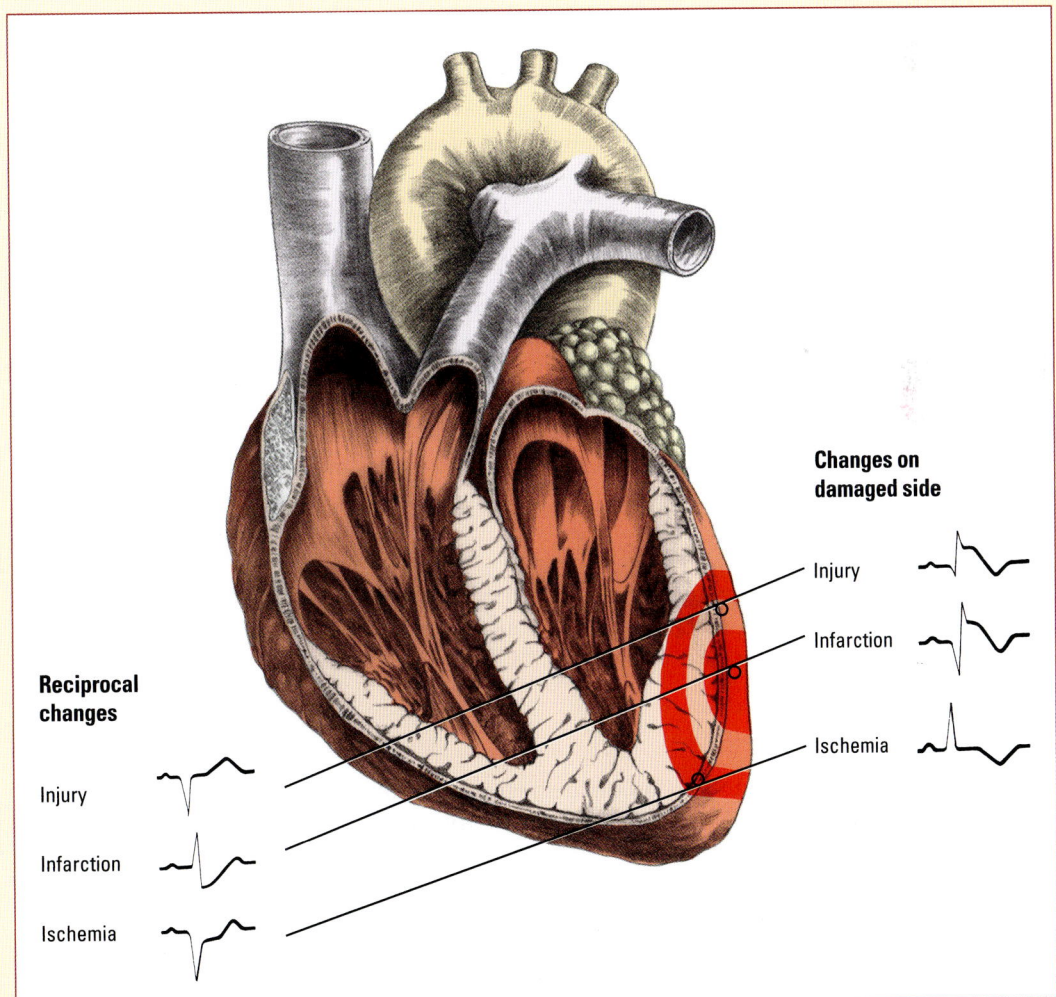

Changes on damaged side
Injury
Infarction
Ischemia

Reciprocal changes
Injury
Infarction
Ischemia

Zone of infarction

The area of myocardial necrosis is called the *zone of infarction*. Scar tissue eventually replaces the dead tissue, and the damage caused is irreversible.

The ECG change associated with a necrotic area is a pathologic Q wave, which results from lack of depolarization. Such Q waves are permanent. MIs that do not produce Q waves are called *non–Q-wave MIs*. (See *Q waves in children*.)

Zone of injury

The zone of infarction is surrounded by the zone of injury, which appears on an ECG as an elevated ST segment. ST-segment elevation results from a prolonged lack of oxygenated blood supplied to the myocardium.

Zone of ischemia

The outermost area is called the *zone of ischemia* and results from an interrupted supply of oxygenated blood. This zone is represented on an ECG by T-wave inversion. Changes in the zones of ischemia or injury are reversible.

From ischemia to injury

Generally, as an MI occurs, the patient experiences chest pain and an ECG shows changes, such as ST-segment elevation, which indicates that myocardial injury is in process. Accompanying changes include flattened or inverted T waves.

Rapid treatment can prevent myocardial necrosis. However, if symptoms persist for more than 6 hours, little can be done to prevent necrosis. That is one of the reasons patients are advised to seek medical attention as soon as symptoms begin.

The telltale Q wave

Q waves can appear hours to days after a MI and signify that an entire thickness of the myocardium has become necrotic. Tall R waves in reciprocal leads may also develop. This type of MI is called a *transmural*, or *Q-wave*, *MI*.

Back to baseline

Knowing how long such changes last can help you determine how long ago an MI occurred. ST segments return to baseline within a few days to 2 weeks. Inverted T waves may persist for several months. Although not every patient who has had an MI develops Q waves, those who do may have them on their ECGs indefinitely.

Ages and stages

Q waves in children

Q waves in leads II, III, aV_F, V_5, and V_6 are normal in children. Q waves in other leads suggest cardiac disease, such as an abnormal left coronary artery.

Mixed signals

Monitoring patients with MI

Remember that specific leads monitor specific walls of the heart. Here's a quick overview of those leads:

• For an anterior wall MI, monitor lead V_1 or MCL_1.

• For a septal wall MI, monitor lead V_1 or MCL_1 to pick up hallmark changes.

• For a lateral wall MI, monitor lead V_6 or MCL_6.

• For an inferior wall MI, monitor lead II.

What to do for an MI?

The most important step you can take for a patient with a MI is to remain vigilant about detecting changes in their condition and ECG. (See *Monitoring patients with MI*, page 294.)

The primary goal of treatment for an MI is to limit the size of the infarction by increasing oxygen supply to the myocardium and decreasing workload. (See *Improving blood flow*.)

In addition to rest, pain relief, and supplemental oxygen, medications such as nitroglycerin, morphine sulfate, beta-adrenergic blockers, calcium channel blockers, angiotensin-converting enzyme inhibitors, and antiarrhythmics are used. Aspirin or glycoprotein IIb/IIIa inhibitors may be used to reduce platelet aggregation. Thrombolytic therapy may also be prescribed to dissolve a thrombus occluding a coronary artery.

Identifying types of MI

The location of the MI is a critical factor in determining the most appropriate treatment and predicting probable complications. Characteristic ECG changes that occur with each type of MI are localized to the leads overlying the infarction site. (See *Locating myocardial damage*.) Here's a look at characteristic ECG changes that occur with different types of MI.

Improving blood flow

Increasing the blood supply to the heart of a patient who has had a MI can help prevent further damage to their heart. In addition to medications, blood flow to the heart can be improved by the following:
- intra-aortic balloon pump
- percutaneous transluminal coronary angioplasty
- atherectomy
- laser treatment
- stent placement
- coronary artery bypass graft

Locating myocardial damage

After you have noted characteristic lead changes of an acute MI, use this chart to identify the areas of damage. Match the lead changes in the second column with the affected wall in the first column and the artery involved in the third column. Column 4 shows reciprocal lead changes.

Wall affected	Leads	Artery involved	Reciprocal changes
Anterior	V_3 to V_4	Left coronary artery, left anterior descending (LAD) artery	II, III, aV_F
Anterolateral	I, aV_L, V_3 to V_6	LAD artery, circumflex artery	II, III, aV_F
Septal	V_1 to V_2	LAD artery	None
Inferior	II, III, aV_F	Right coronary artery	I, aV_L
Lateral	I, aV_L, V_5, V_6	Circumflex artery, branch of left coronary artery	II, III, aV_F
Posterior	V_8, V_9	Right coronary artery, circumflex artery	V_1 to V_4
Right ventricular	V_{4R}, V_{5R}, V_{6R}	Right coronary artery	None

Anterior wall MI

The LAD artery supplies blood to the anterior portion of the left ventricle. The artery supplies blood to the ventricular septum and portions of the right and left bundle branch systems.

When the anterior descending artery becomes occluded, an anterior wall MI occurs. (See *Recognizing an anterior wall MI.*)

Recognizing an anterior wall MI

This 12-lead ECG shows typical characteristics of an anterior wall MI. Note that the R waves don't progress through the precordial leads. Also note the ST-segment elevation in leads V_2 and V_3. As expected, the reciprocal leads II, III, and aV_F show slight ST-segment depression. Axis deviation is normal at +60 degrees.

Lead I

Lead aV_R

Lead V_1

Lead V_4

Lead II

Lead aV_L

Lead V_2

Lead V_5

Lead III

Lead aV_F

Lead V_3

Lead V_6

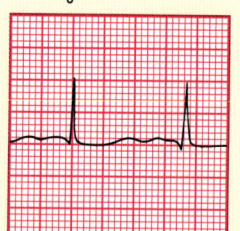

Complications of an anterior wall MI include varying second-degree atrioventricular blocks, bundle branch blocks, ventricular irritability, and left-sided heart failure.

Changing the leads

An anterior wall MI causes characteristic ECG changes in leads V_3 to V_4. The precordial leads show poor R-wave progression because the left ventricle can't depolarize normally. ST-segment elevation and T-wave inversion are also present.

The reciprocal leads for the anterior wall are the inferior leads II, III, and aV_F. They show tall R waves and depressed ST segments.

Septal wall MI

The patient with a septal wall MI has an increased risk for developing a ventricular septal defect. ECG changes are present in leads V_1 and V_2. In those leads, the R wave disappears, the ST segment rises, and the T wave inverts.

Because the LAD artery also supplies blood to the ventricular septum, a septal wall MI commonly accompanies an anterior wall MI. (See *Recognizing an anteroseptal wall MI*, page 298.)

Lateral wall MI

A lateral wall MI is usually caused by a blockage in the left circumflex artery and shows characteristic changes in the left lateral leads I, aV_L, V_5, and V_6. The reciprocal leads for a lateral wall infarction are leads II, III, and aV_F. (See *Recognizing a lateral wall MI*, page 298.)

This type of infarction typically causes premature ventricular contractions and varying degrees of heart block. A lateral wall MI usually accompanies an anterior or inferior wall MI.

Memory jogger

To remember which leads are critical in diagnosing a lateral wall MI, think of the L's in "lateral MI" and "left lateral leads."

Inferior wall MI

An inferior wall MI is usually caused by occlusion of the right coronary artery and produces characteristic ECG changes in the inferior leads II, III, and aV_F and reciprocal changes in the lateral leads I and aV_L. (See *Recognizing an inferior wall MI*, page 298.) It's also called a *diaphragmatic MI* because the heart's inferior wall lies over the diaphragm.

Recognizing an anteroseptal wall MI

This 12-lead ECG shows typical characteristics of an anteroseptal wall MI. Note the poor R-wave progression, the elevated ST segments, and the inverted T waves in leads V_1, V_2, and V_3. Reciprocal changes are seen in leads II, III, and aV_F with depressed ST segments and tall, peaked T waves.

Lead I

Lead aV_R

Lead V_1

Lead V_4

Lead II

Lead aV_L

Lead V_2

Lead V_5

Lead III

Lead aV_F

Lead V_3

Lead V_6

Recognizing a lateral wall MI

This 12-lead ECG shows changes characteristic of a lateral wall MI. In leads I, aV$_L$, V$_5$, and V$_6$, note the pathologic Q waves, the ST-segment elevation, and the T-wave inversion.

Recognizing an inferior wall MI

This 12-lead ECG shows the characteristic changes of an inferior wall MI. In leads II, III, and aV$_F$, note the T-wave inversion, ST-segment elevation, and pathologic Q waves. In leads I and aV$_L$, note the slight ST-segment depression, a reciprocal change. This ECG shows left-axis deviation at -60 degrees.

Patients with an inferior wall MI are at risk for developing sinus bradycardia, sinus arrest, heart block, and premature ventricular contractions. This type of MI occurs either alone or with a lateral wall MI or with a right ventricular MI.

Right ventricular MI

A right ventricular MI usually follows occlusion of the right coronary artery. This type of MI rarely occurs alone. In fact, 40% of all patients with an inferior wall MI also suffer a right ventricular MI.

A right ventricular MI can lead to right-sided heart failure or right-sided block. The classic changes are ST-segment elevation, pathologic Q waves, and inverted T waves in the right precordial leads V$_{4R}$ to V$_{6R}$. (See *Recognizing a right ventricular MI*, page 301.)

Recognizing a right ventricular MI

This 12-lead ECG shows typical characteristics of a right ventricular MI. Note the T-wave inversion in leads V_{3R}, V_{4R}, V_{5R}, and V_{6R}. Pathologic Q waves and ST-segment elevation are also present.

Lead I

Lead aV_R

Lead V_1

Lead V_{3R}

Lead II

Lead aV_L

Lead V_2

Lead V_{4R}

Lead III

Lead aV_F

Lead V_{3R}

Lead V_{5R}

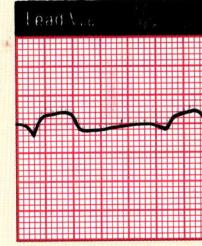

Take the right lead

Identifying a right ventricular MI is difficult without information from the right precordial leads. If these leads aren't available, you can observe leads II, III, and aV_F or watch leads V_1, V_2, and V_3 for ST-segment elevation. If a right ventricular MI has occurred, use lead II to monitor for further damage.

Posterior wall MI

A posterior wall MI is caused by occlusion of either the right coronary artery or the left circumflex arteries. This MI produces reciprocal changes on leads V_1 and V_2.

Classic ECG changes in a posterior wall MI include tall R waves, ST-segment depression, and upright T waves. (See *Recognizing a posterior wall MI.*) Posterior infarctions usually accompany inferior infarctions. Information about the posterior wall and pathologic Q waves that might occur can be obtained from leads V_7 to V_9 using a posterior ECG.

Recognizing a posterior wall MI

This 12-lead ECG shows typical characteristics of a posterior wall MI. Note the tall R waves, the depressed ST segments, and the upright T waves in leads V_1, V_2, and V_3 that represent reciprocal changes. These are reciprocal changes, because the leads that best monitor a posterior wall MI (V_7, V_8, and V_9) aren't on a standard 12-lead ECG.

Lead I

Lead aV$_R$

Lead V$_1$

Lead V$_4$

Lead II

Lead aV$_L$

Lead V$_2$

Lead V$_5$

Lead III

Lead aV$_F$

Lead V$_3$

Lead V$_6$

That's a wrap!

12-Lead ECG interpretation review

Looking at the waves

- *P waves:* Upright; possibly inverted in lead aV$_R$ or biphasic or inverted in leads III, aV$_L$, and V$_1$
- *PR intervals:* Always constant, like QRS-complex durations
- *QRS-complex deflections:* Variable in different leads
- *Q waves:* Possibly pathologic; duration of less than 0.4 seconds when normal
- *T wave:* Slightly rounded and upright; normal deflection upward in leads I, II, and V$_3$ through V$_6$; inverted in leads III, aV$_F$, aV$_R$, aV$_L$, and V$_1$; shouldn't be tall, peaked, or notched
- *ST segments:* should be isoelectric or have minimal deviation

Electrical axis

- Average direction of the heart's electrical activity during ventricular depolarization

Methods of determining axis

- *Quadrant method:* Determines main deflection of QRS complex in leads I and aV$_F$
- *Degree method:* Identifies axis by degrees on the hexaxial system
- *Examination of the waveforms from the six frontal leads:* I, II, III, aV$_R$, aV$_L$, and aV$_F$
- *Normal axis:* Between 0 and +90 degrees (−30 to +90 degrees is acceptable)
- *Left-axis deviation:* Between 0 and −90 degrees
- *Right-axis deviation:* Between +90 and +180 degrees
- *Extreme-axis deviation:* Between +180 and −90 degrees

Disorders affecting 12-lead ECGs
Angina

- *Possible ECG changes:* Peaked or flattened T wave, T-wave inversion, and ST-segment depression with or without T-wave inversion

Bundle branch block

- *QRS complex:* Width increases to greater than 0.12 seconds with bundle branch block.
- *Lead V$_1$ (to the right of heart) and V$_6$ (to the left of heart):* Used to determine whether the block is in the right or left bundle
- *RBBB:* QRS complex has rsR′ pattern and T-wave inversion in lead V$_1$ and widened S wave and upright T wave in lead V$_6$.
- *LBBB:* Wide S wave (which may be preceded by a Q wave or small R wave) and small positive T wave in lead V$_1$; tall, notched R wave or slurred R wave and T-wave inversion in lead V$_6$

Myocardial infarction

- Three pathologic changes on ECG—ischemia, injury, and infarction

Pathologic ECG changes

- *Zone of ischemia:* T-wave inversion
- *Zone of injury:* ST-segment elevation
- *Zone of infarction:* Pathologic Q wave in transmural MI

Locating the MI

- *Anterior wall:* Leads V$_3$ to V$_4$; involves LAD artery
- *Septal wall:* V$_1$ to V$_2$; involves LAD artery

Identifying a right ventricular MI is difficult without the right information from the right precordial leads.

12-Lead ECG interpretation review *(continued)*

- *Inferior wall:* Leads II, III, aV$_F$; involves right coronary artery
- *Lateral wall:* Leads I, aV$_L$, V$_5$, V$_6$; involves left circumflex artery
- *Posterior wall:* Leads V$_7$, V$_8$, V$_9$; involves right coronary or left circumflex arteries
- *Right ventricular wall:* V$_{4R}$, V$_{5R}$, V$_{6R}$; involves right coronary artery

Quick quiz

1. Your patient's ECG shows positively deflected QRS complexes in leads I and aV$_F$. Using the four-quadrant method for determining the electrical axis, you determine that the patient has a(n):

    A. normal axis.
    B. left-axis deviation.
    C. right-axis deviation.
    D. extreme-axis deviation.

Answer: A. If the QRS-complex deflection is positive or upright in both leads, the electrical axis is normal.

2. Your patient's ECG shows a negatively deflected QRS complex in lead I and a positively deflected one in lead aV$_F$. Using the four-quadrant method for determining electrical axis, you determine that the patient has a(n):

    A. normal axis.
    B. left-axis deviation.
    C. right-axis deviation.
    D. extreme-axis deviation.

Answer: C. When lead I points downward and lead aV$_F$ is upright, right-axis deviation exists. Both waves pointing down signals indeterminate-axis deviation.

3. If your patient has a T-wave inversion, ST-segment elevation, and pathologic Q waves in leads II, III, and aV$_F$, suspect an acute MI in the:

    A. anterior wall.
    B. inferior wall.
    C. lateral wall.
    D. septal wall.

Answer: B. Leads II, III, and aV$_F$ face the inferior wall of the left ventricle, so the ECG changes are indicative of an acute inferior wall MI.

4. If a patient's QRS complex has an R' wave in V_1, suspect:
    A. right ventricular hypertrophy.
    B. left ventricular hypertrophy.
    C. LBBB.
    D. RBBB.

Answer: D. In RBBB, depolarization of the right ventricle takes longer than normal, thereby creating an R' wave in lead V_1.

5. Myocardial injury is represented on an ECG by the presence of a(n):
    A. T-wave inversion.
    B. ST-segment elevation.
    C. pathologic Q wave.
    D. ST-segment depression.

Answer: B. ST-segment elevation is the ECG change that corresponds with myocardial injury. It's caused by a prolonged lack of blood supply.

6. On a 12-lead ECG, a posterior wall MI produces:
    A. deep, broad Q waves in leads V_1 through V_4.
    B. inverse or mirror image changes in V_1 and V_2.
    C. raised ST segments in all leads.
    D. poor R-wave progression in the precordial leads.

Answer: B. Leads V_1 and V_2 show reciprocal changes when a posterior wall MI occurs. Look at the mirror images of these leads to determine the presence of a posterior wall MI.

7. An ST segment located 1.5 mm above the baseline is considered:
    A. normal.
    B. slightly depressed.
    C. abnormally elevated.
    D. isoelectric.

Answer: C. ST segments should be isoelectric or have minimal deviation. ST-segment elevation greater than 1 mm above the baseline is considered abnormal.

So far, so good. Now check out the strips on the next page!

Test strips

Okay, it's time to try out a couple of ECG test strips.

1. In the following 12-lead ECG, you'll see an rsR' pattern in lead V_1, as well as T-wave inversion. Looking at lead V_6, you'll note a widened S wave and an upright T wave. These changes indicate:

A. right ventricular MI.
B. LBBB.
C. RBBB.
D. angina.

Answer: C. The rsR' configuration in lead V_1 and the wide S wave in V_6 indicate RBBB.

2. Your patient says he thinks he might have had a heart attack about 3 years ago and had never had it checked with their health care provider. Looking at their admission ECG, you are certain that they sustained a previous MI based on the presence of a(an):

A. pathologic Q waves in leads II, III, and aV_F.
B. inverted T waves in leads I, aV_L, and V_6.
C. depressed ST segments in leads II, aV_L, and V_5.
D. axis between 0 and +90 degrees.

Answer: A. Old damage to the myocardium is indicated by the presence of pathologic Q waves; in this case, in leads II, III, and aV_F. Those findings lead you to suspect the patient suffered an inferior wall MI at some point.

Scoring

⭐⭐⭐   If you answered all nine questions correctly, wow! You have graduated with honors from the School of 12-Lead ECG Interpretation.

⭐⭐   If you answered seven or eight questions correctly, super! You are ready to take a graduate course on 12-lead ECG interpretation.

⭐   If you answered fewer than seven questions correctly, it takes time to become proficient and you're on your way. You will benefit from further review of your notes from 12-Lead ECG Interpretation.

Selected references

Abobaker, A., & Rana, R. M. (2021). V_1 and V_2 pericordial leads misplacement and its negative impact on ECG interpretation and clinical care. *Annals of Noninvasive Electrocardiology, 26*(4), e12844. https://doi.org/10.1111/anec.12844

Cohen, B. J., & Taylor, J. J. (2019). *Memmler's structure and function of the human body* (12th ed.). Wolters Kluwer.

Hampton, J., & Hampton, J. (2019). *The ECG made easy* (9th ed.). Elsevier.

Libby, P., Bonow, R. D., Mann, D. L., Tomaseli, G. F., Bhat, D., Solomon, S. D., & Brunwald, E. (2021). *Brunwald's heart disease: A textbook of cardiovascular medicine* (12th ed.). Saunders Elsevier.

McLaughlin, M. A. (Ed.). (2019). *Cardiovascular care made incredibly easy* (4th ed.). Wolters Kluwer.

Sole, M. L., Klwin, D., & Moseley, M. (2020). *Introduction to critical care nursing* (8th ed.). Mosby Elsevier.

Strauss, D. G., & Shocken, D. D. (2021). *Marriott's practical electrocardiography* (13th ed.). Wolters Kluwer.

Appendices and index

Appendix 1: Practice makes perfect

Questions

1. You're caring for a patient with a history of mitral valve prolapse. Based on your knowledge of the heart's anatomy, you know that the mitral valve is located:
- A. between the left atrium and left ventricl
- B. where the left ventricle meets the aort
- C. between the right atrium and right ventricl
- D. between the right ventricle and pulmonary arter

2. A 45-year-old patient is admitted to your floor for observation after undergoing cardiac catheterization. The test results reveal a blockage in the circumflex artery. The circumflex artery supplies oxygenated blood to which area of the heart?
- A. Anterior wall of the left ventricle
- B. Left atrium
- C. Right bundle branch
- D. Right ventricle

3. Which of the following choices is responsible for slowing heart rate?
- A. Norepinephrine
- B. Vagus nerve
- C. Epinephrine
- D. Isoproterenol

4. Which cycle describes cardiac cells at rest?
- A. Early repolarization
- B. Polarization
- C. Rapid depolarization
- D. Absolute refractory period

5. A patient admitted with an acute myocardial infarction (MI) complains of chest pain. When you look at his ECG monitor, you note a heart rate of 35 beats/min. Which area of his heart has taken over as the heart's pacemaker?
- A. Sinoatrial (SA) node
- B. Atrioventricular (AV) node
- C. Bundle of His
- D. Purkinje fibers

6. Which lead on a cardiac monitor is equivalent to V_1 on a 12-lead ECG?
  A. Lead I
  B. Lead modified chest lead 6 (MCL_6)
  C. Lead aV_F
  D. Lead MCL_1

7. A 37-year-old patient comes to the emergency department (ED) complaining of chest pain that began while he was mowing the lawn. You immediately begin cardiac monitoring and administer oxygen. Next, you obtain a 12-lead ECG. You know that the six limb leads you apply will give you information about which area of the patient's heart?
  A. The frontal plane
  B. The horizontal plane
  C. The vertical plane
  D. The posterior plane

8. A patient with heart failure is transferred to your unit from the medical–surgical unit. Before initiating cardiac monitoring, you must first:
  A. prepare the skin by rubbing it until it reddens.
  B. press the adhesive edge around the outside of the electrode to the patient's chest.
  C. press one side of the electrode against the patient's skin.
  D. attach the leadwire to the electrode before placing it on the patient's chest.

9. A 58-year-old patient is admitted with an acute MI. After you begin cardiac monitoring, you note a baseline that is thick and unreadable. How do you interpret this finding?
  A. Electrical interference
  B. Artifact
  C. Wandering baseline
  D. Weak signal

10. What does the horizontal axis of an ECG represent?
  A. Amplitude
  B. Time
  C. Electrical voltage
  D. Heart rate

11. A 65-year-old patient diagnosed with angina is admitted to your telemetry unit. You begin cardiac monitoring and record a rhythm strip. Using the eight-step method of rhythm strip interpretation, what should you do first?
  A. Calculate the heart rate.
  B. Evaluate the P wave.
  C. Check the rhythm.
  D. Measure the PR interval.

12. A 72-year-old patient calls you to his room because he's experiencing substernal chest pain that radiates to his jaw. You record a rhythm strip and monitor his vital signs. Which portion of the patient's ECG complex may become elevated or depressed indicating myocardial damage?

    A. T wave
    B. ST segment
    C. QRS complex
    D. P wave

13. A 76-year-old patient with heart failure is receiving furosemide (Lasix) 40 mg IV twice daily. When you look at his rhythm strip, you note prominent U waves. Which condition may have caused U waves to appear on your patient's rhythm strip?

    A. Hypokalemia
    B. Hypocalcemia
    C. Worsening heart failure
    D. Pericarditis

14. An 80-year-old patient with a history of atrial fibrillation is admitted with digoxin toxicity. When you assess his rhythm strip using the 10-times method, you note that his heart rate is 40 beats/min. Based on this finding, you should:

    A. check the patient's pulse and correlate it with the heart rate on the rhythm strip.
    B. recheck the heart rate on the rhythm strip using the sequence method.
    C. record another rhythm strip and reassess the heart rate on the rhythm strip.
    D. recheck the heart rate on the rhythm strip using the 1,500 method.

15. A patient with a history of paroxysmal atrial tachycardia develops digoxin toxicity. Because digoxin toxicity may cause prolongation of the PR interval, you must monitor his rhythm strip closely. What's the duration of a normal PR interval?

    A. 0.06 to 0.10 seconds
    B. 0.12 to 0.20 seconds
    C. 0.24 to 0.30 seconds
    D. 0.36 to 0.44 seconds

16. A patient is admitted to your telemetry unit with a diagnosis of sick sinus syndrome. Which medication should you keep readily available to treat a symptomatic event?

    A. Isoproterenol
    B. Verapamil
    C. Lidocaine
    D. Atropine

17. A 45-year-old patient is admitted with an acute MI. In the ED, he received nitroglycerin and morphine to treat his chest pain, and he's currently pain-free. His monitor reveals sinus tachycardia at a rate of 123 beats/min. Which statement is true regarding sinus tachycardia after acute MI?
   A. Sinus tachycardia is a normal response that typically abates after the first 24 hours.
   B. Sinus tachycardia is a poor prognostic sign because it may be associated with massive heart damage.
   C. Sinus tachycardia is a typical response to morphine administration.
   D. Sinus tachycardia is a sign that the heart is starting to heal.

18. A patient who has been taking digoxin (Lanoxin) suddenly develops the rhythm shown. What's your interpretation of the rhythm?

   A. Normal sinus rhythm
   B. Sinus arrhythmia
   C. Sinus bradycardia
   D. Junctional escape rhythm

19. A patient develops sinus bradycardia. Which symptoms indicate that his cardiac output is falling?
   A. Hypertension and further drop in heart rate
   B. Hypotension and dizziness
   C. Increased urine output and syncope
   D. Warm, dry skin, and hypotension

20. A patient admitted 2 days ago with an acute MI suddenly develops premature atrial contractions (PACs). What is the most likely cause of this arrhythmia in this patient?
   A. Increased caffeine intake
   B. Impending cardiogenic shock
   C. Developing heart failure
   D. Imminent cardiac arrest

21. A patient diagnosed with heart failure is admitted to your telemetry unit. He complains of seeing yellow-green halos around visual images. He also states that he's been nauseated and unable to eat for the past few days. Based on these findings you suspect:
   A. digoxin toxicity.
   B. atrial fibrillation.
   C. worsening heart failure.
   D. MI.

22. A patient returns to your unit after cardiac surgery in sinus tachycardia. As you perform your assessment of the patient, you note that his cardiac monitor shows a new onset atrial fibrillation at a rate of 160 beats/min. The patient suddenly begins complaining of chest pain. Based on these findings, what's the best treatment?
   A. Digoxin administration
   B. Defibrillation
   C. Direct current cardioversion (DCCV)
   D. Flecainide administration

23. A 32-year-old patient with a history of Wolff-Parkinson-White (WPW) syndrome is admitted to your floor after gallbladder surgery. Which ECG characteristics are typical in a patient with WPW syndrome?
   A. Prolonged PR interval and narrowed QRS complex
   B. Prolonged PR interval and presence of a delta wave
   C. Shortened PR interval and narrowed QRS complex
   D. Widened QRS complex and presence of a delta wave

A slurred QRS complex is referred to as a delta wave.

24. A 68-year-old patient with a history of heart failure is receiving digoxin. At the beginning of your shift, you record the patient's rhythm strip shown in the image. You interpret this rhythm as:

   A. junctional tachycardia.
   B. wandering pacemaker.
   C. accelerated junctional rhythm.
   D. sinus tachycardia.

25. A patient with a history of chronic obstructive pulmonary disease is admitted to your floor with hypoxemia. You begin cardiac monitoring, which reveals the rhythm shown in the image. You interpret this rhythm as:

   A. premature junctional contractions.
   B. wandering pacemaker.
   C. accelerated junctional rhythm.
   D. premature atrial contractions (PACs).

26. A patient is admitted to your unit with digoxin toxicity. You record a rhythm strip and note that the rhythm is regular, the rate is 80 beats/min, and the P waves are inverted in lead II and occur before each QRS complex. Based on these findings, you interpret the rhythm as:

    A. accelerated junctional rhythm.
    B. junctional tachycardia.
    C. junctional escape rhythm.
    D. paroxysmal atrial tachycardia.

27. A patient with an acute MI develops an arrhythmia. You record the rhythm strip shown in the image and identify the arrhythmia as:

    A. idioventricular rhythm.
    B. junctional escape rhythm.
    C. premature junctional contractions.
    D. sinus bradycardia.

28. The same patient with the arrhythmia identified in question 27 is hypotensive. You must immediately administer which of the following agents to increase his heart rate?

    A. Lidocaine
    B. Isoproterenol
    C. Atropine
    D. Amiodarone

29. A patient with a low magnesium level develops an arrhythmia. You record the rhythm strip shown in the image and identify the arrhythmia as:

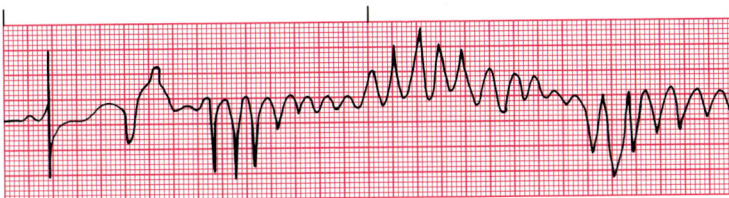

    A. monomorphic ventricular tachycardia.
    B. ventricular fibrillation.
    C. paroxysmal supraventricular tachycardia.
    D. torsades de pointes.

30. A patient with an acute anterior wall MI develops third-degree heart block. His blood pressure is 78/44 mm Hg and he's complaining of dizziness. You should immediately administer atropine and:
   A. follow with a dose of isoproterenol.
   B. apply a transcutaneous pacemaker.
   C. place the patient in Trendelenburg position.
   D. prepare for synchronized cardioversion.

31. An 86-year-old patient is found in his apartment without heat on a cold winter day. He's admitted to your unit with hypothermia. You begin cardiac monitoring, which displays the rhythm shown in the image. You document this strip as:

   A. normal sinus rhythm with first-degree AV block.
   B. second-degree AV block Type 1.
   C. sinus tachycardia.
   D. junctional tachycardia.

32. You're caring for a patient who developed complications after an acute MI requiring transvenous pacemaker insertion. His monitor alarm sounds and the rhythm strip shown in the image is recorded. You interpret this rhythm as which type of pacemaker malfunctions?

   A. Failure to capture
   B. Failure to pace
   C. Undersensing
   D. Oversensing

33. A patient admitted to the cardiac care unit with digoxin toxicity required transvenous pacemaker insertion. While assessing the patient, you note the rhythm shown in the image on the patient's monitor. This rhythm strip displays:

    A. oversensing.
    B. failure to sense.
    C. failure to pace.
    D. undersensing.

34. Your patient complains that his heart is skipping beats. You immediately record a rhythm strip from his cardiac monitor and take his vital signs. Based on the rhythm strip shown in the image, you should notify the practitioner of:

    A. failure to sense.
    B. oversensing.
    C. pacemaker-mediated tachycardia.
    D. failure to pace.

35. When teaching a patient with a newly inserted permanent pacemaker, the following information is most important:
    A. avoid computed tomography scans.
    B. hiccups are normal for the first few days after pacemaker insertion.
    C. avoid tight clothing.
    D. magnetic resonance imaging scans are safe.

36. You're caring for a 75-year-old patient who's receiving oral procainamide to control supraventricular tachycardia. Before discharge, you should instruct the patient:
    A. to avoid chewing the drug, which may cause him to get too much of the drug at once.
    B. that lupuslike symptoms are normal and will cease 2 to 3 weeks after initiation of therapy.
    C. that a bitter taste is common.
    D. that he may crush the extended-release tablet if it's difficult to swallow.

37. A patient returns to your floor from the postanesthesia care unit after undergoing a right lower lobectomy. When you begin cardiac monitoring, you note the rhythm strip shown in the image. Which drug will the practitioner most likely prescribe to rapidly convert this rhythm?

    A. Propafenone
    B. Digoxin
    C. Atropine
    D. Ibutilide

38. You note that your patient develops a prolonged QT interval on his rhythm strip. You notify the practitioner immediately because you know that prolongation of the QT interval places the patient at risk for what?
    A. Atrial fibrillation
    B. Junctional tachycardia
    C. Polymorphic ventricular tachycardia
    D. Atrial flutter

39. A 74-year-old patient is admitted to your floor from the ED with syncope. You note the rhythm shown in the image when you record a rhythm strip from his cardiac monitor. Based on this rhythm strip, you should question an order for which drug on the patient's chart?

    A. Warfarin
    B. Verapamil
    C. Epinephrine
    D. Atropine

40. A 36-year-old patient with a history of heart transplantation is admitted to your floor for observation after an appendectomy. If the patient develops symptomatic bradycardia, which drug is indicated?
    A. Atropine
    B. Isoproterenol
    C. Dopamine
    D. Propranolol

41. The surgeon orders a preoperative 12-lead ECG for your patient who is scheduled for a thoracotomy in the morning. Using your knowledge of 12-lead ECGs, which leads are bipolar?

    A. aV_R, aV_L, and aV_F

    B. I, II, and III

    C. V_1, V_2, and V_3

    D. V_4, V_5, and V_6

42. Each of the 12 leads of an ECG views the heart from a different angle. Lead I views which area of the heart?

    A. Inferior wall

    B. Anterior wall

    C. Posterior wall

    D. Lateral wall

43. The practitioner orders a signal-averaged ECG for a patient who sustained an acute MI. Why is this test typically ordered?

    A. To locate posterior wall damage

    B. To identify whether the patient is at risk for sudden death from sustained ventricular tachycardia

    C. To identify whether the patient has suffered damage to his right ventricle

    D. To identify left bundle branch block in an anterior wall MI

44. You're caring for a patient with a history of angina who calls you into his room because he's experiencing chest pain. His admission orders included a 12-lead ECG with each episode of chest pain. You immediately retrieve the ECG machine. To ensure proper placement, where should you place lead V_1?

    A. Over the fourth intercostal space at the right sternal border

    B. Over the fourth intercostal space at the left sternal border

    C. Over the fifth intercostal space at the left anterior axillary line

    D. Over the fifth intercostal space at the left midclavicular line

45. A 12-lead ECG is ordered for a 32-year-old patient who comes to the ED complaining of chest pain. You know that a 12-lead ECG is necessary to assess conduction of the:

    A. right ventricle.

    B. right and left ventricles.

    C. left ventricle.

    D. right and left atria.

46. You're caring for a 72-year-old patient admitted with unstable angina. He calls you into his room and complains of chest pain that he rates an 8 on a scale of 0 to 10 (10 being the worst). You immediately obtain a 12-lead ECG. Which ECG change would you expect with angina?

    A. Pathologic Q wave

    B. T-wave inversion

    C. Widened QRS complex

    D. Poor R-wave progression

47. A patient's 12-lead ECG reveals left axis deviation. Left axis deviation is considered normal in?
  A. Infants
  B. Small children
  C. Pregnant women
  D. Healthy adults

48. A 38-year-old patient is admitted with a diagnosis of unstable angina. Which statement is true about unstable angina?
  A. The pain is typically triggered by exertion or stress.
  B. The pain is typically relieved by rest.
  C. The pain typically lasts less than 2 minutes.
  D. The pain may occur while the patient is sleeping.

49. After experiencing substernal chest pain for about 4 hours, a patient drives himself to the ED. He's triaged immediately and a 12-lead ECG is obtained. Which change on the patient's ECG is associated with myocardial necrosis?
  A. Pathologic Q waves
  B. T-wave inversion
  C. ST-segment elevation
  D. Narrowed QRS complex

50. When examining your patient's 12-lead ECG, you notice a bundle branch block. Which leads should you check to determine whether the block is in the right or left bundle?
  A. V_1 and V_6
  B. II and aV_F
  C. V_4 and V_5
  D. I and III

51. You obtain a telemetry strip on a patient after coronary artery bypass surgery. After interpreting the rhythm strip shown in the image, which arrhythmia should you document?

  A. Atrial flutter
  B. Second-degree AV block Type II
  C. Sinus arrhythmia
  D. Third-degree AV block

52. You're caring for a patient with an evolving anterolateral wall MI. While examining the patient's 12-lead ECG, you would expect to note changes in which leads? (Select all that apply.)

    A. Lead I

    B. Lead III

    C. Lead aV_F

    D. Lead V_4

    E. Lead V_6

53. As part of a preoperative assessment, you begin preparation for a 12-lead ECG. Using the figure, identify the area on the patient's chest where you would place lead V_1.

54. While interpreting the rhythm strip shown in the image for a patient who was just admitted to the telemetry unit, you document the PR interval as how many seconds?

_____ seconds

Answers

1. A. The bicuspid valve, commonly called the *mitral valve*, is located between the left atrium and left ventricle.

2. B. The circumflex artery supplies oxygenated blood to the lateral walls of the ventricle, the left atrium, and the left posterior fasciculus of the left bundle branch.

3. B. The vagus nerve carries impulses that slow the heart rate and the conduction of impulses through the AV node and ventricles.

4. B. Polarization describes cardiac cells at rest.

5. D. If the Purkinje fibers take over as the heart's pacemaker, impulses are typically discharged at a rate of 20 to 40 beats/min.

6. D. Lead MCL_1 is the equivalent to V_1 on a 12-lead ECG.

7. A. The six limb leads—leads I, II, III, aV_R, aV_L, and aV_F—provide information about the heart's frontal plane.

8. A. Before initiating cardiac monitoring, you must first prepare the patient's skin. Use a special rough patch on the back of the electrode, a dry washcloth, or a gauze pad to briskly rub each site until the skin reddens.

9. A. Electrical interference appears on the ECG as a baseline that's thick and unreadable. Electrical interference is caused by electrical power leakage. It may also occur because of interference from other equipment in the room or improperly grounded equipment.

10. B. The horizontal axis of the ECG strip represents time.

11. C. Using the eight-step method of rhythm strip interpretation, you should check the rhythm first and then calculate the rate. Next, evaluate the P wave, check out the PR interval and the QRS complex, examine the T wave, measure the QT interval, and, finally, check for ectopic beats and other abnormalities.

12. B. A change in the ST segment may indicate myocardial damage. A ST segment may become either elevated or depressed.

13. A. The U wave isn't present on every rhythm strip. A prominent U wave may be due to hypokalemia, hypercalcemia, or digoxin toxicity.

14. A. Although you can use the 10-times method, the 1,500 method, or the sequence method to determine heart rate, you shouldn't rely on these methods. Always check a pulse to correlate it with the heart rate on the ECG.

15. B. The normal duration of a PR interval is 0.12 to 0.20 seconds.

16. D. Atropine or epinephrine may be administered for symptomatic bradycardia that's caused by sick sinus syndrome. Therefore, you should keep these drugs readily available.

17. B. Sinus tachycardia occurs in about 30% of patients after acute MI and is considered a poor prognostic sign because it may be associated with massive heart damage.

18. B. The rhythm strip shows sinus arrhythmia. If sinus arrhythmia develops suddenly in the patient taking digoxin, the patient may be experiencing digoxin toxicity.

19. B. When sinus bradycardia is symptomatic, the resulting drop in cardiac output produces such signs and symptoms as hypotension and dizziness.

20. C. In a patient with an acute MI, PACs can serve as an early sign of heart failure or an electrolyte imbalance.

21. A. The patient with digoxin toxicity may develop arrhythmias, blurred vision, hypotension, increased severity of heart failure, yellow-green halos around visual images, anorexia, nausea, and vomiting.

22. C. If the patient with atrial fibrillation complains of chest pain, emergency measures, such as DCCV, are necessary. Beta-blockers or calcium channel blockers may be used to control the ventricular response in patients with atrial fibrillation who are without symptoms. Antiarrhythmic medications may be helpful to decrease recurrence.

23. D. WPW syndrome causes a shortened PR interval (less than 0.10 seconds) and a widened QRS complex (greater than 0.10 seconds). The beginning of the QRS complex may appear slurred. This hallmark sign is referred to as a *delta wave.*

24. A. The rhythm strip reveals junctional tachycardia. The rhythm is regular, the rate is 110 beats/min, a P wave occurs after each QRS complex, and the PR interval isn't measurable.

25. B. The rhythm strip reveals a wandering pacemaker. The key characteristics are the varying shapes of the P waves.

26. A. Based on these findings, the patient's rhythm strip reveals accelerated junctional rhythm.

27. A. The rhythm strip reveals idioventricular rhythm.

28. C. The agent of choice for the treatment of idioventricular rhythm is atropine. A pacemaker may be necessary after atropine administration.

29. D. The rhythm strip shows torsades de pointes.

30. B. If the patient's cardiac output is inadequate (low blood pressure and dizziness), you should immediately administer atropine and apply a transcutaneous pacemaker. The patient may need a transvenous pacemaker until the block resolves. If the block doesn't resolve, he'll need a permanent pacemaker.

31. A. You should document in your notes that the patient's monitor reveals normal sinus rhythm with first-degree AV block. Hypothermia is one cause of this arrhythmia.

32. A. The rhythm strip shows the pacemaker's failure to capture. The ECG pacemaker spike isn't followed by a QRS complex.

33. C. The rhythm strip reveals the pacemaker's failure to pace. After two paced beats, there's no apparent pacemaker activity on the ECG. Begin cardiopulmonary resuscitation (CPR).

34. A. The ECG pacemaker spikes fall where they shouldn't, indicating a failure to sense.

35. C. You should instruct the patient to avoid tight clothing or direct pressure over the pulse generator, to avoid magnetic resonance imaging scans and certain other diagnostic studies, and to notify the practitioner if he feels confused, lightheaded, or short of breath. The patient should also notify the practitioner if he has palpitations, hiccups, or a rapid or unusually slow heart rate.

36. A. Warn the patient taking oral procainamide not to chew it because this might cause a release of too much of the drug at once. Lupuslike symptoms are associated with long-term use of procainamide and may require discontinuation of the drug. A bitter taste is also an adverse effect of procainamide. The extended-release tablet should not be crushed.

37. D. This rhythm strip reveals atrial fibrillation. Ibutilide is used for rapid conversion of recent-onset atrial fibrillation or flutter to sinus rhythm.

38. C. Prolongation of the QT interval is a sign that the patient is predisposed to developing polymorphic ventricular tachycardia.

39. B. The rhythm strip reveals sick sinus syndrome. Verapamil should be avoided in sick sinus syndrome or second- or third-degree AV block without a pacemaker and in atrial fibrillation or flutter because of WPW syndrome.

40. B. Isoproterenol is the drug of choice for treating symptomatic bradycardia in patients who have undergone heart transplantation. The vagal nerve dissection that occurs during heart transplantation surgery renders atropine ineffective in these patients.

41. B. The 12 leads include three bipolar limb leads (I, II, and III), three unipolar augmented limb leads (aV_R, aV_L, and aV_F), and six unipolar precordial leads (V_1, V_2, V_3, V_4, V_5, and V_6).

42. D. Lead I views the lateral wall of the heart.

43. B. Signal-averaged ECG helps identify patients at risk for sudden death from sustained ventricular tachycardia. The test uses a computer to identify late electrical potentials that can't be detected by a 12-lead ECG.

44. A. Lead V_1 should be placed over the fourth intercostal space at the right sternal border.

45. C. A 12-lead ECG is used to assess left ventricular conduction activity. A right-sided ECG is necessary to assess right ventricular conduction activity.

46. B. Classic ECG changes associated with angina include a peaked T wave, flattened T wave, T-wave inversion, ST-segment depression with T-wave inversion, and ST-segment depression without T-wave inversion.

47. C. Left axis deviation is a normal finding in pregnant women. Right axis deviation is normal in infants and small children.

48. D. Unstable angina is more easily provoked and may occur while the patient is sleeping, causing him to awaken. It's also unpredictable and tends to worsen over time. In stable angina, pain is triggered by exertion or stress and is commonly relieved by rest. Each episode follows a similar pattern.

49. A. The area of myocardial necrosis is called the *zone of infarction*. The ECG change associated with a necrotic area is a pathologic Q wave. The zone of injury shows up on an ECG as an elevated ST segment. The zone of ischemia is represented by T-wave inversion.

50. A. After you identify a bundle branch block, examine lead V_1, which lies to the right of the heart, and lead V_6, which lies to the left of the heart. These leads will tell you if the block is in the right or left bundle.

51. D. The rhythm strip reveals third-degree AV block. Characteristics of this arrhythmia include a regular atrial rhythm along with a regular but slow ventricular rhythm, an absence of a relationship between P waves and QRS complexes, and P and R waves that march across the strip in rhythm.

52. A, D, E. In an anterolateral wall MI, ECG changes occur in leads I, aV_L, V_4, V_5, and V_6.

53. Lead V_1 should be placed over the fourth intercostal space at the right sternal border.

54. 0.14. The PR interval is measured from the beginning of the P wave to the beginning of the QRS complex. The normal duration of the PR interval is 0.12 to 0.20 seconds.

Appendix 2: Brushing up on interpretation skills

Introduction

Use these sample rhythm strips as a practical way to brush up on your ECG interpretation skills. Record the rhythm, rates, and waveform characteristics in the blank spaces provided, and then compare your findings with the answers beginning on page 354.

Questions

1.

Atrial rhythm:_____

Ventricular rhythm:_____

Atrial rate:_____

Ventricular rate:_____

P wave:_____

PR interval:_____

QRS complex:_____

T wave:_____

QT interval:_____

Other:_____

Interpretation:_____

_____

2.

Atrial rhythm:_____

Ventricular rhythm:_____

Atrial rate:_____

Ventricular rate:_____

P wave:_____

PR interval:_____

QRS complex:_____

T wave:_____

QT interval:_____

Other:_____

Interpretation:_____

_____

3.

Atrial rhythm:_____

Ventricular rhythm:_____

Atrial rate:_____

Ventricular rate:_____

P wave:_____

PR interval:_____

QRS complex:_____

T wave:_____

QT interval:_____

Other:_____

Interpretation:_____

_____

4.

Atrial rhythm:_____

Ventricular rhythm:_____

Atrial rate:_____

Ventricular rate:_____

P wave:_____

PR interval:_____

QRS complex:_____

T wave:_____

QT interval:_____

Other:_____

Interpretation:_____

_____

5.

Atrial rhythm:_____

Ventricular rhythm:_____

Atrial rate:_____

Ventricular rate:_____

P wave:_____

PR interval:_____

QRS complex:_____

T wave:_____

QT interval:_____

Other:_____

Interpretation:_____

_____

6.

Atrial rhythm:_____

Ventricular rhythm:_____

Atrial rate:_____

Ventricular rate:_____

P wave:_____

PR interval:_____

QRS complex:_____

T wave:_____

QT interval:_____

Other:_____

Interpretation:_____

_____

7.

Atrial rhythm:_____

Ventricular rhythm:_____

Atrial rate:_____

Ventricular rate:_____

P wave:_____

PR interval:_____

QRS complex:_____

T wave:_____

QT interval:_____

Other:_____

Interpretation:_____

_____

8.

Atrial rhythm:_____

Ventricular rhythm:_____

Atrial rate:_____

Ventricular rate:_____

P wave:_____

PR interval:_____

QRS complex:_____

T wave:_____

QT interval:_____

Other:_____

Interpretation:_____

_____

9.

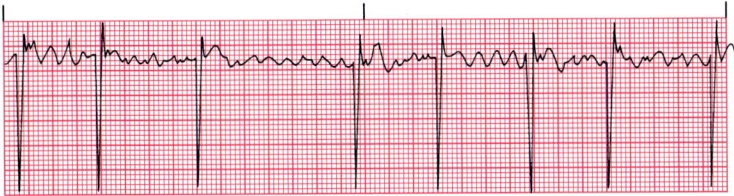

Atrial rhythm:_____
Ventricular rhythm:_____
Atrial rate:_____
Ventricular rate:_____
P wave:_____
PR interval:_____
QRS complex:_____
T wave:_____
QT interval:_____
Other:_____
Interpretation:_____
_____

10.

Atrial rhythm:_____
Ventricular rhythm:_____
Atrial rate:_____
Ventricular rate:_____
P wave:_____
PR interval:_____
QRS complex:_____
T wave:_____
QT interval:_____
Other:_____
Interpretation:_____
_____

11.

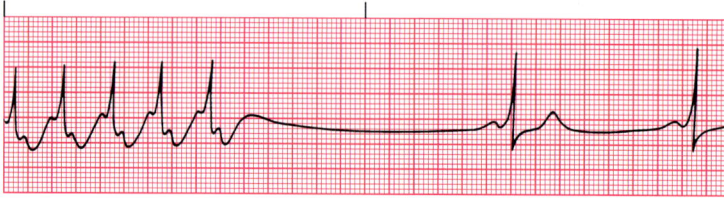

Atrial rhythm:_____
Ventricular rhythm:_____
Atrial rate:_____
Ventricular rate:_____
P wave:_____
PR interval:_____
QRS complex:_____
T wave:_____
QT interval:_____
Other:_____
Interpretation:_____

_____

12.

Atrial rhythm:_____
Ventricular rhythm:_____
Atrial rate:_____
Ventricular rate:_____
P wave:_____
PR interval:_____
QRS complex:_____
T wave:_____
QT interval:_____
Other:_____
Interpretation:_____

_____

13.

Atrial rhythm:_____

Ventricular rhythm:_____

Atrial rate:_____

Ventricular rate:_____

P wave:_____

PR interval:_____

QRS complex:_____

T wave:_____

QT interval:_____

Other:_____

Interpretation:_____

_____

14.

Atrial rhythm:_____

Ventricular rhythm:_____

Atrial rate:_____

Ventricular rate:_____

P wave:_____

PR interval:_____

QRS complex:_____

T wave:_____

QT interval:_____

Other:_____

Interpretation:_____

_____

15.

Atrial rhythm:_____

Ventricular rhythm:_____

Atrial rate:_____

Ventricular rate:_____

P wave:_____

PR interval:_____

QRS complex:_____

T wave:_____

QT interval:_____

Other:_____

Interpretation:_____

_____

16.

Atrial rhythm:_____

Ventricular rhythm:_____

Atrial rate:_____

Ventricular rate:_____

P wave:_____

PR interval:_____

QRS complex:_____

T wave:_____

QT interval:_____

Other:_____

Interpretation:_____

_____

17.

Atrial rhythm:_____

Ventricular rhythm:_____

Atrial rate:_____

Ventricular rate:_____

P wave:_____

PR interval:_____

QRS complex:_____

T wave:_____

QT interval:_____

Other:_____

Interpretation:_____

_____

18.

Atrial rhythm:_____

Ventricular rhythm:_____

Atrial rate:_____

Ventricular rate:_____

P wave:_____

PR interval:_____

QRS complex:_____

T wave:_____

QT interval:_____

Other:_____

Interpretation:_____

_____

19.

Atrial rhythm:_____

Ventricular rhythm:_____

Atrial rate:_____

Ventricular rate:_____

P wave:_____

PR interval:_____

QRS complex:_____

T wave:_____

QT interval:_____

Other:_____

Interpretation:_____

_____

20.

Atrial rhythm:_____

Ventricular rhythm:_____

Atrial rate:_____

Ventricular rate:_____

P wave:_____

PR interval:_____

QRS complex:_____

T wave:_____

QT interval:_____

Other:_____

Interpretation:_____

_____

21.

Atrial rhythm:_____

Ventricular rhythm:_____

Atrial rate:_____

Ventricular rate:_____

P wave:_____

PR interval:_____

QRS complex:_____

T wave:_____

QT interval:_____

Other:_____

Interpretation:_____

_____

22.

Atrial rhythm:_____

Ventricular rhythm:_____

Atrial rate:_____

Ventricular rate:_____

P wave:_____

PR interval:_____

QRS complex:_____

T wave:_____

QT interval:_____

Other:_____

Interpretation:_____

_____

23.

Atrial rhythm:_____
Ventricular rhythm:_____
Atrial rate:_____
Ventricular rate:_____
P wave:_____
PR interval:_____
QRS complex:_____
T wave:_____
QT interval:_____
Other:_____
Interpretation:_____
_____

24.

Atrial rhythm:_____
Ventricular rhythm:_____
Atrial rate:_____
Ventricular rate:_____
P wave:_____
PR interval:_____
QRS complex:_____
T wave:_____
QT interval:_____
Other:_____
Interpretation:_____
_____

25.

Atrial rhythm:_____

Ventricular rhythm:_____

Atrial rate:_____

Ventricular rate:_____

P wave:_____

PR interval:_____

QRS complex:_____

T wave:_____

QT interval:_____

Other:_____

Interpretation:_____

_____

26.

Atrial rhythm:_____

Ventricular rhythm:_____

Atrial rate:_____

Ventricular rate:_____

P wave:_____

PR interval:_____

QRS complex:_____

T wave:_____

QT interval:_____

Other:_____

Interpretation:_____

_____

27.

Atrial rhythm:_____

Ventricular rhythm:_____

Atrial rate:_____

Ventricular rate:_____

P wave:_____

PR interval:_____

QRS complex:_____

T wave:_____

QT interval:_____

Other:_____

Interpretation:_____

_____

28.

Atrial rhythm:_____

Ventricular rhythm:_____

Atrial rate:_____

Ventricular rate:_____

P wave:_____

PR interval:_____

QRS complex:_____

T wave:_____

QT interval:_____

Other:_____

Interpretation:_____

_____

29.

Atrial rhythm:_____

Ventricular rhythm:_____

Atrial rate:_____

Ventricular rate:_____

P wave:_____

PR interval:_____

QRS complex:_____

T wave:_____

QT interval:_____

Other:_____

Interpretation:_____

_____

30.

Atrial rhythm:_____

Ventricular rhythm:_____

Atrial rate:_____

Ventricular rate:_____

P wave:_____

PR interval:_____

QRS complex:_____

T wave:_____

QT interval:_____

Other:_____

Interpretation:_____

_____

31.

Atrial rhythm:_____

Ventricular rhythm:_____

Atrial rate:_____

Ventricular rate:_____

P wave:_____

PR interval:_____

QRS complex:_____

T wave:_____

QT interval:_____

Other:_____

Interpretation:_____

_____

32.

Atrial rhythm:_____

Ventricular rhythm:_____

Atrial rate:_____

Ventricular rate:_____

P wave:_____

PR interval:_____

QRS complex:_____

T wave:_____

QT interval:_____

Other:_____

Interpretation:_____

_____

33.

Atrial rhythm:_____

Ventricular rhythm:_____

Atrial rate:_____

Ventricular rate:_____

P wave:_____

PR interval:_____

QRS complex:_____

T wave:_____

QT interval:_____

Other:_____

Interpretation:_____

_____

34.

Atrial rhythm:_____

Ventricular rhythm:_____

Atrial rate:_____

Ventricular rate:_____

P wave:_____

PR interval:_____

QRS complex:_____

T wave:_____

QT interval:_____

Other:_____

Interpretation:_____

_____

35.

Atrial rhythm:_____

Ventricular rhythm:_____

Atrial rate:_____

Ventricular rate:_____

P wave:_____

PR interval:_____

QRS complex:_____

T wave:_____

QT interval:_____

Other:_____

Interpretation:_____

_____

36.

Atrial rhythm:_____

Ventricular rhythm:_____

Atrial rate:_____

Ventricular rate:_____

P wave:_____

PR interval:_____

QRS complex:_____

T wave:_____

QT interval:_____

Other:_____

Interpretation:_____

_____

37.

Atrial rhythm:_____

Ventricular rhythm:_____

Atrial rate:_____

Ventricular rate:_____

P wave:_____

PR interval:_____

QRS complex:_____

T wave:_____

QT interval:_____

Other:_____

Interpretation:_____

_____

38.

Atrial rhythm:_____

Ventricular rhythm:_____

Atrial rate:_____

Ventricular rate:_____

P wave:_____

PR interval:_____

QRS complex:_____

T wave:_____

QT interval:_____

Other:_____

Interpretation:_____

_____

39.

Atrial rhythm:_____

Ventricular rhythm:_____

Atrial rate:_____

Ventricular rate:_____

P wave:_____

PR interval:_____

QRS complex:_____

T wave:_____

QT interval:_____

Other:_____

Interpretation:_____

_____

40.

Atrial rhythm:_____

Ventricular rhythm:_____

Atrial rate:_____

Ventricular rate:_____

P wave:_____

PR interval:_____

QRS complex:_____

T wave:_____

QT interval:_____

Other:_____

Interpretation:_____

_____

41.

Atrial rhythm:_____

Ventricular rhythm:_____

Atrial rate:_____

Ventricular rate:_____

P wave:_____

PR interval:_____

QRS complex:_____

T wave:_____

QT interval:_____

Other:_____

Interpretation:_____

_____

42.

Atrial rhythm:_____

Ventricular rhythm:_____

Atrial rate:_____

Ventricular rate:_____

P wave:_____

PR interval:_____

QRS complex:_____

T wave:_____

QT interval:_____

Other:_____

Interpretation:_____

_____

43.

Atrial rhythm:_____

Ventricular rhythm:_____

Atrial rate:_____

Ventricular rate:_____

P wave:_____

PR interval:_____

QRS complex:_____

T wave:_____

QT interval:_____

Other:_____

Interpretation:_____

_____

44.

Atrial rhythm:_____

Ventricular rhythm:_____

Atrial rate:_____

Ventricular rate:_____

P wave:_____

PR interval:_____

QRS complex:_____

T wave:_____

QT interval:_____

Other:_____

Interpretation:_____

_____

45.

Atrial rhythm:_____

Ventricular rhythm:_____

Atrial rate:_____

Ventricular rate:_____

P wave:_____

PR interval:_____

QRS complex:_____

T wave:_____

QT interval:_____

Other:_____

Interpretation:_____
_____

46.

Atrial rhythm:_____

Ventricular rhythm:_____

Atrial rate:_____

Ventricular rate:_____

P wave:_____

PR interval:_____

QRS complex:_____

T wave:_____

QT interval:_____

Other:_____

Interpretation:_____
_____

47.

Atrial rhythm:_____

Ventricular rhythm:_____

Atrial rate:_____

Ventricular rate:_____

P wave:_____

PR interval:_____

QRS complex:_____

T wave:_____

QT interval:_____

Other:_____

Interpretation:_____

_____

48.

Atrial rhythm:_____

Ventricular rhythm:_____

Atrial rate:_____

Ventricular rate:_____

P wave:_____

PR interval:_____

QRS complex:_____

T wave:_____

QT interval:_____

Other:_____

Interpretation:_____

_____

49.

Atrial rhythm:_____

Ventricular rhythm:_____

Atrial rate:_____

Ventricular rate:_____

P wave:_____

PR interval:_____

QRS complex:_____

T wave:_____

QT interval:_____

Other:_____

Interpretation:_____

50.

Atrial rhythm:_____

Ventricular rhythm:_____

Atrial rate:_____

Ventricular rate:_____

P wave:_____

PR interval:_____

QRS complex:_____

T wave:_____

QT interval:_____

Other:_____

Interpretation:_____

_____

51.

Atrial rhythm:_____

Ventricular rhythm:_____

Atrial rate:_____

Ventricular rate:_____

P wave:_____

PR interval:_____

QRS complex:_____

T wave:_____

QT interval:_____

Other:_____

Interpretation:_____

_____

52.

Atrial rhythm:_____

Ventricular rhythm:_____

Atrial rate:_____

Ventricular rate:_____

P wave:_____

PR interval:_____

QRS complex:_____

T wave:_____

QT interval:_____

Other:_____

Interpretation:_____

_____

53.

Atrial rhythm:_____

Ventricular rhythm:_____

Atrial rate:_____

Ventricular rate:_____

P wave:_____

PR interval:_____

QRS complex:_____

T wave:_____

QT interval:_____

Other:_____

Interpretation:_____

_____

54.

Atrial rhythm:_____

Ventricular rhythm:_____

Atrial rate:_____

Ventricular rate:_____

P wave:_____

PR interval:_____

QRS complex:_____

T wave:_____

QT interval:_____

Other:_____

Interpretation:_____

_____

Answers

1.

Atrial rhythm: Regular, except for missing PQRST complex
Ventricular rhythm: Regular, except for missing PQRST complex
Atrial rate: 40 beats/min; underlying rate 50 beats/min
Ventricular rate: 40 beats/min
P wave: Normal size and configuration; absent during pause
PR interval: 0.20 seconds
QRS complex: 0.08 seconds
T wave: Normal configuration; absent during pause
QT interval: 0.40 seconds
Other: None
Interpretation: Sinus arrest

2.

Atrial rhythm: Irregular
Ventricular rhythm: Irregular
Atrial rate: 60 beats/min; underlying rate 88 beats/min
Ventricular rate: 90 beats/min
P wave: None with premature ventricular contractions (PVCs); present with QRS complexes
PR interval: 0.16 seconds
QRS complex: Underlying rate 0.08 seconds; 0.16 seconds with PVCs
T wave: Normal configuration; opposite direction with PVCs
QT interval: 0.42 seconds
Other: None
Interpretation: Normal sinus rhythm with trigeminal PVCs

3.

Atrial rhythm: Regular
Ventricular rhythm: Regular
Atrial rate: 125 beats/min
Ventricular rate: 125 beats/min
P wave: Normal size and configuration
PR interval: 0.14 seconds
QRS complex: 0.08 seconds
T wave: Normal configuration
QT interval: 0.32 seconds
Other: None
Interpretation: Sinus tachycardia

4.

Atrial rhythm: Irregular
Ventricular rhythm: Irregular
Atrial rate: 60 beats/min; underlying rate 71 beats/min

Ventricular rate: 70 beats/min
P wave: None with PVC; present with QRS complexes
PR interval: 0.16 seconds
QRS complex: 0.08 seconds; 0.14 seconds with PVC
T wave: Normal configuration
QT interval: 0.40 seconds
Other: None
Interpretation: Normal sinus rhythm with PVC

5.
Atrial rhythm: Irregular
Ventricular rhythm: Irregular
Atrial rate: 40 beats/min; underlying rate 70 beats/min
Ventricular rate: 70 beats/min
P wave: None with PVCs; present with QRS complexes
PR interval: 0.16 seconds
QRS complex: 0.08 seconds; 0.16 seconds with PVCs
T wave: Normal configuration
QT interval: 0.40 seconds
Other: None
Interpretation: Normal sinus rhythm with run of PVCs

6.
Atrial rhythm: Absent
Ventricular rhythm: Chaotic
Atrial rate: Absent
Ventricular rate: Undetermined
P wave: Absent
PR interval: Unmeasurable
QRS complex: Indiscernible
T wave: Indiscernible
QT interval: Not applicable
Other: None
Interpretation: Ventricular fibrillation

7.
Atrial rhythm: Regular
Ventricular rhythm: Regular
Atrial rate: 90 beats/min; underlying rate 107 beats/min
Ventricular rate: 110 beats/min
P wave: Present in normal QRS complexes
PR interval: 0.16 seconds
QRS complex: 0.08 seconds
T wave: Normal configuration
QT interval: 0.32 seconds
Other: Random pacemaker spikes
Interpretation: Sinus tachycardia with pacemaker failure to sense

8.

Atrial rhythm: Unmeasurable
Ventricular rhythm: Regular
Atrial rate: Unmeasurable
Ventricular rate: Paced rate 40 beats/min; pacer fires at 75 beats/min
P wave: Absent
PR interval: Unmeasurable
QRS complex: Unmeasurable
T wave: Unmeasurable
QT interval: Unmeasurable
Other: None
Interpretation: Paced rhythm with failure to capture

9.

Atrial rhythm: Irregular
Ventricular rhythm: Irregular
Atrial rate: Indiscernible
Ventricular rate: 80 beats/min
P wave: Absent; fine fibrillation waves present
PR interval: Indiscernible
QRS complex: 0.08 seconds
T wave: Indiscernible
QT interval: Unmeasurable
Other: None
Interpretation: Atrial fibrillation

10.

Atrial rhythm: Regular
Ventricular rhythm: Irregular
Atrial rate: 50 beats/min
Ventricular rate: 40 beats/min
P wave: Normal; some not followed by QRS complexes
PR interval: 0.16 seconds and constant (may be prolonged)
QRS complex: 0.08 seconds
T wave: Normal configuration; absent if QRS complexes are absent
QT interval: 0.40 seconds
Other: None
Interpretation: Second-degree atrioventricular (AV) block type II, also known as Mobitz II

11.

Atrial rhythm: Irregular
Ventricular rhythm: Irregular
Atrial rate: 60 beats/min
Ventricular rate: 70 beats/min
P wave: Rate and configuration vary
PR interval: Varies with rhythm

QRS complex: 0.10 seconds
T wave: Configuration varies
QT interval: Configuration varies
Other: None
Interpretation: Sick sinus syndrome

12.
Atrial rhythm: Regular
Ventricular rhythm: Regular
Atrial rate: 110 beats/min
Ventricular rate: 110 beats/min
P wave: Normal size and configuration
PR interval: 0.16 seconds
QRS complex: 0.10 seconds
T wave: Normal configuration
QT interval: 0.36 seconds
Other: None
Interpretation: Sinus tachycardia

13.
Atrial rhythm: Regular
Ventricular rhythm: Regular
Atrial rate: 270 beats/min
Ventricular rate: 70 beats/min
P wave: Saw-tooth edged
PR interval: Unmeasurable
QRS complex: 0.10 seconds
T wave: Unidentifiable
QT interval: Unidentifiable
Other: None
Interpretation: Atrial flutter (4:1 block)

14.
Atrial rhythm: Irregular
Ventricular rhythm: Irregular
Atrial rate: About 110 beats/min
Ventricular rate: About 110 beats/min
P wave: Size and configuration vary
PR interval: Rate varies
QRS complex: 0.08 seconds
T wave: Inverted
QT interval: 0.22 seconds
Other: None
Interpretation: Multifocal atrial tachycardia

15.
Atrial rhythm: Irregular
Ventricular rhythm: Irregular
Atrial rate: 100 beats/min

Ventricular rate: 100 beats/min
P wave: Normal size and configuration, except during premature beat
PR interval: 0.16 seconds; unmeasurable for premature beat
QRS complex: 0.06 seconds
T wave: Normal configuration
QT interval: 0.36 seconds
Other: None
Interpretation: Sinus tachycardia with PVCs

16.
Atrial rhythm: Unmeasurable
Ventricular rhythm: Unmeasurable
Atrial rate: Unmeasurable
Ventricular rate: Unmeasurable
P wave: Absent
PR interval: Unmeasurable
QRS complex: Unmeasurable
T wave: Absent
QT interval: Unmeasurable
Other: None
Interpretation: Asystole

17.
Atrial rhythm: Unmeasurable
Ventricular rhythm: Unmeasurable; fibrillatory waves present
Atrial rate: Unmeasurable
Ventricular rate: Unmeasurable
P wave: Absent
PR interval: Absent
QRS complex: Unmeasurable
T wave: Opposite direction of QRS complex
QT interval: Absent
Other: None
Interpretation: Ventricular fibrillation

18.
Atrial rhythm: Regular
Ventricular rhythm: Irregular
Atrial rate: 75 beats/min
Ventricular rate: 50 beats/min
P wave: Normal size and configuration
PR interval: Lengthens with each cycle until dropped
QRS complex: 0.06 seconds
T wave: Normal configuration
QT interval: 0.38 seconds
Other: None
Interpretation: Second-degree AV block type I, also known as Mobitz I
or Wenckebach

19.

Atrial rhythm: Regular
Ventricular rhythm: Regular
Atrial rate: 90 beats/min
Ventricular rate: 30 beats/min
P wave: Normal size and configuration, except when hidden within T wave
PR interval: Rate varies
QRS complex: 0.16 seconds
T wave: Normal configuration
QT interval: 0.56 seconds
Other: None
Interpretation: Third-degree AV block, also known as complete heart block

20.

Atrial rhythm: Regular
Ventricular rhythm: Regular
Atrial rate: 60 beats/min
Ventricular rate: 60 beats/min
P wave: Normal size and configuration
PR interval: 0.36 seconds
QRS complex: 0.08 seconds
T wave: Normal configuration
QT interval: 0.40 seconds
Other: None
Interpretation: Normal sinus rhythm with first-degree AV block

21.

Atrial rhythm: Regular
Ventricular rhythm: Regular
Atrial rate: 35 beats/min
Ventricular rate: 35 beats/min
P wave: Normal configuration
PR interval: 0.18 seconds
QRS complex: 0.12 seconds
T wave: Normal configuration
QT interval: 0.44 seconds
Other: None
Interpretation: Sinus bradycardia

22.

Atrial rhythm: Irregular
Ventricular rhythm: Irregular
Atrial rate: 50 beats/min
Ventricular rate: 50 beats/min
P wave: Normal configuration

PR interval: 0.20 seconds
QRS complex: 0.08 seconds
T wave: Normal configuration
QT interval: 0.52 seconds
Other: None
Interpretation: Sinus bradycardia with premature atrial contraction (PAC)

23.
Atrial rhythm: Irregular
Ventricular rhythm: Irregular
Atrial rate: Unmeasurable
Ventricular rate: 60 beats/min
P wave: Not present
PR interval: Unmeasurable
QRS complex: 0.06 seconds
T wave: Flattened
QT interval: Unmeasurable
Other: None
Interpretation: Junctional escape rhythm

24.
Atrial rhythm: Regular
Ventricular rhythm: Regular
Atrial rate: Unmeasurable
Ventricular rate: 38 beats/min
P wave: Absent
PR interval: Unmeasurable
QRS complex: 0.04 seconds
T wave: Normal configuration
QT interval: 0.44 seconds
Other: None
Interpretation: Junctional bradycardia

25.
Atrial rhythm: Regular
Ventricular rhythm: Regular
Atrial rate: 68 beats/min
Ventricular rate: 43 beats/min
P wave: Normal configuration
PR interval: Unmeasurable
QRS complex: 0.12 seconds
T wave: Normal configuration
QT interval: Unmeasurable
Other: P wave no correlation with QRS complex
Interpretation: Third-degree AV block, also known as complete heart block

26.
Atrial rhythm: Regular
Ventricular rhythm: Regular
Atrial rate: 100 beats/min
Ventricular rate: 100 beats/min
P wave: Normal initially, then becomes inverted with shortened PR interval
PR interval: 0.14 seconds initially, then unmeasurable
QRS complex: 0.08 seconds
T wave: Normal configuration
QT interval: 0.36 seconds
Other: None
Interpretation: Sinus tachycardia leading to junctional tachycardia

27.
Atrial rhythm: Not present
Ventricular rhythm: Regular
Atrial rate: Not present
Ventricular rate: 30 beats/min
P wave: Absent
PR interval: Unmeasurable
QRS complex: Abnormal
T wave: Abnormal configuration
QT interval: Unmeasurable
Other: None
Interpretation: Idioventricular rhythm

28.
Atrial rhythm: Irregular
Ventricular rhythm: Irregular
Atrial rate: 280 beats/min
Ventricular rate: 110 beats/min
P wave: Flutter waves
PR interval: Unmeasurable
QRS complex: 0.08 seconds
T wave: Indiscernible
QT interval: Unmeasurable
Other: None
Interpretation: Atrial flutter with variable block

29.
Atrial rhythm: Regular
Ventricular rhythm: Regular
Atrial rate: 94 beats/min
Ventricular rate: 94 beats/min
P wave: Inverted
PR interval: 0.12 seconds

QRS complex: 0.08 seconds
T wave: Inverted
QT interval: 0.30 seconds
Other: None
Interpretation: Junctional rhythm with slightly accelerated heart rate

30.
Atrial rhythm: Irregular
Ventricular rhythm: Irregular
Atrial rate: 70 beats/min
Ventricular rate: 70 beats/min
P wave: Normal
PR interval: 0.16 seconds
QRS complex: 0.10 seconds
T wave: Biphasic
QT interval: 0.38 seconds
Other: None
Interpretation: Sinus arrhythmia

31.
Atrial rhythm: Irregular
Ventricular rhythm: Irregular
Atrial rate: 60 beats/min
Ventricular rate: 60 beats/min
P wave: Variable configurations
PR interval: 0.16 seconds
QRS complex: 0.10 seconds
T wave: Inverted
QT interval: 0.36 seconds
Other: None
Interpretation: Wandering pacemaker

32.
Atrial rhythm: Irregular
Ventricular rhythm: Irregular
Atrial rate: 180 beats/min
Ventricular rate: 100 beats/min
P wave: Abnormal; slight saw-tooth appearance
PR interval: Unmeasurable
QRS complex: 0.10 seconds
T wave: Abnormal configuration
QT interval: Unmeasurable
Other: None
Interpretation: Atrial flutter with varying conduction ratios

33.
Atrial rhythm: Irregular
Ventricular rhythm: Irregular

Atrial rate: 88 beats/min
Ventricular rate: 88 beats/min
P wave: Normal
PR interval: 0.16 seconds
QRS complex: 0.08 seconds
T wave: Normal
QT interval: 0.40 seconds
Other: ST-segment depression
Interpretation: Normal sinus rhythm with PACs

34.
Atrial rhythm: Slightly irregular
Ventricular rhythm: Slightly irregular
Atrial rate: 110 beats/min
Ventricular rate: 110 beats/min
P wave: P-wave shape different for multiple P waves
PR interval: Unmeasurable
QRS complex: 0.08 seconds
T wave: Indiscernible
QT interval: Unmeasurable
Other: None
Interpretation: Multifocal atrial tachycardia

35.
Atrial rhythm: Regular
Ventricular rhythm: Irregular
Atrial rate: 80 beats/min
Ventricular rate: 60 beats/min
P wave: Biphasic
PR interval: 0.12 seconds
QRS complex: 0.12 seconds
T wave: Normal
QT interval: 0.34 seconds
Other: Two P waves without QRS complex
Interpretation: Second-degree atrioventricular (AV) block type II, also
known as Mobitz II

36.
Atrial rhythm: Absent
Ventricular rhythm: Absent
Atrial rate: Absent
Ventricular rate: Absent
P wave: Absent
PR interval: Unmeasurable
QRS complex: Absent
T wave: Absent
QT interval: Unmeasurable
Other: None
Interpretation: Asystole

37.
Atrial rhythm: Irregular
Ventricular rhythm: Irregular
Atrial rate: 60 beats/min
Ventricular rate: 120 beats/min
P wave: Biphasic when present
PR interval: 0.16 seconds
QRS complex: 0.10 seconds
T wave: Elevated
QT interval: 0.40 seconds when measurable
Other: None
Interpretation: Normal sinus rhythm with PVCs and couplets

38.
Atrial rhythm: Indiscernible
Ventricular rhythm: Regular
Atrial rate: Indiscernible
Ventricular rate: 38 beats/min
P wave: Indiscernible
PR interval: Unmeasurable
QRS complex: 0.36 seconds
T wave: Indiscernible
QT interval: Unmeasurable
Other: None
Interpretation: Idioventricular rhythm

39.
Atrial rhythm: Regular
Ventricular rhythm: Irregular
Atrial rate: 70 beats/min
Ventricular rate: 140 beats/min
P wave: Normal with sinus beats
PR interval: 0.14 seconds
QRS complex: 0.08 seconds
T wave: Distorted
QT interval: Unmeasurable
Other: None
Interpretation: Normal sinus rhythm with PVCs occurring every other beat, also known as ventricular bigeminy

40.
Atrial rhythm: Irregular
Ventricular rhythm: Irregular
Atrial rate: Indiscernible
Ventricular rate: 100 beats/min
P wave: Indiscernible
PR interval: Unmeasurable
QRS complex: 0.08 seconds

T wave: Flattened
QT interval: Unmeasurable
Other: None
Interpretation: Atrial fibrillation

41.
Atrial rhythm: Irregular
Ventricular rhythm: Irregular
Atrial rate: Indiscernible
Ventricular rate: 150 beats/min
P wave: None
PR interval: Unmeasurable
QRS complex: 0.04 seconds in nonpaced beats
T wave: Flattened
QT interval: Unmeasurable
Other: ST-segment depression
Interpretation: Atrial fibrillation with ventricular pacing

42.
Atrial rhythm: None
Ventricular rhythm: Chaotic
Atrial rate: None
Ventricular rate: Unmeasurable
P wave: Indiscernible
PR interval: Unmeasurable
QRS complex: Unmeasurable
T wave: Indiscernible
QT interval: Unmeasurable
Other: None
Interpretation: Ventricular fibrillation

43.
Atrial rhythm: Not visible
Ventricular rhythm: Regular
Atrial rate: Indiscernible
Ventricular rate: 150 beats/min
P wave: Not visible
PR interval: Unmeasurable
QRS complex: 0.12 seconds
T wave: Normal
QT interval: 0.24 seconds
Other: None
Interpretation: Junctional tachycardia

44.
Atrial rhythm: Irregular
Ventricular rhythm: Irregular
Atrial rate: 80 beats/min

Ventricular rate: 80 beats/min
P wave: Normal configuration
PR interval: 0.22 seconds
QRS complex: 0.10 seconds
T wave: Normal configuration
QT interval: 0.38 seconds
Other: None
Interpretation: First-degree AV block with bigeminal PACs

45.
Atrial rhythm: Regular
Ventricular rhythm: Regular
Atrial rate: 150 beats/min
Ventricular rate: 150 beats/min
P wave: Peaked
PR interval: 0.12 seconds
QRS complex: 0.08 seconds
T wave: Flattened
QT interval: 0.24 seconds
Other: None
Interpretation: Atrial tachycardia

46.
Atrial rhythm: Regular
Ventricular rhythm: Regular
Atrial rate: 79 beats/min
Ventricular rate: 79 beats/min
P wave: Normal configuration
PR interval: 0.16 seconds
QRS complex: 0.08 seconds
T wave: Normal configuration
QT interval: 0.40 seconds
Other: None
Interpretation: Normal sinus rhythm

47.
Atrial rhythm: None
Ventricular rhythm: Regular
Atrial rate: Indiscernible
Ventricular rate: 60 beats/min
P wave: Not present
PR interval: Unmeasurable
QRS complex: 0.06 seconds
T wave: Normal configuration
QT interval: 0.32 seconds
Other: None
Interpretation: Junctional escape rhythm

48.
Atrial rhythm: Indiscernible
Ventricular rhythm: Chaotic
Atrial rate: Unmeasurable
Ventricular rate: Greater than 300 beats/min
P wave: Indiscernible
PR interval: Unmeasurable
QRS complex: Abnormal
T wave: Indiscernible
QT interval: Unmeasurable
Other: None
Interpretation: Ventricular tachycardia

49.
Atrial rhythm: Regular
Ventricular rhythm: Regular
Atrial rate: 60 beats/min
Ventricular rate: 60 beats/min
P wave: Inverted
PR interval: 0.08 seconds
QRS complex: 0.12 seconds
T wave: Normal configuration
QT interval: 0.44 seconds
Other: None
Interpretation: Junctional escape rhythm

50.
Atrial rhythm: Unmeasurable
Ventricular rhythm: Irregular
Atrial rate: Unmeasurable
Ventricular rate: Unmeasurable
P wave: Absent
PR interval: Absent
QRS complex: Unmeasurable
T wave: Indiscernible
QT interval: Unmeasurable
Other: Continuous switching of ventricular rhythm between positive
and negative directions
Interpretation: Torsades de pointes

51.
Atrial rhythm: Regular
Ventricular rhythm: Regular
Atrial rate: 107 beats/min; pacemaker generated
Ventricular rate: 107 beats/min; pacemaker generated
P wave: Follows pacer spike
PR interval: 0.12 seconds
QRS complex: 0.06 seconds

T wave: Normal configuration
QT interval: 0.28 seconds
Other: Sinus tachycardia with pacemaker spikes
Interpretation: AV pacing

52.
Atrial rhythm: Regular
Ventricular rhythm: Irregular
Atrial rate: 80 beats/min
Ventricular rate: 60 beats/min
P wave: Normal configuration
PR interval: 0.24 seconds
QRS complex: 0.12 seconds
T wave: Normal configuration
QT interval: 0.38 seconds
Other: Dropped ventricular beats
Interpretation: Normal sinus rhythm with second-degree AV block type II (Mobitz II)

53.
Atrial rhythm: Irregular
Ventricular rhythm: Irregular
Atrial rate: 70 beats/min
Ventricular rate: 80 beats/min
P wave: Normal configuration but absent on premature beats
PR interval: 0.20 seconds
QRS complex: 0.08 seconds
T wave: Flattened
QT interval: Unmeasurable
Other: None
Interpretation: Normal sinus rhythm with premature junctional complexes

54.
Atrial rhythm: Regular
Ventricular rhythm: Regular
Atrial rate: 50 beats/min
Ventricular rate: 50 beats/min
P wave: Normal configuration
PR interval: 0.16 seconds
QRS complex: 0.12 seconds
T wave: Normal configuration
QT interval: 0.44 seconds
Other: None
Interpretation: Sinus bradycardia

Introduction

Differentiating ECG rhythm strips can often be a tricky proposition, especially when waveform patterns appear strikingly similar. These pairs of rhythm strips are among the most challenging to interpret. Test your knowledge and skill by correctly identifying each rhythm strip; answers begin on page 373.

Questions

1.

Rhythm strip A

Rhythm strip A is:_____

Rhythm strip B

Rhythm strip B is:_____

2.

Rhythm strip A

Rhythm strip A is:_____

Rhythm strip B

Rhythm strip B is:_____

3.

Rhythm strip A

Rhythm strip A is:_____

Rhythm strip B

Rhythm strip B is:_____

4.

Rhythm strip A

Rhythm strip A is:_____

Rhythm strip B

Rhythm strip B is:_____

5.

Rhythm strip A

Rhythm strip A is:_____

Rhythm strip B

Rhythm strip B is:_____

6.

Rhythm strip A

Rhythm strip A is:_____

Rhythm strip B

Rhythm strip B is:_____

7.

Rhythm strip A

Rhythm strip A is:_____

Rhythm strip B

Rhythm strip B is:_____

Answers

1.

Rhythm strip A: Atrial fibrillation

Rhythm strip B: Multifocal atrial tachycardia (MAT)

To help you decide whether a rhythm is atrial fibrillation or the similar MAT, focus on the presence of P waves as well as the atrial and ventricular rhythms. You may find it helpful to look at a longer (greater than 6 seconds) rhythm strip.

Atrial fibrillation

- Carefully look for discernible P waves before each QRS complex.
- If you can't clearly identify P waves, fibrillatory (f) waves appear in place of P waves, and the rhythm is irregular, then the rhythm is probably atrial fibrillation.
- Carefully look at the rhythm, focusing on the R-R intervals. Remember that one of the hallmarks of atrial fibrillation is an irregularly irregular rhythm.

Multifocal atrial tachycardia

- P waves are present in MAT. Keep in mind, however, that the shape of the P waves will vary, with at least three different P-wave shapes visible in a single rhythm strip.
- You should be able to see most, if not all, of the various P-wave shapes repeat.
- Although the atrial and ventricular rhythms are irregular, the irregularity generally isn't as pronounced as in atrial fibrillation.

2.

Rhythm strip A: Atrial fibrillation
Rhythm strip B: Junctional rhythm

At times, it can be easy to mistake atrial fibrillation for junctional rhythm. Here's how to tell the two apart.

Atrial fibrillation

- Examine lead II, which provides a clear view of atrial activity. Look for fibrillatory (f) waves, which appear as a wavy line. These waves indicate atrial fibrillation. The rhythm is irregular with atrial fibrillation.
- Chronic atrial fibrillation tends to have fine or small f waves and a controlled ventricular rate (less than 100 beats/min).

Junctional rhythm

- Junctional rhythm is always regular.
- Examine lead II. The P wave may occur before, be hidden in, or occur after the QRS complex (see preceding the rhythm strip). If visible, the P wave is inverted; if the P wave is before the QRS complex, the PR interval is less than 0.12 seconds.

3.

Rhythm strip A: Wandering pacemaker
Rhythm strip B: Premature atrial contraction (PAC)

Because PACs are commonly encountered, it's possible to mistake wandering pacemaker for PACs unless the rhythm strip is carefully examined. In such cases, you may find it helpful to look at a longer (greater than 6 seconds) rhythm strip.

Wandering pacemaker

- Carefully examine the P waves. You must be able to identify at least three different shapes of P waves (see the preceding rhythm strip) in wandering pacemaker.
- The atrial rhythm varies slightly, with an irregular P-P interval. The ventricular rhythm also varies slightly, with an irregular R-R interval. The changing site of impulse formation accounts for the slight variations in the rhythm.

Premature atrial contraction

- The PAC occurs earlier than the sinus P wave, with an abnormal configuration when compared with a sinus P wave. It's possible to see multifocal PACs, which originate from multiple ectopic pacemaker sites in the atria. In this setting, the P waves have different shapes.
- With the exception of the irregular atrial and ventricular rhythms that result from the PAC, the underlying rhythm is usually regular.

4.

Rhythm strip A: Accelerated idioventricular rhythm
Rhythm strip B: Accelerated junctional rhythm

Idioventricular rhythms and junctional rhythms appear similar but have different causes. To distinguish between the two, closely examine the duration of the QRS complex and then look for P waves.

Accelerated idioventricular rhythm
- The QRS duration will be greater than 0.12 seconds.
- The QRS complex will have a wide and bizarre configuration.
- P waves are usually absent.
- The ventricular rate is generally between 40 and 100 beats/min.

Accelerated junctional rhythm
- The QRS duration and configuration are usually normal.
- Inverted P waves generally occur before or after the QRS complex. However, remember that P waves may also be buried within QRS complexes.
- The ventricular rate is typically between 60 and 100 beats/min.

5.

Rhythm strip A: Ventricular tachycardia, specifically ventricular flutter (V-flutter)

Rhythm strip B: Torsades de pointes

Ventricular tachycardia or V-flutter result from the rapid, regular, repetitive beating of the ventricles. It's produced by a single ventricular, monomorphic focus firing at a rapid rate of 250 to 350 beats/min. The hallmark of this arrhythmia is its smooth sine-wave appearance. If you were to turn the strip upside down, it looks the same. Overall, it's a form of ventricular tachycardia that demonstrates a loss of organized electrical activity.

Torsades de pointes is a variant form of ventricular tachycardia, with a rapid ventricular rate that varies between 250 and 350 beats/min. It's characterized by QRS complexes that gradually change back and forth, with the amplitude of each successive complex gradually increasing, and then decreasing. This results in an overall outline of the rhythm commonly described as *spindle shaped.*

The illustrations shown here highlight key differences between the two arrhythmias.

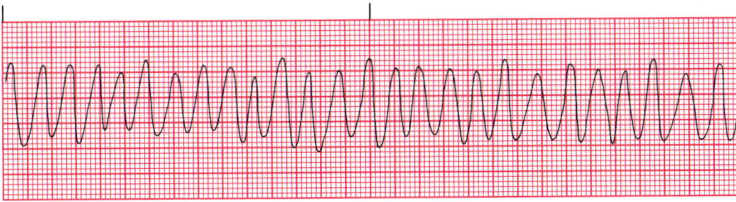

Ventricular tachycardia or V-flutter
- Smooth sine-wave appearance

Torsades de pointes
- Spindle-shaped appearance

6.

Rhythm strip A: Nonconducted PAC
Rhythm strip B: Second-degree atrioventricular (AV) block type II, also known as Mobitz II

You'll see conducted sinus beats marching in a row, all with the same PR interval followed by a blocked sinus P wave (P wave without a QRS following it). Note the pause following the blocked P wave that, when measured, equals two times the length of the sinus cycle. To differentiate a nonconducted PAC from a second-degree AV block type II, Mobitz II, look for constancy of the P-P interval. It's important to correctly identify a PAC from an AV block. High-degree AV blocks can lead to life-threatening consequences.

Nonconducted PAC
- If the P-P interval, including the extra P wave, isn't constant, it's a nonconducted PAC.

Second-degree AV block type II
- If the P-P interval is constant, including the extra P wave, it's a second-degree AV block type II.

7.

Rhythm strip A: Intermittent ventricular pacing
Rhythm strip B: Premature ventricular contraction (PVC)

Knowing whether your patient has a pacemaker will help you avoid mistaking a ventricular-paced beat for a PVC. If your facility uses a monitoring system that eliminates artifacts, make sure the monitor is set up correctly for a patient with a pacemaker. Otherwise, the pacemaker spikes may be eliminated as well.

Intermittent ventricular pacing

- The paced ventricular complex will have a pacemaker spike preceding it (see the pacemaker spike before the down-sloping ventricular beat in the preceding strip). You may need to look in different leads for a bipolar pacemaker spike because it's small and may be difficult to see.
- The paced ventricular complex of a properly functioning pacemaker won't occur early or prematurely. It will occur only when the patient's own ventricular rate falls below the rate set for the pacemaker.

Premature ventricular contraction

- PVCs will occur prematurely and won't have pacemaker spikes preceding them.

Nonconducted PACs are usually benign but second-degree AV blocks type II can be life-threatening.

Appendix 4: Quick guide to arrhythmias

Sinus arrhythmia

Cut along the dotted lines to test your strength with quick-review cards.

Features
- Rhythm irregular; varies with respiratory cycle
- P and R-R intervals shorter during inspiration, longer during expiration
- Normal P wave preceding each QRS complex

Treatment
- Typically, no treatment necessary; possible correction of underlying cause

Sinus bradycardia

Features
- Rhythm regular
- Rate less than 60 beats/min
- Normal P wave preceding each QRS complex
- Normal QRS complex
- QT interval may be prolonged

Treatment
- No treatment needed if patient is without symptoms; if drugs are the cause, consider discontinuing the offensive agent
- For low cardiac output, dizziness, weakness, altered level of consciousness, or low blood pressure, consider a temporary or permanent pacemaker and pharmacological therapy: atropine, dopamine, or epinephrine

Sinus tachycardia

Features
- Rhythm regular
- Atrial and ventricular rates greater than 100 beats/min
- Normal P wave preceding each QRS complex
- Normal QRS complex
- QT interval commonly shortened

Treatment
- No treatment necessary if patient is asymptomatic
- Correction of underlying cause
- Beta-adrenergic blocker or calcium-channel blocker administration, if cardiac ischemia occurs

Sinus arrest

Features
- Rhythm normal, except for missing PQRST complexes
- P wave is periodically absent with entire PQRST complexes missing; when present, normal P wave precedes each QRS complex

Treatment
- Treatment may not be required for pauses less that 6 seconds in asymptomatic patients
- Note the frequency of pauses and the time of day these pauses occur. Often pauses will occur during sleep, which is a nocturnal pause for most. In which case, consider the presence of obstructive sleep apnea; the patient may need a referral to sleep medicine
- For mild symptoms, consider discontinuing drugs that slow the heart rate
- Atropine administration if patient is symptomatic
- Temporary or permanent pacemaker for repeated episodes

Premature atrial contractions

Features
- Premature, abnormal P waves (differ in configuration from normal P waves)
- QRS complexes after P waves, except in blocked premature atrial contractions (PACs)
- P wave often buried or identified in preceding T wave

Treatment
- No treatment needed if patient is asymptomatic
- Treatment of underlying cause; avoidance of triggers (caffeine or smoking) and use of stress-reduction measures
- Consider beta-adrenergic blockers or calcium channel blockers if PACs occur frequently or heart rate is fast
- If bothersome with high supraventricular ectopic burden, consider catheter ablation

Atrial tachycardia

Features
- Typically a regular rhythm
- Rate 150 to 250 beats/min
- P waves regular but hidden in preceding T wave; precede QRS complexes
- Usually has sudden onset and termination

Treatment
- Vagal stimulation and adenosine administration
- Consider calcium channel blocker, beta-adrenergic blocker, amiodarone, procainamide or sotalol
- Atrial overdrive pacing
- If other treatment fails, synchronized direct current cardioversion (DCCV) may be considered
- Consider catheter ablation with recurrence

Atrial flutter

Features
- Atrial rhythm regular; ventricular rhythm variable
- Atrial rate 250 to 400 beats/min; ventricular rate depends on degree of atrioventricular (AV) block
- Sawtooth P-wave configuration of fibrillatory waves (F waves)

Treatment
- Beta-adrenergic blockers or calcium channel blockers if patient is stable and heart function is normal
- Amiodarone, dofetilide, dronedarone, flecainide, propafenone, sotalol arrhythmia are some antiarrhythmics used to treat this arrhythmia
- Synchronized DCCV immediately if patient is unstable
- The decision to cardiovert is determined based on whether the overall atrial flutter burden is high as measured on an internal loop recorder, cardiac device, or continuous cardiac monitor (such as a Holter or cardiac event monitor)
- Anticoagulation before cardioversion is important for stroke prevention
- Of note, if the patient has not been anticoagulated for several weeks before synchronized cardioversion or if the person has missed any doses of a prescribed anticoagulant, a transesophageal echocardiogram (TEE) will be performed before DCCV to check for any thrombus in the left atrial appendage (LAA). If a clot is found, the synchronized DCCV will be deferred in selected patients out of concern that the clot may embolize
- Consider catheter ablation with recurrence

Atrial fibrillation

Features
- Atrial and ventricular rhythms are grossly irregular
- Atrial rate greater than 400 beats/min; ventricular rate varies
- No P waves; replaced by fine fibrillatory waves

Treatment
- Consider calcium channel blockers or beta-adrenergic blockers if patient is stable
- Amiodarone, dofetilide, dronedarone, flecainide, propafenone, sotalol arrhythmia are some antiarrhythmic agents used to treat this arrhythmia
- If the patient is symptomatic or unstable evidenced by a rapid ventricular rate, chest discomfort, myocardial ischemia on the ECG, the decision to administer intravenous push (IVP) antiarrhythmic agents and synchronized DCCV is immediate
- When the rhythm offers a controlled ventricular rate and the patient is stable, anticoagulation is prescribed along with rate control agents
- The overall atrial fibrillation burden is determined by using an internal loop recorder, cardiac device, or continuous cardiac monitor (such as a Holter or cardiac event monitor)
- Anticoagulation before cardioversion is important for stroke prevention
- Of note, if the patient has not been anticoagulated for several weeks before synchronized cardioversion or if the person has missed any doses of a prescribed anticoagulant, a TEE will be performed before DCCV to check for any thrombus in the LAA. If a clot is found, the synchronized DCCV will be deferred in selected patients out of concern that the clot may embolize
- Consider catheter ablation with recurrence

Wandering pacemaker

Features
- Rhythm irregular
- PR interval varies
- P waves change in configuration, indicating origin in sinoatrial node, atria, or AV junction (*Hallmark:* At least three different P-wave configurations)

Treatment
- No treatment needed if patient is asymptomatic
- Treatment of underlying causes if patient is symptomatic

Premature junctional contractions

Features
- Rhythm irregular
- P waves before, hidden in, or after QRS complexes; inverted if visible
- PR interval less than 0.12 seconds, if P wave precedes QRS complex
- QRS configuration and duration normal

Treatment
- No treatment if patient is without symptoms
- Correction of underlying cause
- Discontinue heart rate control agents, if appropriate.
- Possible elimination of caffeine

Junctional tachycardia

Features
- Rhythm regular
- Rate 100 to 200 beats/min
- P waves before, hidden in, or after QRS complexes; inverted if visible

Treatment
- Correction of underlying cause
- Discontinuation of digoxin, if appropriate
- Vagal maneuvers, adenosine, amiodarone, beta-adrenergic blockers, or calcium channel blockers to slow rate
- Follow advanced cardiac life support (ACLS) protocol: tachycardia with pulse
- Possible pacemaker insertion
- Consider catheter ablation with recurrence

Junctional escape rhythm

Features
- Rhythm regular
- Rate 40 to 60 beats/min
- P waves before, hidden in, or after QRS complexes; inverted if visible
- PR interval less than 0.12 seconds (measurable only if P wave appears before QRS complex)

Treatment
- Treatment of underlying cause
- Atropine administration for symptomatic slow rate
- Pacemaker insertion if refractory to drugs
- Discontinue heart rate control agents, if appropriate
- Consider catheter ablation with recurrence

First-degree AV block

Features
- Rhythm regular
- PR interval greater than 0.20 seconds
- P wave preceding each QRS complex; QRS complex normal

Treatment
- Cautious use of digoxin, calcium channel blockers, and beta-adrenergic blockers
- Correction of underlying cause

Second-degree AV block type I (Mobitz I, Wenckebach)

Features
- Atrial rhythm regular
- Ventricular rhythm irregular
- Atrial rate exceeds ventricular rate
- PR interval progressively, but only slightly, longer with each cycle until a P wave appears without a QRS complex (dropped beat)

Treatment
- Treatment of underlying cause
- Atropine administration or temporary pacemaker, for symptomatic bradycardia
- Discontinue or reduce heart rate control agents, if appropriate

Second-degree AV block type II (Mobitz type II)

Features
- Atrial rhythm regular
- Ventricular rhythm possibly irregular, varying with degree of block
- QRS complexes periodically absent

Treatment
- Treatment of underlying cause
- Atropine, dopamine, or epinephrine administration, for symptomatic bradycardia (atropine may worsen ischemia with myocardial infarction [MI])
- Temporary or permanent pacemaker
- Discontinue heart rate control agents, if appropriate

Third-degree AV block (complete heart block)

Features
- Atrial and ventricular rhythms regular
- Ventricular rate is 40 to 60 beats/min (AV node origin); less than 40 beats/min (Purkinje system origin)
- No relationship between P waves and QRS complexes representing a lack of conduction between the atria and ventricles
- QRS complex normal (originating in AV node) or wide and bizarre (originating in Purkinje system)

Treatment
- Treatment of underlying cause
- Atropine, dopamine, or epinephrine for symptomatic bradycardia (don't use atropine with wide QRS complexes)
- Temporary or permanent pacemaker
- Discontinue heart rate control agents

Premature ventricular contractions

Features
- Underlying rhythm regular; P wave absent with premature ventricular contractions (PVCs)
- Ventricular rhythm irregular during PVC
- QRS premature, usually followed by compensatory pause
- QRS complex wide and bizarre, duration greater than 0.12 seconds
- Premature QRS complexes occurring singly, in pairs, or in threes; possibly unifocal or multifocal
- Most ominous when clustered, multifocal, and with R wave on T pattern

Treatment
- If warranted, procainamide, lidocaine, or amiodarone administration
- Treatment of underlying cause, such as hypokalemia, hypomagnesemia, or hypoxia

- Remove triggers, such as alcohol, caffeine, stress, tobacco, or stimulants
- Beta-blockers or calcium channel blockers
- The overall PVC burden is determined by using an internal loop recorder, cardiac device, or continuous cardiac monitor (such as a Holter or cardiac event monitor)
- Consider catheter ablation

Ventricular tachycardia

Features
- Ventricular rate 100 to 250 beats/min
- QRS complexes wide and bizarre; duration greater than 0.12 seconds
- P waves indiscernible

Treatment
- Monomorphic ventricular tachycardia (VT) with pulse: Follow ACLS protocol
- Polymorphic VT with normal QT interval: Follow ACLS protocol
- Polymorphic VT with prolonged QT interval: Stop drugs that may prolong QT interval and treat electrolyte imbalances
- Pulselessness: Initiate cardiopulmonary resuscitation (CPR) and follow ACLS protocol
- In nonurgent circumstances, consider catheter ablation and an automated implantable internal cardioverter defibrillator (AICD)
- Consider genetic testing

Ventricular fibrillation

Features
- Ventricular rhythm rapid and chaotic
- QRS wide and irregular; no visible P waves

Treatment
- CPR and unsynchronized defibrillation or automated external defibrillator (AED): Follow ACLS protocol
- Drug therapy: epinephrine, amiodarone, or lidocaine
- Advanced airway: endotracheal intubation
- Treat underlying conditions, such as acidosis, cardiac tamponade, myocardial ischemia, hypoxia, hypothermia, hypoglycemia, tension pneumothorax, hemothorax, thrombosis, or chest trauma.
- In nonurgent circumstances, consider AICD if at risk for recurrent ventricular fibrillation
- Consider genetic testing

Asystole

Features
- No atrial or ventricular rate or rhythm
- No discernible P waves, QRS complexes, or T waves

Treatment
- Follow ACLS protocol
- Endotracheal intubation
- Transcutaneous pacemaker
- Treatment of underlying cause

aberrant conduction: abnormal pathway of an impulse traveling through the heart's conduction system

ablation: catheter cryoablation or radiofrequency employed to eradicate irritable foci in the heart; used to prevent tachyarrhythmias

afterload: resistance that the left ventricle must work against to pump blood through the aorta

amplitude: height of a waveform

arrhythmia: disturbance of the normal cardiac rhythm from the abnormal origin, discharge, or conduction of electrical impulses

artifact: waveform interference in an ECG tracing that results from patient movement, electrical interference, or poorly functioning equipment

atrial kick: amount of blood pumped into the ventricles as a result of atrial contraction; contributes approximately 30% of total cardiac output

automaticity: ability of a cardiac cell to initiate an impulse on its own

bigeminy: premature beat occurring every other beat; alternates with normal QRS complexes

biotransformation: series of chemical changes of a substance as a result of enzyme activity; end result of drug biotransformation may be active or inactive metabolites

biphasic: complex containing both an upward and a downward deflection; usually seen when the electrical current is perpendicular to the observed lead

Brugada syndrome: a heritable arrhythmia syndrome with a characteristic electrocardiographic pattern and increased risk of sudden cardiac death due to polymorphic ventricular tachycardia

bundle branch block: slowing or blocking of an impulse as it travels through one of the bundle branches

capture: successful pacing of the heart, represented on the ECG tracing by a pacemaker spike followed by a P wave or QRS complex

cardiac output: amount of blood ejected from the left ventricle per minute; normal value is 4 to 8 L/min

cardioversion: restoration of normal rhythm using synchronized, direct electrical current or drug therapy

carotid sinus massage: manual pressure applied to the carotid sinus to slow the heart rate

circus reentry: delayed impulse in a one-way conduction pathway in which the impulse remains active and reenters the surrounding tissues to produce another impulse

compensatory pause: period following a premature contraction during which the heart regulates itself, allowing the sinoatrial node to resume normal conduction

conduction: transmission of electrical impulses through the myocardium

conductivity: ability of one cardiac cell to transmit an electrical impulse to another cell

contractility: ability of a cardiac cell to contract after receiving an impulse

couplet: pair of premature beats occurring together

defibrillation: termination of fibrillation by asynchronized, electrical shock

deflection: direction of a waveform, based on the direction of a current

depolarization: response of a myocardial cell to an electrical impulse that causes movement of ions across the cell membrane, which triggers myocardial contraction

diastole: phase of the cardiac cycle when both atria (atrial diastole) or both ventricles (ventricular diastole) are at rest and filling with blood

ECG complex: waveform representing electrical events of one cardiac cycle; consists of five main waveforms (labeled P, Q, R, S, and T), a sixth waveform (labeled U) that occurs under certain conditions, the PR and QT intervals, and the ST segment

ectopic beat: contraction that occurs as a result of an impulse generated from a site other than the sinoatrial node

electrical axis: direction of the depolarization waveform as seen in the frontal leads

enhanced automaticity: condition in which pacemaker cells increase the firing rate above their inherent rate

excitability: ability of a cardiac cell to respond to an electrical stimulus

extrinsic: not inherently part of the cardiac electrical system

idiopathic ventricular fibrillation: the absence of any identifying structural or genetic abnormalities to explain ventricular fibrillation or out-of-hospital cardiac arrest

indicative leads: leads that have a direct view of an infarcted area of the heart

intrinsic: naturally occurring electrical stimulus from within the heart's conduction system

inverted: negative or downward deflection on an ECG

late electrical potentials: cardiac electrical activity that occurs after depolarization; predisposes the patient to ventricular tachycardia

lead: perspective of the electrical activity in a particular area of the heart through the placement of electrodes on the chest wall

monomorphic: form of ventricular tachycardia in which the QRS complexes have a uniform appearance from beat to beat

multiform or multifocal: type of premature ventricular contractions that have differing QRS configurations as a result of their origin from different irritable sites in the ventricle

nonsustained ventricular tachycardia: ventricular tachycardia that lasts less than 30 seconds

pacemaker: group of cells that generates impulses to the heart muscle or a battery-powered device that delivers an electrical stimulus to the heart to cause myocardial depolarization

paroxysmal: episode of an arrhythmia that starts and stops suddenly

polymorphic: type of ventricular tachycardia in which the QRS complexes change from beat to beat

preload: stretching force exerted on the ventricular muscle by the blood it contains at the end of diastole

proarrhythmia: rhythm disturbance caused or made worse by drugs or other therapy

quadrigeminy: premature beat occurring every fourth beat that alternates with three normal QRS complexes

reciprocal leads: leads that take a view of an infarcted area of the heart opposite that taken by indicative leads

reentry mechanism: failure of a cardiac impulse to follow the normal conduction pathway; instead, it follows a circular path

refractory: type of arrhythmia that doesn't respond to usual treatment measures

refractory period: brief period during which excitability in a myocardial cell is depressed

repolarization: recovery of the myocardial cells after depolarization during which the cell membrane returns to its resting potential

retrograde depolarization: depolarization that occurs backward toward the atrium instead of downward toward the ventricles; results in an inverted P wave

rhythm strip: length of ECG paper that shows multiple ECG complexes representing a picture of the heart's electrical activity in a specific lead

Stokes–Adams attack: sudden episode of lightheadedness or loss of consciousness caused by an abrupt slowing or stopping of the heartbeat

sustained ventricular tachycardia: type of ventricular tachycardia that lasts longer than 30 seconds

systole: phase of the cardiac cycle when both of the atria (atrial systole) or the ventricles (ventricular systole) are contracting

trigeminy: premature beat occurring every third beat that alternates with two normal QRS complexes

triplet: three premature beats occurring together

uniform or unifocal: type of premature ventricular contraction that has the same or similar QRS configuration and that originates from the same irritable focus in the ventricle

vagal stimulation: pharmacologic or manual stimulation of the vagus nerve to slow the heart rate

Valsalva maneuver: technique of forceful expiration against a closed glottis; used to slow the heart rate

Wolff-Parkinson-White syndrome: paroxysmal supraventricular tachycardia due to an abnormal continuity between the atrium and the ventricle referred to as an accessory pathway

Index

Note: i refers to an illustration; *t* refers to a table.

393

Note: i refers to an illustration; *t* refers to a table.

Note: i refers to an illustration; t refers to a table.

Note: i refers to an illustration; *t* refers to a table.

Note: i refers to an illustration; *t* refers to a table.

Note: i refers to an illustration; *t* refers to a table.

Note: i refers to an illustration; *t* refers to a table.

Note: i refers to an illustration; *t* refers to a table.

Note: i refers to an illustration; *t* refers to a table.